AMBULATORY MONITORING
and Blood Pressure Variability

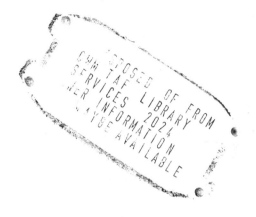

'For Janet'

AMBULATORY MONITORING
and Blood Pressure Variability

Thomas G Pickering, MD, DPhil, FRCP

Professor of Medicine, Cardiovascular Center,
The New York Hospital – Cornell Medical Center, New York

With contributions by
Carl Pieper, PhD,

The New York Hospital – Cornell Medical Center, New York

and
Clyde B Schechter, MD,

Department of Community Medicine, Mount Sinai School of Medicine,
New York

SCIENCE
PRESS ■

© Copyright 1991 by Science Press Ltd, 34-42
Cleveland Street, London W1P 5FB

British Library Cataloguing in Publication data
Pickering, Thomas G.
Ambulatory monitoring and blood pressure variability.
    1. Man. Blood. Hypertension
    I. Title II. Pieper, Carl III. Schechter, Clyde B.
    616.132

ISBN 1-870026-71-3 Part 1
ISBN 1-870026-57-8 Part 2
ISBN 1-870026-62-4 Part 1 & Part 2 Set
ISBN 1-870026-82-9 Single volume

Project editor: Caroline Black
Text editors: Lucinda Reed Harding and Ulla Parker
Illustration: Mai-Ling Wong, Paul Bernson, Giles Newport
Computer Graphics: Gary Brown, John Cheung, Giles Newport
Typesetting: Danielle Budd
Index: Doreen Blake
Printed in Hong Kong by Excel Printing

Contents

Acknowledgements

I should like to thank my colleagues who provided many helpful comments and criticisms of the manuscript. In addition to Carl Pieper and Clyde Schechter, these were Ray Murray, Gary James, Bill Gerin, Dick Devereux, Peter Schnall, Yvette Schlussel and Katherine Warren. My wife, Janet, also provided much constructive criticism.

My secretary Helen Del Duca gave her tireless support throughout the period of writing.

And last, but not least, my particular thanks are due to Dorothy Carmine, who did all the word processing with unfailing patience and good humour, and without whom this book would not have been possible.

Abbreviations

AAMI	Association for the Advancement of Medical Instrumentation
ADH	antidiuretic hormone
ADP	adenosine diphosphate
AHA	American Heart Association
ANF	atrial natriuretic factor
AUC	area under the curve
BHAT	Beta-Blocker Heart Attack Trial
BHS	British Hypertension Society
CHD	coronary heart disease
CPAP	continuous positive airway pressure
CVP	central venous pressure
DBP	diastolic blood pressure
ECG	electrocardiogram
EEG	electroencephalogram
FDA	Food and Drug Administration
FES	foil electret sensor
FPA	fibrinopeptide A
G theory	generalizability theory
HDFP	Hypertension Detection and Follow-Up Program
HR	heart rate
JNC	Joint National Committee
LVH	left ventricular hypertrophy
MBP	mean blood pressure
MILIS	Multicenter Investigation of Limitation of Infarct Size Trial
MRFIT	Multiple Risk Factor Intervention Trial
MSNA	muscle sympathetic nerve activity
NAG	N-acetyl-glucosaminidase
NHANES	National Health and Nutrition Examination Survey
PAI	plasminogen activator inhibitor
QALY	quality-adjusted life year
REM	rapid eye movement
RMSSD	root of the mean squared successive differences
SBP	systolic blood pressure
SDD	standard deviation of the differences
SHR	spontaneously hypertensive rat
t-PA	tissue-type plasminogen activator

Foreword

This book was written to fill a void. Its themes are a technique (ambulatory monitoring) and a concept (the importance of blood pressure variability). The two are, of course, related, because science advances not only by the development of new techniques to answer specific questions, but also by the fact that these same techniques often raise more questions than they answer. Ambulatory blood pressure monitoring was first developed over 30 years ago, but has only gained recognition in the last 10 years, and is now seeing rapid growth. I believe that in the next 10 years it will become a standard clinical procedure for the evaluation of hypertensive patients.

At the time of writing there is no book providing a comprehensive review of the subject, although at least two proceedings of conferences on ambulatory blood pressure monitoring have been published. My objectives in writing it were to provide a comprehensive review of the literature in the area, and also to discuss topics of relevance to the understanding of blood pressure variability and its consequences. Parts of the book will be of more interest to the practising clinician, while others are oriented more towards researchers.

Most medical texts these days are a compilation of chapters written by various authors, which is in many cases an inevitable consequence of the increasing specialization of science and of 'knowing more and more about less and less.' This book is somewhat unusual in that it is, for the most part, the work of a single author. This has the potential advantage of ensuring a consistency of coverage of the different topics, but also the disadvantage of reflecting one person's prejudices. My own prejudice, as becomes clear in the second half, is to favour the investigation of the role that behavioural factors play in the diagnosis and development of hypertension, although I have little enthusiasm for the 'reactivity hypothesis'. Furthermore, I believe that hypertension is primarily a disorder of the tonic regulation of blood pressure, rather than its short-term variability or reactivity.

For the last two chapters, which deal with the cost-effectiveness of ambulatory monitoring and data analysis, I have sought the help of two colleagues, Clyde Schechter and Carl Pieper, who are better qualified than I am.

I would conclude that the opinions expressed herein are solely those of myself and my co-authors.

1 Introduction

Of all the measurements made in clinical medicine, blood pressure is one of the most important and regularly performed, but at the same time is one of the most unreliable. The inherent variability of blood pressure poses a problem for the clinician attempting to classify a patient as normotensive or hypertensive, and also a challenge for the research worker trying to explain it. When Stephen Hales measured blood pressure in a struggling horse in 1733 [1], he recorded a level of 8 feet 3 inches, which translates into 190 mmHg. Thus, on the very first occasion that blood pressure was measured, a reasonably accurate, but very unrepresentative, reading was obtained. Hales recognized that blood pressure was not a fixed entity, and wrote:

> '...even in the same animal the force of the blood in its vessels, is continually varying, according to the different kinds and quantities of food, the various distances of time after taking food, the more or less plethoric state of the blood vessels, also from exercise, rest, different states of vigour or vivacity of the animal, and many other circumstances, which may conduce to vary the force of the blood: for the healthy state of animals is not confined to the scanty limits, of one determinate degree of vital vigour in the blood: but the allwise Framer of these admirable machines has so ordered it, as that their healthy state shall not be disturbed by every little variation of this force, but has made it consistent with a very considerable latitude in the variation of it.'

The main theme of this book is the assessment and interpretation of such variations. Nearly 50 years ago Ayman and Goldshine [2] described their experience with 34 hypertensive patients who had been trained to record their blood pressure at home, or have it measured by a family member. Almost without exception, the patients recorded lower pressures than the physicians obtained in their clinic, in some cases by as much as 70/36 mmHg. Furthermore, such differences persisted over a 6-month period of observation. The authors suggested that the measurement of blood pressure by the patient might have three advantages over conventional clinic measurements. The first was a better understanding of the factors that influence blood pressure; the second an improved prediction of prognosis; and the third a better way of evaluating treatment. Their observations received little attention at the time, but have major implications today, the most important of which is that some patients may be misclassified as being hypertensive on the basis of their clinic readings[1] if their pressures are normal outside the clinic. While clinic pressures remain the gold standard for most physicians, there is increasing acceptance that this standard may be flawed, and that pressures measured outside the clinic may improve the reliability of the diagnosis in the individual patient.

One of the reasons why the observations of Ayman and Goldshine were largely ignored was that no one knew what to make of them. Today, there are two pressing reasons for taking them more seriously. The first is that we now know, beyond any reasonable doubt, that subjects with very mild elevations in pressure are at increased risk of developing cardiovascular morbidity as a result of their blood pressure, and that this risk can, in some cases, be reduced by antihypertensive treatment. Hence, the way in which blood pressure is measured assumes increasing importance. The second reason is the increased availability of devices for measuring blood pressure outside the physician's clinic, both as a result of the development of non-invasive ambulatory blood pressure monitoring, and by the marketing of electronic monitors designed for self-monitoring of blood pressure at home. Such devices are likely to give blood pressure readings that are different from the conventional clinic readings, and one of the main purposes of this book is to review what these readings mean.

What is hypertension?

A favourite theory of Sir George Pickering [3], my father, was that hypertension is not a discrete entity to be defined in a binary fashion, but rather a quantity to be expressed as a number, on the grounds that it is continuously distributed in the population, and that there is a curvilinear relationship between blood pressure and cardiovascular risk. He took great delight in indicating that the 'dividing line' separating normotension and hypertension was nothing more than artefact, and frequently highlighted the fact that the dividing lines suggested by other workers ranged from as low as 120/80 mmHg to as high as 180/110 mmHg. The crux of his argument was that blood pressure is distributed unimodally in the population, and that its inheritance is polygenic. Put another way, it is not possible to define a distinct 'hypertensive' population. Two analogous situations are body weight and blood cholesterol, both of which are distributed in a continuous way and are also, therefore, best defined quantitatively rather than qualitatively. In the case of blood cholesterol there is evidence for a number of distinct genetic forms [4], and it is conceivable that what we currently describe as essential hypertension is, in fact,

---

[1]The term 'clinic readings' is used throughout this book, and refers to conventional sphygmomanometer measurements made in a clinic setting by a physician or nurse. 'Office' and 'casual' readings are synonymous terms.

a number of discrete genetic entities with a varying contribution of environmental influences.

The fact that normotension and hypertension cannot be rigidly defined on the basis of a single level of blood pressure has important consequences when considering ambulatory, or home, monitoring of blood pressure. While these techniques may enable a more precise estimate of an individual's 'true' level of blood pressure, there is no reason why they should provide any better separation between normal and abnormal levels. Such estimates must also be dealt with quantitatively, rather than qualitatively.

The concept of the dividing line involves two separate issues. One is theoretical, and concerns the question whether there are two populations with different levels of blood pressure. The other is practical, and concerns the level of blood pressure at which the benefits of treatment outweigh the risks of no treatment. There is no *a priori* reason why, if it were possible to draw a dividing line in each of these two cases, it would occur at the same level of blood pressure. In fact, it is not even theoretically possible to define a single point at which treatment should be started, since blood pressure is only one of several factors determining the level of risk: the same level of pressure in two individuals may be associated with quite different levels of risk.

Hypertension as a public health problem

According to the Joint National Committee on the Detection, Evaluation, and Treatment of High Blood Pressure, as many as 58 million people in the United States have high blood pressure (defined as a pressure exceeding 140/90 mmHg) or are taking antihypertensive medication [5]. This number is based on the United States National Health and Nutrition Examination Survey (NHANES) of 1976–1982 in 16 204 people aged between 18 and 74 years [6]. Since the distribution of blood pressure in the general population is roughly normal with a skew at the upper end of the range, choosing a higher dividing line for defining hypertension will give a much lower prevalence of hypertension. Furthermore, the estimate of 58 million was based on three measurements of blood pressure made on a single occasion, and it is well recognized that the apparent prevalence of hypertension would be less if measurements on more than one occasion were used: in the Charlottesville blood pressure survey [7] 20% of subjects had elevated blood pressure on the first visit, which decreased to 9% after a second visit. One of the findings common to many clinical trials of the treatment of mild hypertension is that many patients in the placebo treatment groups who are classified as being hypertensive after the initial screening (usually over two or three visits) become normotensive during the course of the trial [8].

The distribution of hypertension is uneven across the population. In the NHANES it was more common in blacks (38.2% of the population) than in whites (28.8%). Men show a somewhat higher overall prevalence of hypertension than women (33.0 versus 26.8%), but above the age of 55 years it becomes more common in women. The prevalence increases progressively with age.

The NHANES also found that just over half of all hypertensive individuals (53.9%) were aware that they had high blood pressure; 33% were on medication, and only 11% had their pressure adequately controlled (below 140/90 mmHg).

The vast majority of these hypertensive individuals had blood pressures in the range of mild hypertension (defined as a systolic pressure between 140 and 159 mmHg, and a diastolic pressure below 90 mmHg), which together constituted 22.7% of the general population. Only 1.6% came into the moderate hypertension range (diastolic pressure between 105 and 114 mmHg), and 0.6% were classified as having severe hypertension (diastolic pressure above 115 mmHg).

The risks associated with hypertension

There is convincing evidence that the risk of cardiovascular morbidity increases progressively with higher blood pressures (Fig. 1.1). Despite the fact that hypertension is often defined by the level of diastolic pressure, this relationship is, if anything, stronger for systolic than for diastolic pressure [9]. The gradient of risk is apparent at all levels of pressure; there is a doubling of risk even in the range between 80 and 89 mmHg of diastolic pressure [10], although Anderson has re-analysed the Framingham study data and concluded that there is a 'dog's leg' in the curve relating risk and diastolic pressure, such that there is an appreciable increase of risk at 90 mmHg [11].

The increased risk is mainly attributable to stroke and coronary heart disease (CHD). Indeed, for the former, blood pressure is by far the most important risk factor, whereas for the latter smoking and cholesterol are equally important.

At what level of risk should we be concerned? The life insurance companies, which provided much of the initial evidence that hypertension confers increased risk, begin to increase premiums at a relative risk of 1.2–1.4 [12]. The National High Blood Pressure Education Program Working Group recommended that a relative risk of 1.5–2.0 is a level of public health concern [10]. The answer to the question really depends on two things: the absolute level of risk, and what can be done to reduce it. Thus, a doubling of an exceedingly low level of risk is not necessarily of concern, since the absolute level is still very small. Furthermore, while lowering diastolic pressure from 90 to 80 mmHg might conceivably lower risk, in practice the costs and side effects of such a recommendation would be prohibitive.

The importance of systolic pressure

It is puzzling that diastolic pressure is commonly regarded as being more important clinically than systolic

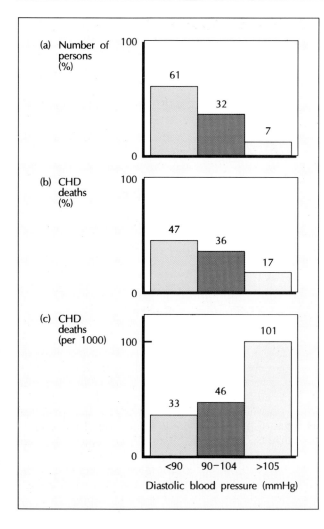

Fig. 1.1. The risk of cardiovascular morbidity increases progressively with higher blood pressure. Using data from the Framingham Study, grouping the population in tertiles according to the level of diastolic blood pressure is problematical with mild hypertensive subjects. Most 'hypertensive' patients have mild hypertension (a), and although their level of risk is only slightly increased (c), their greater number means that they account for the majority of coronary heart disease (CHD) deaths in hypertensives (b).

pressure. A large number of epidemiological studies [9,13] reviewed in a recent publication from the Multiple Risk Factor Intervention Trial (MRFIT) [14] have shown, almost without exception, that systolic pressure is a more important determinant of risk than diastolic pressure, whether it be for all-cause mortality, CHD, congestive heart failure, or stroke. This is well illustrated in Fig. 1.2, which is from a 20-year prospective study of Italian men [15].

The focus on diastolic pressure appears to date from the Veterans Administration Trial [16] showing the benefits of treating hypertension, which enrolled patients on the basis of their diastolic pressures. Most of the subsequent therapeutic trials have continued this practice [17], and it is therefore not clear to what extent benefits of treatment would relate to systolic pressure rather than diastolic pressure.

The reason why systolic pressure should be more important than diastolic pressure is not hard to explain. Physical and biological materials are much more susceptible to stress when it is intermittent rather than static, and in viscous materials such as arteries, internal stresses are greater when the deforming stress occurs at faster rates [18]. On this basis, we might anticipate the rate of change in arterial pressure to be a more important determinant of vascular damage than its mean level. Systolic pressure would be more affected by this than diastolic pressure.

While it is generally assumed that the average level of pressure over time is what causes vascular damage, it should be remembered that little or no information is available on the pathological significance of the transient peaks and troughs in blood pressure which are inevitable in daily life, and even less on the significance of the shape of the waveform itself (Fig. 1.3). Evidence that blood pressure variability is important is presented in Chapter 13.

The paradox of mild hypertension: treatment benefits the population, but not the individual patient

In the past 10 years or so a number of large-scale clinical trials have shown that treatment of mild hypertension can benefit the population at risk. In an excellent review of these findings, McMahon et al. [17] concluded that the incidence of stroke can be significantly reduced (by about 40%), while for myocardial infarction there was an insignificant reduction (of about 8%): overall, the net benefit was 10%. In the Hypertension Detection and Follow-up Program (HDFP), of which the main results were published in 1979 [19], overall mortality was reduced by approximately 20% (from 7.4 to 5.9%) in patients whose diastolic pressure at the time of entry to the trial was between 90 and 104 mmHg. From the point of view of the individual patient, however, these results look very different. Thus, of 100 patients treated, approximately one patient is protected from a morbid event, while six patients experience a morbid event despite being treated. Another 10 patients experience side effects from the treatment, and all 100 patients will have had to bear the cost of treatment. Thus, the vast majority of patients with mild hypertension can expect to derive no benefit from treatment: hence the paradox.

This dilemma could be resolved in two ways, which are not mutually exclusive. One would be to develop treatment which is cheap and free of side effects. If, for example, one could be immunized against cardiovascular disease in the same way as against polio or diphtheria, there would be no argument that all at-risk individuals should be treated. Similarly, if a mild reduction of sodium intake was universally effective, the same recommendation could be made. Unfortunately, while the newer forms of treatment, such as calcium antagonists and angiotensin converting enzyme inhibitors, may have somewhat fewer

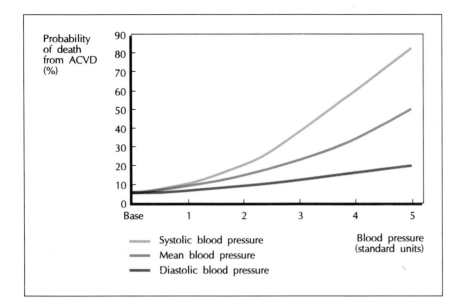

Fig. 1.2. The relationship between three measures of blood pressure (systolic, mean, diastolic) and the probability of death from atherosclerotic cardiovascular disease (ACVD) over 20 years in a study of Italian men. The levels of blood pressure are expressed in standard deviations, starting from a 'base' given by low levels corresponding to the same probability of death. Reproduced with permission [15].

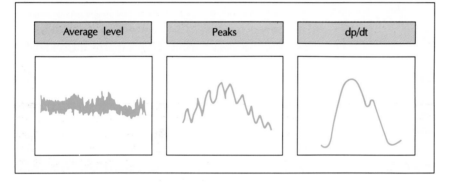

Fig. 1.3. Three possible factors contributing to the vascular damage caused by high blood pressure. Reproduced with permission from Pickering, *Circulation* 1987, 76 (suppl 1): 77–78.

side effects than beta blockers and diuretics, they are also considerably more expensive.

The other way out of the dilemma is to improve the stratification of risk within the hypertensive population. It is known from epidemiological studies that only a small proportion of patients with mild hypertension will suffer a morbid event as a result of their blood pressure. The corollary of this is that at the other end of the spectrum there is also a group of patients who are at low risk and hence do not need treatment. Since blood pressure itself is the major risk factor for cardiovascular disease, it is reasonable to suppose that more reliable measurements of an individual's 'true' level of blood pressure may give a more reliable estimate of prognosis.

The development of ambulatory monitoring

Non-invasive ambulatory monitoring of blood pressure first became a practical reality in the 1960s, with the development and application of the Remler recorder (Remler, Brisbane, California, USA) by Allen Hinman and Maurice Sokolow. Many of the issues discussed in this book

were originally raised by these investigators in a trio of classic papers [20–22], and are still pertinent today. The first of these papers [20] described an early version of the recorder, which was relatively bulky, and required the patient to inflate the cuff manually. The second [21] described the application of the recorder in hypertensive patients. It included a photograph of an attractive young woman wearing a Dior suit and white gloves more reminiscent of the 1950s than the 1960s[2], and the recorder, which consisted of two cases (one worn on each hip), a cuff and inflating bulb, and a pair of signal lights clipped to the subject's blouse to indicate when she should take a reading. By today's standards, this was a very cumbersome device, but it provided excellent data. This paper established the enormous variability of blood pressure during the day (sleep recordings were, of course, impossible to take), as shown in Fig. 1.4. It also demonstrated that casual pressures tend to be higher than ambulatory pressures in the majority of patients.

The third paper of the trio, published in 1966 [22], showed that the ambulatory pressures, recorded over 2–3 days, correlated more closely with target organ damage than the casual pressures. This relationship was closer for the average level of pressure than either the highest or the

---

[2]Dr Dorothee Perloff, Sokolow's long-time associate, has another version of this photograph, which she sometimes shows at medical meetings, but which was presumably deemed unsuitable for a serious cardiology journal. It shows the same young woman wearing, in addition to the blood pressure monitor, a bikini, and holding a beach ball. Whether she actually went to the beach in this get-up seems doubtful.

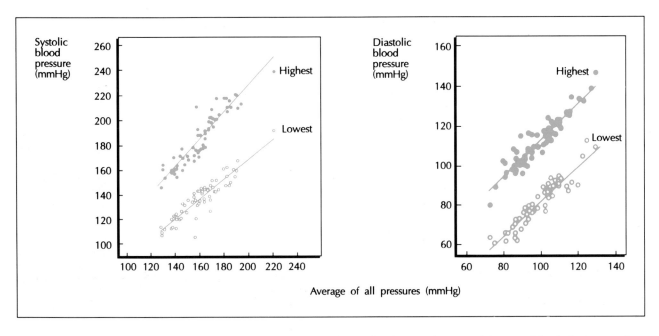

Fig. 1.4. The range of blood pressure (highest and lowest) occurring during the day as a function of the overall level of pressure. There is only a modest increase in blood pressure lability in hypertensive subjects. Reproduced with permission [21].

lowest readings. This paper provides the cornerstone of the evidence that ambulatory recordings may have greater clinical validity than casual readings.

I wrote to Dr Sokolow to ask him about his early work on the development of ambulatory monitoring, and he replied as follows:

'We had published our work on the natural history of untreated hypertension, which was published in *Circulation* in 1961 (Sokolow M, Perloff DP: The prognosis of essential hypertension treated conservatively. *Circulation* 1961, 23:697). At that time we were struck by the fact that although the mortality rate rose as the blood pressure increased in groups of patients, there were substantial numbers of exceptions to the rule. Some patients with equivalent elevated pressures survived whereas other died. In thinking about the possible reasons, it occurred to me that other than the associated presence of coronary disease the most likely was the fact that the office pressure was not representative of the pressure during the person's ordinary life and that if we could obtain ambulatory pressures we would have a better handle on the situation. Allen Hinman, an internist practicing in town, wanted to work with us in our hypertension clinic and I put him to work thinking about how to get an ambulatory portable device. He was interested in gadgets and engineering and was eager to proceed. At the same time, we were doing research on the role of social and psychological factors in hypertension, and an excellent psychologist, Dr Margaret Singer, was working with us. Her husband was a physics professor at Berkeley, and we enlisted his support in designing the apparatus. He is the one who came up with the original design. We then approached Robert Gray, who was an old friend of mine, who was the president of Remler Corporation. He agreed to manufacture the equipment. In addition to Dr Hinman, Dr Arthur Bickford and Dr Bernard Engle, who were working in our unit, did the original testing, with me supervising the effort, and Hinman published the results of that preliminary work. In the semifinal draft, Hinman had a footnote thanking me for the original conception of the idea, for pushing the development of the ambulatory recording and for supervising the early clinical testing, but this somehow got left off in the final paper. Following the original paper by Hinman and the two associates, I then took over the project and used it in our hypertensive patients for clinical evaluation; our 1966 paper in *Circulation* predicted the findings in all the subsequent ones (Sokolow M, Werdegar D, Kain KH, Hinman AT: Relationship between the level of blood pressure measured casually and by portable recorders and severity of complications in essential hypertension. *Circulation* 1966, 34:279). In that paper we showed that there was a significant differences between the office and the ambulatory pressures in 85% of patients and that the ambulatory pressures were more closely related to the target organ damage than were the office pressures. We also showed that for an given office pressure, the ambulatory pressure would vary considerably and one could not predict the ambulatory pressure from the office pressure in an individual patient. We also demonstrated the reliability of the apparatus and with it showed the marked variability of the blood pressure over the course of the day. Using the log that the patient kept, we were also able to analyze those factors during the day which were responsible for elevation of pressure, such as a negative affect, anger, as well as activity. We also showed that contrary to the usual assumption, the blood pressure throughout the day was often higher in the morning than at the end of the day. When the patient was alone his pressure was lower than when he was with other people. We have a lot of psychological data that we have not put together primarily because I was ready to retire and because of some personal tragedies. Our long-term aim was to determine whether ambulatory or office pressure was the more reliable in predicting prognosis; we demonstrated that ambulatory pressures were and published our findings in the *JAMA* in 1983. Some years ago Dr Hinman went to Japan and talked to a number of electronic firms there as well as some of the first in the US trying to persuade them to make an automatic apparatus to automate the decoding, to decrease the size of the recorder, and to make other improvements. Each one said it would cost more than $1 million to design such an apparatus. The NIH subsequently sent a request for proposals to develop such an apparatus; they awarded none of them because the minimum estimated cost was $1 million. During this time, NASA came to us and used our Remler apparatus to determine the blood pressure in the astronauts during their flight. They miniaturized it and promised to give us one but never did.'

At the same time that this work was being conducted in San Francisco, Frank Stott, working in my father's department in Oxford, was developing a non-invasive recorder which was fully automatic, and hence could measure blood pressure changes during sleep [23]. This machine, which was not portable, but could be wheeled to a patient's bedside, also demonstrated the large spontaneous variability of blood pressure over a 24-hour period. Rather than developing a non-invasive ambulatory recorder, Stott took the bold move of producing an intra-arterial recorder. This device, which was the forerunner of the Oxford Medilog recorder (Oxford Instruments, Oxford, UK), recorded pressure from a nylon catheter in the brachial artery. The arterial pressure trace was recorded on film, with a light galvanometer, and the catheter was perfused with heparinized saline from a chamber pressurized with cigarette lighter fluid. This work resulted in another classic paper by Bevan, Honour and Stott in 1969 [24]. Figure 1.5, reproduced from this paper, was originally commented on, in the typically terse manner of scientific reporting, as follows:

'Arterial pressure, plotted at 5 min intervals, of subject A.B. The period of sleep is shown by the horizontal bar. The high pressures shown at 16.00 and 24.00 hours are due to a painful stimulus and coitus respectively.'

My father subsequently disclosed what really happened [25]:

'Figure 1 [Fig. 1.5] shows the results obtained in Dr. Bevan with this device. Between 15.00 and 16.00 hours he was standing listening to me conducting a ward round. His arterial pressure was surprisingly low, reaching 80/50 mmHg. He was clearly bored, perhaps almost asleep. The head nurse stuck a pin into his behind, and his pressure rose abruptly to 150/70 mmHg.

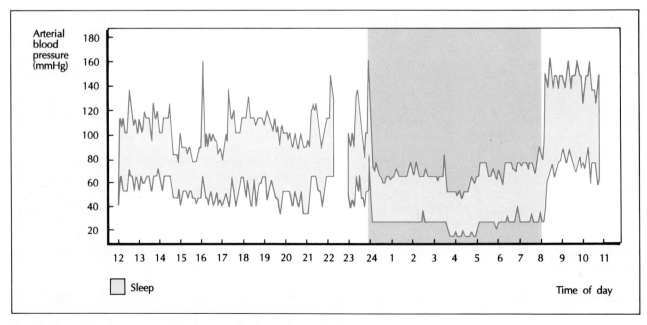

Fig. 1.5. Diurnal blood pressure profile of a normal subject obtained with intra-arterial ambulatory monitoring. Reproduced with permission [24].

The abrupt rise at 24.00 hours represented the effect of coitus. This was followed by sleep during which his arterial pressure was grossly reduced, falling as low as 55/30 mmHg. The pressure rose to relatively high levels after waking at 8.00 hours during the time that he was helping to get his children off to school.'

After this there was further work done on the phenomenology of blood pressure variability using the intra-arterial technique, which was generally regarded as a rather esoteric research tool. The pioneering work of Sokolow's group with the non-invasive method was not, however, followed up during the 1970s, although the Remler recorder was commercially available. At the end of the 1970s, there were two notable incidents: Del Mar Avionics (Del Mar Avionics, Irvine, California, USA) introduced the first fully automatic non-invasive monitor, the Pressurometer II, which was actually no less bulky and no more reliable than the Remler recorder, and in 1979 the results of the first of a series of clinical trials (the HDFP trial) showing the benefits of treating patients with mild hypertension were published [19]. The later Pressurometer III is shown in Fig. 1.6. Since that time there has been a dramatic increase in the variety and number of non-invasive recorders available, spurred on partly by developments in technology, but also by increasing concerns that the mass treatment of mild hypertension is no panacea.

The concept of the 'true' blood pressure

When dealing with a phenomenon as variable as blood pressure, physicians are continually faced with a problem: if a pressure of 155/95 mmHg is recorded on one occasion, and 135/85 mmHg on another, which reading is correct? What is the patient's real blood pressure? It is unsatisfactory to say that both readings are correct (although this may well be the case), particularly if the two readings were taken under similar circumstances without any overt changes in the patient's condition. For both practical and conceptual reasons we need some method of attaching a single number to that patient's blood pressure. This we may refer to as the 'true' blood pressure, which we can conceive as the average level of pressure over a prolonged period of time around which short-term fluctuations occur. The majority of measurements made for clinical purposes are, in effect, attempts to estimate the true pressure, but can at best only be approximations of it, because of both the inherent variability of blood pressure and measurement error.

An important question is the length of time over which the true pressure should be defined. This cannot be rigidly set, for the simple reason that the true pressure may change over time (e.g. as a result of antihypertensive

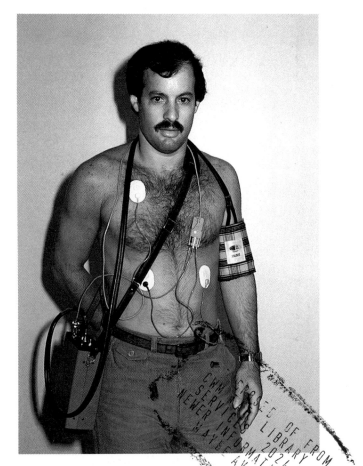

Fig. 1.6. The DelMar Avionics Pressurometer III, one of the earlier non-invasive ambulatory monitors.

treatment) but we would normally think of it in terms of weeks or months. Thus, the closest estimate of true pressure would be obtained by a series of 24-hour beat-to-beat blood pressure recordings using a technique which is highly accurate and which does not itself alter blood pressure (a condition which none of the available invasive or non-invasive blood pressure monitors currently satisfies).

The concept of the true blood pressure has appeal at a number of different levels. Mathematically it is useful in models of blood pressure screening and cost-effectiveness analysis (reviewed in Chapter 15); physiologically, it can be regarded as the set-point about which short-term fluctuations in blood pressure are regulated; and pathologically, it is the level of pressure which determines the extent of vascular damage associated with hypertension.

Blood pressure monitoring for studying the influence of behavioural factors

Ambulatory monitoring, because it provides the capability of measuring blood pressure during normal daily activities, provides a unique opportunity to evaluate the effects of behavioural or psychological factors. In the past this has been attempted, almost exclusively, in the rather artificial circumstances of a laboratory: it is doubtful whether such results can be generalized. There are three distinct ways in which behaviour may influence blood pressure, all of which will be reviewed in the ensuing chapters. First, there is no question that the measurement of clinic pressure is greatly affected by the doctor–patient relationship; second, there is also no question that acute changes of mood can change blood pressure. The third possibility, which is the most intriguing and the least certain, is that behavioural factors can contribute to the development of sustained hypertension.

One of the major limitations of studies of the role of behavioural factors has been their focus on short-term changes in blood pressure. A huge literature has developed on reactivity testing, in which the cardiovascular and humoral responses to a variety of behavioural stressors are measured under standardized conditions. The emphasis of this approach is on the response to the stimulus, rather than on the baseline level. One of the themes of this book, however, is that what distinguishes the hypertensive individual from the normotensive individual is the difference in the baseline or true level of blood pressure rather than its variability or reactivity. It is also proposed that the control of the baseline levels is separate from the control of variability. The sympathetic nervous system is the most likely mediator of any behaviourally induced increases in blood pressure, and it is noteworthy that while there is considerable evidence for an increase in the tonic or baseline level of sympathetic activity, there is no evidence for a phasic change.

Hypertension is thus a 'baseline disorder', not a disorder of reactivity. The focus of behavioural studies should, therefore, be on behavioural factors that affect the resting level of pressure, rather than on its reactivity. A convincing demonstration of a role for behavioural factors in the development of hypertension will, therefore, only be obtained by showing an effect on the true level of blood pressure, not on the short-term fluctuations.

References

1. HALES S. In *Classics in Arterial Hypertension* edited by Ruskin A. Springfield: Charles C. Thomas, 1956, pp 5–29.
2. AYMAN D, GOLDSHINE AD. Blood pressure determinations by patients with essential hypertension: the difference between clinic and home readings before treatment. *Am J Med Sci* 1940, 200:465–470.
3. PICKERING GW: *High Blood Pressure*. London: Churchill, 1968.
4. BERG K. Genetics of coronary heart disease. *Prog Med Genet* 1983, 5:35–90.
5. The 1988 Report of the Joint National Committee on the Detection, Evaluation, and Treatment of High Blood Pressure. *Arch Intern Med* 1988, 148:1023–1038.
6. Hypertension prevalence and the status of awareness, treatment, and control in the United States: final report of the Subcommittee on Definition and Prevalence of the 1984 Joint National Committee. *Hypertension* 1985, 7:457–468.
7. CAREY RM, AYERS CR: Labile hypertension. Precursor of sustained essential hypertension? *Am J Med* 1976, 61:811–814.
8. MIALL WE, BRENNAN PJ: Observations on the natural history of mild hypertension in the control groups of clinical trials. In *Mild Hypertension: Natural History and Management* edited by Gross F, Strasser T. Chicago: Pitman/Year Book Medical Publishers, 1979, pp 38–46.
9. KANNEL WB, WOLF PA, MCGEE DL, DAWBER TR, MCNAMARA PM, CASTELLI WP: Systolic pressure, arterial rigidity and risk of stroke. The Framingham Study. *JAMA* 1981, 245:1225–1229.
10. Final Report of the Working Group on Risk and High Blood Pressure. An epidemiological approach to describing risk associated with blood pressure levels. *Hypertension* 1985, 7:641–651.
11. ANDERSON TW: Re-examination of some of the Framingham blood presure data. *Lancet* 1978, ii:1139–1141.
12. *The Underwriting Significance of Hypertension for the Life Insurance Industry*. Bethesda: National Heart and Lung Institute, 1974, DHEW publication no. (NIH) 74–426.
13. KANNEL WB, CASTELLI WP, MCNAMARA PM, MCKEE PA, FEINLEIB M: Role of blood pressure in the development of congestive heart failure. The Framingham Study. *N Engl J Med* 1972, 287:781–787.
14. RUTAN GH, KULLER LH, NEATON JD, WENTWORTH DN, MCDONALD RH, MCFATE-SMITH W: Mortality associated with diastolic hypertension and isolated systolic hypertension among men screened for multiple-risk factor intervention trial. *Circulation* 1988, 77:504–514.
15. MENOTTI A, SECCARECCIA F, GIAMPAOLI S, GIULI B: The predictive role of systolic, diastolic, and mean blood pressures on cardiovascular and all causes of death. *J Hypertens* 1989, 7:595–599.
16. Veterans Administration Cooperative Study Group on Antihypertensive Agents: Effects of treatment on morbidity in hypertension. II. Results of patients with diastolic pressure averaging 90 through 114 mmHg. *JAMA* 1970, 213:1143–1145.
17. MCMAHON SW, CUTLER JA, FURBERG CD, PAYNE GH: The effects of drug treatment for hypertension on morbidity and mortality for cardiovacular disease: a review of randomized controlled trials. *Prog Cardiovasc Dis* 1986, **19** (suppl 1): 99–118.
18. O'ROURKE MF: Basic concepts for the understanding of large arteries in hypertension. *J Cardiovasc Pharmacol* 1985, 7 (suppl):S14–S21.
19. Hypertension Detection and Follow-up Program Cooperative Group: Five year findings of the Hypertension Detection and Follow-up Program. II. Mortality by race, sex, and age. *JAMA* 1979, 242:2572–2577.
20. HINMAN AT, ENGEL BT, BICKFORD AF: Portable blood pressure recorder: accuracy and preliminary use in evaluating intradaily variations in pressure. *Am Heart J* 1962, 63:663–668.
21. KAIN HK, HINMAN AT, SOKOLOW M: Arterial blood pressure measurements with a portable recorder in hypertensive patients. I. Variability and correlation with 'casual' pressure. *Circulation* 1964, 30:882–892.
22. SOKOLOW M, WERDEGAR D, KAIN HK, HINMAN AT: Relationship between level of blood pressure measured casually and by portable recorders and severity of complications in essential hypertension. *Circulation* 1966, 34:279–298.
23. RICHARDSON DW, HONOUR AJ, FENTON GW, STOTT FH, PICKERING GW: Variation in arterial pressure throughout the day and night. *Clin Sci* 1964, 26:445–460.
24. BEVAN AT, HONOUR AJ, STOTT FH: Direct arterial pressure recording in unrestricted man. *Clin Sci* 1969, 36:329–344.
25. PICKERING GW: Hypertension. Definitions, natural histories, and consequences. In *Hypertension Manual* edited by Laragh JH. New York: Yorke, 1973, pp 3–30.

2   Blood pressure measurement

For most hypertensive patients, a mildly elevated level of blood pressure is the only abnormality that can be detected on routine examination. Since it is beyond dispute that blood pressure is not a fixed entity, its measurement is often the single most important component in the evaluation of the hypertensive patient. The problem is compounded by the fact that management decisions may be based on differences in blood pressure of 5 mmHg or less. Hence, small differences in the recorded blood pressure may determine whether or not treatment is recommended for a particular patient.

As a result of the overriding importance of blood pressure one might think that physicians would take particular care in its measurement. Unfortunately, but perhaps not surprisingly, this is not the case: a recent survey of 114 physicians in Newfoundland found that none followed all the recommended procedures of the American Heart Association (AHA) [1].

There are three main sources of error in the measurement procedure. First, there are inherent inaccuracies in both invasive and non-invasive methods (particularly the latter); second, there are potential errors due to blood pressure variability, so that the pressure measured at one instance may give a poor estimate of an individual's 'true' level of pressure. This variability is reviewed in Chapter 4. The third source of error is due to the elevation of pressure which may occur in the clinic setting, and is reviewed in Chapter 7.

The purpose of this chapter is to review the techniques currently available for the measurement of blood pressure. Much of the rest of the book will examine whether the readings that are obtained are representative of the true blood pressure. While invasive recording made directly from the artery is widely accepted as the most accurate method (the 'gold standard'), in this chapter we will describe a new non-invasive method (the K_2 method), which may be more accurate than many fluid-filled intra-arterial recordings.

With rare exceptions, the clinical measurement of blood pressure is performed non-invasively, traditionally by an observer with a stethoscope but increasingly by automatic or semi-automatic devices. Most of these use either the Korotkoff sound or the oscillometric techniques, although there are other methods that have recently become available.

The arterial pressure wave and the determinants of systolic pressure

Progressive changes occur as the arterial pressure wave proceeds to the peripheral circulation, with an increase in pulse pressure and the maximal rate of rise (dP/dt). Mean pressure changes very little but there is an in-

crease in systolic pressure and a slight decrease in diastolic pressure [2]. For a person with an aortic pressure of 122/81 mmHg the corresponding pressure might be 131/79 mmHg in the brachial artery and 136/77 mmHg in the radial artery. These latter two sites are the most commonly used for intra-arterial recording. The relationship between peripheral (radial) and central (aortic) pulse pressure is similar during rest and exercise (radial being about 46% greater than aortic in both conditions). However, during upright tilt the radial pulse pressure may be 65% greater than the aortic pulse pressure [3].

The simplest model of the arterial tree is the 'Windkessel', which can be likened to an expansible chamber (the large arteries) into which the heart pumps, with a narrow outlet of variable resistance (the arterioles) [4]. In this model, an increase in the peripheral resistance raises the level of mean arterial pressure without altering the shape of the pressure wave, while a decrease in compliance raises the pulse pressure without altering the mean pressure. Ventricular ejection (stroke volume) is the other major determinant of the pulse pressure.

This model does not take into consideration the other major determinant of the shape of the pressure wave — wave reflection from the periphery. The effects of this are shown schematically in Fig. 2.1, in which the

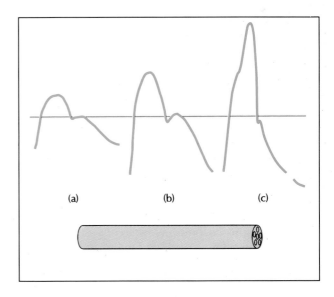

Fig. 2.1. Hypothetical pressure waves at the input of a tubular model of the arterial tree, shown at the bottom of the figure. (a) Normal compliance and timing of wave reflection; (b) decreased compliance but normal timing of wave reflection; (c) decreased compliance with early wave reflection. Reproduced with permission [4].

arterial tree is considered as a tube with a partially closed end from which the incident pressure wave is reflected.

The normal waveform (Fig. 2.1a) has a secondary diastolic wave after the incisura, which is attributable to wave reflection from the peripheral end of the tube. When the compliance of the tube is reduced the pulse pressure is increased (Fig. 2.1b). However, the decreased compliance will also increase pulse wave velocity, so that the reflected wave will return to the central circulation sooner, and will now augment the pressure wave before the incisura, as shown in Fig. 2.1c. The net effect of this will be to produce a late systolic peak, which is a characteristic feature of the arterial pressure waveform in hypertensive individuals, and in elderly normotensive individuals [5].

A more mathematical description of these phenomena is to regard the pressure wave as having two major determinants: ventricular ejection and input impedance. The latter may be regarded as the dynamic component of the peripheral resistance, and is itself determined by the two dynamic factors described above — arterial compliance and wave reflection.

The increased systolic pressure in more peripheral arteries is a consequence of peripheral wave reflection, with a summation of the incident and reflected waves [6]. The systolic pressure gradient between central and peripheral arteries may be less marked in older and more hypertensive subjects. However, because the stiffer arteries conduct the pulse wave quicker and more effectively, the augmentation of the systolic peak by the reflected wave in the more central arteries is more pronounced [7,8]. Since arterial stiffness is partly dependent on vascular tone, it changes in different situations, with the result that the relationship between central and peripheral systolic pressure can also change. O'Rourke and colleagues [9] have shown that arterial vasodilator therapy (which reduces arterial stiffness and hence wave reflection) can lower systolic pressure in the central aorta by as much as 25 mmHg without any change in the brachial artery systolic pressure.

Intra-arterial recording

Although measurement of intra-arterial pressure is generally accepted as the gold standard of blood pressure recording, its clinical use is limited by virtue of its invasiveness. However, it is often used for the evaluation of non-invasive blood pressure recorders. While intraarterial recording is potentially the most accurate method for measuring blood pressure, its accuracy may be limited by the frequency response of the recording system. Such recordings are commonly made with a long, thin, fluid-filled line connecting the artery and the transducer. This coupling may adversely affect the fidelity of the intraarterial pressure being recorded, often taking the form of an overshoot in systolic pressure. In addition, such lines may contain small air bubbles, and these factors may interact to cause substantial damping and distortion of the signal [10]. The best coupling is provided by short, stiff tubing.

The limitations of fluid-filled recording systems for measuring intra-arterial pressure have been well reviewed by

Bruner *et al.* [11]. They state that the accurate recording of any waveform requires a system with a resonant frequency at least five times higher than the highest frequency component of the waveform. In the case of the arterial pressure wave this is about 5 Hz, so that a system with a resonant frequency of at least 25 Hz is needed. The majority of recording systems in clinical use have a low resonant frequency (ranging from 8 to 25 Hz), and are under-damped. The closer the resonant frequency of the system is to the frequency of the pressure wave the more the system will tend to resonate, resulting in amplification of the recorded wave. Kravetz *et al.* [12] showed that a system with a resonant frequency of 8 Hz amplified brachial artery systolic pressure by 27%.

It is now possible to obtain catheter-tipped transducers of sufficiently small size to be inserted into the brachial artery, which avoid these problems and give recordings that are free of artefact. Figure 2.2 compares measurements of intra-arterial pressure made with a conventional fluid-filled system and a Millar solid-state catheter-tipped transducer (Millar Instruments, Houston, Texas, USA).

Non-invasive techniques for measuring blood pressure

Korotkoff sound technique

Despite continued efforts to find a superior method, the technique first described by Korotkoff in 1905 [13] remains the most widely used, both for clinical measurement of blood pressure and for automatic recorders. The classic description of the five phases of the Korotkoff sounds was first proposed by Ettinger in 1907 [14], and has been faithfully reproduced since then in every description of the method. Not to be left out, we will repeat it here. The phases are:

(1) a clear tapping sound that gradually increases in intensity;

(2) a murmur or swishing noise of variable duration;

(3) murmur disappears and a clear sound increasing in intensity appears;

(4) muffling or a soft blowing quality;

(5) disappearance of sound.

This classification is hallowed by time, if nothing else. It has, so far as we are aware, no scientific validity or practical utility, with the exception of phases 4 and 5.

The origin of the Korotkoff sounds has been a subject of debate for many years. The two most popular theories are that they are caused by pressure-induced movement of the arterial wall, or by turbulent flow through the compressed arterial lumen. However, both may be true: McCutcheon and Rushmer [15] showed that there are two components, an initial transient sound due to wall movement, followed by a more prolonged compression

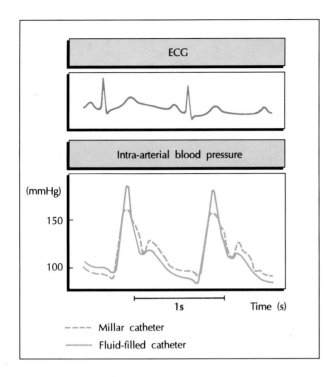

Fig. 2.2. Simultaneous intra-arterial measurements from the brachial artery using both a fluid-filled catheter and a Millar solid-state catheter-tipped transducer. Note the overshoot from the fluid-filled system due to under-damping.

murmur associated with an increase in flow. Dock [16], using a model with isolated segments of artery, concluded that the sounds were due to a sudden tautening of the arterial wall.

Comparisons of auscultatory and intra-arterial blood pressure

Several studies have compared measurements taken by the auscultatory Korotkoff sound method and intra-arterial recordings. Figure 2.3 summarizes the findings of 12 studies which reported average differences between direct measurement of pressure recorded from the brachial artery and the Korotkoff sound method [17–28]. The range of discrepancies is quite striking: the authors of one study commented that the difference between the two methods might be as much as 25 mmHg in some individuals [21]. These results show that the Korotkoff sound method tends to give values for systolic pressure that are lower than the intra-arterial pressure, and diastolic values that are higher, but there is no obvious superiority for phase 5 over phase 4. The discrepancies between the two methods cannot be attributed to differences in arm circumference or skinfold thickness [20,21]. Ragan and Bordley [17], in one of the pioneering studies of this series, made the interesting observation that, in subjects with normal sized arms, the agreement between the two methods was very close when the intra-arterial pressure wave showed 'a relatively full pulse' with a rounded peak. When, however, the pulse was of 'an

empty, peaked type', with a sharp initial systolic peak, the auscultatory readings were too low. These observations were confirmed by Thomson and Doupe [29], who measured the 'peakedness' of the intra-arterial pressure wave by its duration at 15 mmHg below the systolic peak. They found a close agreement between the peakedness and the error of the auscultatory measurement. Both investigators made the plausible suggestion that such brief peaks in pressure may be insufficient to open the occluded artery and hence generate a Korotkoff sound. An alternative explanation is that such peaks are artefacts due to under-damping.

Author	Systolic pressure	Diastolic pressure	
		Phase 4	Phase 5
Ragan and Bordley [17] (NT)	−2.0	−8.0	−
(HT)	6.0	−9.0	−
Kotte et al. [18] (NT)	0.0	−6.0	−
(HT)	5.0	−8.0	−
Roberts et al. [19]	3.2	−2.3	−9.0
Holland and Humerfelt [20]	24.6	5.3	13.0
Breit and O'Rourke [21]	3.1	−17.9	−6.0
Hunyor et al. [22]	10.0	−	−8.0
O'Callaghan et al. [27]	7.0	−	−10.4
Pregnancy			
Gould et al. [23]	−0.8	−	11.3
Raftery and Ward [24]	5.4	−11.1	−6.6
Ginsburg and Duncan [25]	−6.4	−	−15.0
Elderly			
Finnegan et al. [26]	5.2	−	−8.2
O'Callaghan et al. [27]	4.4	−	−9.2
Vardan et al. [28]	−2.6	−	−17.8

Fig. 2.3. Average differences (mmHg) between intra-arterial and Korotkoff sound measurements of blood pressure (brachial artery).

The human ear can only detect vibrations above a frequency of around 20 Hz. In fact, as shown in Figure 2.4, most of the energy that is generated under a sphygmomanometer cuff during blood pressure measurement is below the audible range, and shows no sudden change at systolic or diastolic pressure, in contrast with the more abrupt changes in energy above 20 Hz.

There is still no universal agreement about which phase of the Korotkoff sounds should be used for recording diastolic pressure: as shown in Fig. 2.3, there is no clear superiority of phase 4 or 5 when compared with the intra-arterial diastolic pressure.

The official recommendation of the AHA was formerly to report both the fourth and fifth phases [30], but more recently it has recommended using the fifth phase, ex-

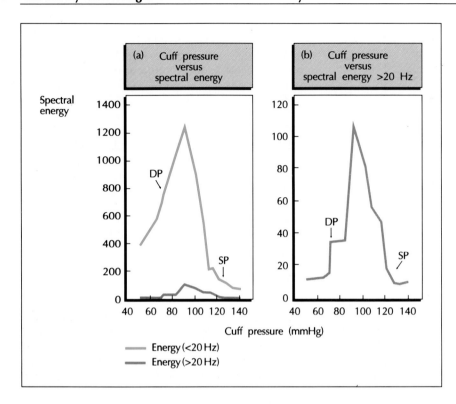

Fig. 2.4. Recordings obtained with a high-fidelity transducer placed under a sphygmomanometer cuff during deflation. In (a) the spectral energy of the signal has been separated into components above and below 20 Hz (note that most of the energy is below this level); (b) shows an amplified plot of the energy above 20 Hz, corresponding to the audible Korotkoff sounds. With the oscillometric technique, low-frequency vibrations in the cuff are detected. DP, diastolic pressure (auscultatory): SP, systolic pressure (auscultatory).

cept in children [31]. Most of the large-scale clinical trials which have evaluated the benefits of treating hypertension have used the fifth phase. However, the Framingham study, which has given us much of our knowledge about the risks associated with hypertension, used the fourth phase. Most people today use the fifth phase.

Sources of error with the auscultatory method

A number of factors may lead to inaccuracies with the Korotkoff sound technique.

Cuff size

The size of the cuff relative to the diameter of the arm is critical. Maxwell *et al.* [32] compared readings in obese subjects taken with the three generally available cuff sizes for adults, and recommended that the appropriate cuff size be selected according to the arm diameter. In their study, however, simultaneous intra-arterial pressures were not obtained. In general, the error can be reduced by using a large adult-sized cuff for all except the skinniest arms. This was first shown by King in normotensive young men [33]. Comparisons between direct and indirect pressures were made using both a standard cuff (26 × 13 cm) and a long cuff (42 × 13 cm). The longer cuff gave many fewer readings which were more than 20 mmHg different from the intra-arterial readings. In another study by van Montfrans *et al.* [34] the effects of using six different cuff sizes (ranging from 12 × 23 cm to 14 × 38 cm) were compared with intra-arterial pressures in obese and non-obese adults. In the non-obese subjects

it made little difference which cuff size was used, while in the obese subjects any cuffs bigger than 12 × 23 cm or 12 × 30 cm gave similar readings. These authors concluded that satisfactory results would be obtained by using a 14 × 38 cm cuff in all adults. Somewhat similar conclusions were reached by Russell *et al.* [35], who compared pressures taken with a standard and a large adult cuff with pressures recorded directly from the femoral artery. They found that both cuffs underestimated systolic pressure by about the same amount; for diastolic pressure the large cuff was more accurate, while the standard cuff underestimated it. Russell *et al.* also recommended using a large cuff for routine blood pressure measurement in adults. Finally, Linfors *et al.* [36] evaluated the consequences of using three different cuff sizes (standard, large, and thigh size) in 470 patients with a variety of arm sizes. In non-obese patients with an arm circumference of less than 35 cm, the blood pressure recorded was the same whichever cuff size was used. However, in obese patients with larger arms there was a considerable difference, with higher pressures being recorded using the smaller cuffs. Thus, 44% of these patients had systolic pressures above 140 mmHg with the standard cuff, 32% with the large cuff, and 28% with the thigh cuff. The problems associated with using different-sized cuffs for different-sized arms are even more pronounced in children, as described below.

In the United States, the most widely advocated protocol for the selection of the appropriate cuff size is that recommended by the AHA [31] (see Fig. 2.5). Surprisingly, these recommendations bear little relationship to what is actually available. The Baum Company, who proudly hail themselves as the 'Blood Pressure Standard the World Over' have quite different criteria, and their available cuff

Cuff type	Recommended—AHA (1988)*		Available—Baum†	
	Arm circumference (cm)	Cuff size (cm)	Arm circumference (cm)	Cuff size (cm)
Newborn	<7.5	3 × 5	<5	2.5 × 5
Infant	7.5–13	5 × 8	10–19	6 × 12
Child	13–20	8 × 1	18–26	9 × 18
Adult	24–32	13 × 24	25–35	12 × 23
Large adult	32–42	17 × 32	33–47	15 × 33
Thigh	>42	20 × 42	>46	18 × 33

*American Heart Association; †W.A. Baum Company, Copiague, New York, USA.

Fig. 2.5. Recommended and available cuff sizes for auscultatory measurement of blood pressure.

sizes do not match those recommended by the AHA, as also shown in Fig. 2.5. The British Hypertension Society (BHS) noted that although most commercially available adult cuffs are only 23 cm long, 35 cm long cuffs should be used for normal and lean arms and 42 cm cuffs are recommended for muscular and obese arms [37]. In the light of the evidence reviewed above, their recommendations should give more accurate readings than those of the AHA.

Arm position

Blood pressure measurements are also influenced by the position of the arm. Mitchell *et al.* [38] compared the blood pressures obtained with the arm in three positions; horizontal, at 45° to the trunk, and hanging down. As shown in Fig. 2.6, there was a progressive increase in the blood pressure, of about 5–6 mmHg, as the arm was moved down. Similar differences were recorded by Webster *et al.* [39]. These changes are exactly what would be expected from the changes in hydrostatic pressure.

These findings have important implications for ambulatory monitoring: serious errors in the recorded pressure will occur if the position of the upper arm varies while readings are being taken. During the day this can be prevented by ensuring that the arm is always parallel to the trunk. However, problems will occur at night when the subject is sleeping on his/her side. Schwan and Pavek [40] studied subjects in four supine positions while blood pressure was being recorded using an ambulatory monitor on the left arm. As shown in Fig. 2.7 blood pressure was 10 mmHg lower when lying on the right side (with the monitored arm above heart level) than when lying on the left side (when the monitored arm was below heart level). This observation may explain some of the variance in blood pressure seen during sleep when measured non-invasively.

Observer error and observer bias

Both error and bias by the observer are important sources of error when conventional sphygmomano-

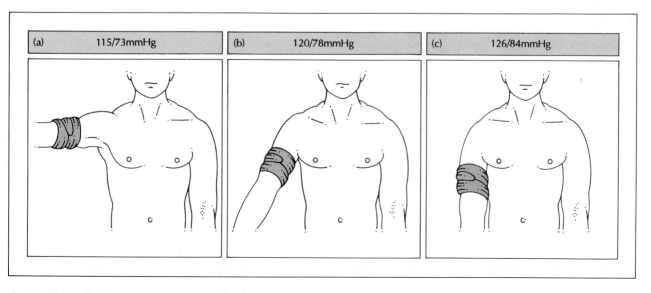

Fig. 2.6. Effects of different arm positions on blood pressure. Based on the data of Mitchell *et al.* [38].

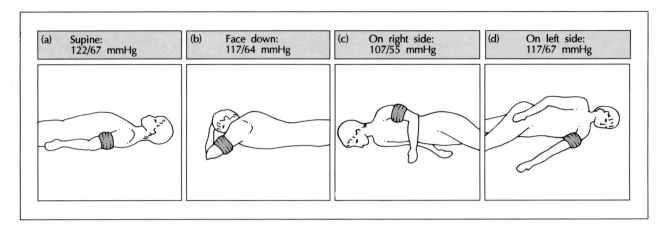

| (a)   Supine:
122/67 mmHg | (b)   Face down:
117/64 mmHg | (c)   On right side:
107/55 mmHg | (d)   On left side:
117/67 mmHg |

Fig. 2.7. Blood pressure measurements in different positions. Reproduced with permission [40].

meters are used. Differences in auditory acuity between observers may lead to consistent errors, and digit preference is very common, with most observers recording a disproportionate number of readings ending in five or zero [41]. A particularly flagrant example of digit preference is illustrated in Fig. 2.8, which shows the results of a study of blood pressure during pregnancy [42]. The clinic staff recorded diastolic pressures of 60 mmHg with monotonous regularity, while the project coordinator, using a Hawksley random-zero device (Baum, Copiague, New York, USA), recorded higher and more variable pressures.

In a large population survey conducted by 19 nurses, who had all received 2 weeks' training in blood pressure measurement, the average values of blood pressure recorded by individual observers were found to vary by as much as 5–10 mmHg [43]. The level of pressure that is recorded may also be profoundly influenced by behavioural factors related to the effects of the observer on the subject, the best known of which is the presence of a physician. It has been known for more than 50 years that blood pressures recorded by a physician can be as much as 30 mmHg higher than pressures taken by the patient at

home, using the same technique and in the same posture [44]. Physicians also record higher pressures than nurses or technicians [45,46]. In our own population of patients with mild hypertension (diastolic pressures between 90 and 104 mmHg), we have estimated that approximately 20% have 'white coat' hypertension, that is, pressures that are persistently high when in the presence of a physician, but normal at other times [46], as discussed in more detail in Chapter 7.

Other factors that influence the pressure that is recorded may include both the race and sex of the observer; Comstock [47] found that men tended to have higher pressures when these were taken by a woman than when taken by a man, while the opposite was true for women. Similar findings have been reported recently by McCubbin et al. [48]. Whether or not the person taking the blood pressure is of the same race as the subject is also important [49].

The extent to which inter-observer differences in blood pressure are due to differences in technique, as opposed to the white coat effect, can be assessed by having two observers take simultaneous readings with a double-headed stethoscope.

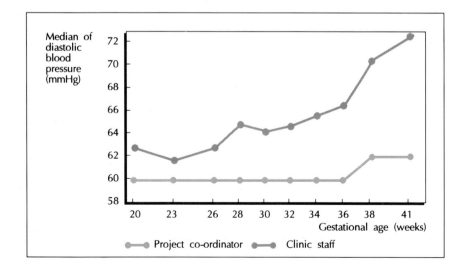

Fig. 2.8. Median values of diastolic pressure in pregnant women obtained in an obstetrics clinic by clinic staff and by a project coordinator using a Hawksley random-zero sphygmomanometer. Reproduced with permission from Villar et al., Am J Obstet Gynecol 1989, 161:1019–1024.

Rate of cuff inflation and deflation

This was investigated systematically by King [50] using an electric pump to inflate and deflate the cuff at different rates. The rate of inflation had no significant effect on the blood pressure, but with very slow rates of deflation (2 mmHg/s or less) the intensity of the Korotkoff sounds was diminished, resulting in the recording of slightly higher diastolic pressures. This effect has been attributed to venous congestion reducing the rate of blood flow during very slow deflation [51]. The generally recommended deflation rate is 2–3 mmHg/s.

The rate of inflation and deflation is of crucial importance during self-monitoring of blood pressure, because the isometric exercise involved in inflating the cuff produces a transient elevation in pressure of about 10 mmHg [52]. While this only lasts for about 20 s, if the cuff is deflated too soon the pressure may not have returned to baseline, and a spuriously high systolic pressure will be recorded.

Auscultatory gap

This phenomenon has a venerable history, having been recognized by Krylov in 1906 [53] only a year after Korotkoff first described the auscultatory technique. It can be defined as the loss and reappearance of Korotkoff sounds that occur during cuff deflation between systolic and diastolic pressures, in the absence of cardiac arrhythmias. Thus, if its presence is not recognized, it may lead to the registration of spuriously high diastolic pressures or low systolic pressures.

Its origins have remained something of a mystery, but we have recently used the K_2 technique (described below) to show that there are in fact three types of auscultatory gap [54]. Two are due to phasic changes in arterial pressure. The most common type (which we have called G1) occurs when there is a transient decrease in blood pressure following the registration of systolic pressure, so that Korotkoff sounds are no longer heard, but reappear as the pressure rises again, as shown in Fig. 2.9. The mirror image of this (G2) occurs with a transient increase in pressure when the cuff is just above diastolic pressure. The third type (G3) is not due to any sudden change in pressure, but is seen in patients who have a poorly developed K_2 (see below), which results in barely audible Korotkoff sounds.

The auscultatory gap may pose a problem for automatic recorders which operate by the Korotkoff sound technique, and results in gross errors in the measurement of diastolic pressure [55]. Oscillometric devices are less susceptible to this problem [55].

Cuff-inflation hypertension

Although in most patients the act of inflating a sphygmomanometer cuff does not itself change the blood pressure, as shown by intra-arterial [56] and Finapres

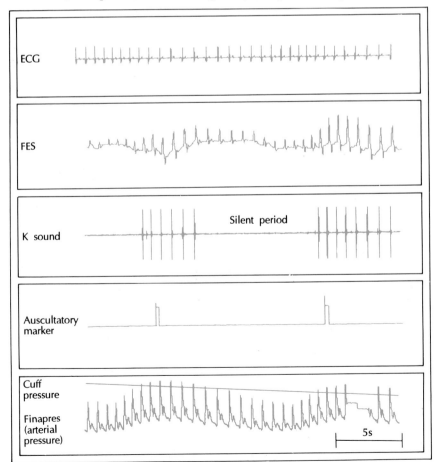

Fig. 2.9. Auscultatory gap (G1 type) caused by a transient change in arterial pressure. Traces are: ECG; foil electret sensor (FES) — a transducer under the cuff; K sound (detected from a microphone placed in a stethoscope earpiece); auscultatory marker showing appearance of sounds heard by observer; cuff pressure; and arterial pressure measured non-invasively by a Finapres device. Reproduced with permission from Blank *et al.* (manuscript in preparation).

(Ohmeda, Madison, Wisconsin, USA) [52] recordings, in occasional patients there may be a transient but substantial increase (of up to 40 mmHg) coinciding with cuff inflation [57]. An example is shown in Fig. 2.10.

This condition appears to be distinct from white coat hypertension, where the increase in pressure both precedes the act of inflation and outlasts it. The blood pressure pattern shown in Fig. 2.10 can be contrasted with Fig. 7.8, which shows white coat hypertension. It should also be distinguished from the transient increase in blood pressure which occurs during self-measurement, due to the muscular act of inflating the cuff (see Fig. 2.10).

Technical sources of error

There are also technical sources of error with the auscultatory method, although these are usually much less when a mercury column is used than with many of the semi-automatic methods (see below). These include the following: the position of the column should be at approximately the level of the heart; the mercury should read zero when no pressure is applied; and it should fall freely when the pressure is reduced (this may not occur if the mercury is not clear or if the pin-hole connecting the mercury column to the atmosphere is blocked). With aneroid meters, it is essential that they are checked against a mercury column both at zero pressure and when pressure is applied to the cuff. Surveys of such devices used in clinical practice have shown that they are frequently inaccurate [58].

Random-zero sphygmomanometer

Some of the sources of observer error, such as digit preference, may be reduced by the use of a random-zero (Hawksley) sphygmomanometer [59]. This device is a mercury sphygmomanometer whose zero point may be varied randomly; after a reading is taken, the zero value is subtracted from it to give the true reading. The elimination of digit preference is more apparent than real, however, because although it may not appear in the final value, digit preference may still occur when the pressures are read off the mercury column. This device does not, of course, eliminate the more subtle psychosocial effects due to the interaction of the observer and the subject.

Two studies have compared the random-zero device with readings obtained simultaneously from a conventional mercury sphygmomanometer, using a single cuff connected to the two devices [60,61]. In both cases the random-zero device gave consistently lower readings (by 1–3 mmHg for systolic pressure, and 2–3 mmHg for diastolic pressure). These differences may be due to the increased height of the mercury column in the random-zero manometer tube [60].

Oscillometric technique

This was first demonstrated by Marey[1] in 1876 [62], and it was subsequently shown that when the oscillations of pressure in a sphygmomanometer cuff are recorded during gradual deflation, the point of maximal oscillation corresponds to the mean intra-arterial pressure [63,64]. The oscillations begin at approximately systolic pressure and continue below diastolic pressure (see Fig. 2.11), so that systolic and diastolic pressure can only be estimated indirectly according to some empirically derived algorithm. One advantage of this method is that no transducer needs to be placed over the brachial artery, so that placement of the cuff is not critical. As shown in Fig. 2.12, two studies using the Dinamap automatic recorder (Critikon, Tampa, Florida, USA) [65,66], which works on the oscillometric principle, have shown excellent agreement between intra-arterial and oscillometric measurement, particularly when compared with the rather poor results using the auscultatory technique (Fig. 2.5). Another study using a different oscillometric device (The Takeda 751; A and D Engineering, Tokyo, Japan) also found that the agreement with intra-arterial readings was as good as for auscultatory measurement [67]. Yelderman and Ream [68] compared mean arterial pressure measured directly from the radial artery with oscillometrically determined mean pressure from the brachial artery during anaesthesia, and found remarkably close agreement between the two, with an average difference of 1 ± 6 mmHg. Furthermore, the correlation coefficients for the within-subject changes were also close ($r = 0.87$ on average). The oscillometric technique has recently been used successfully in ambulatory blood pressure monitors (such as the Spacelabs recorders, Spacelabs, Redmond, Washington, USA). It should be pointed out that different brands of oscillometric recorders use different algorithms, and there is no generic oscillometric technique.

Other potential advantages of the oscillometric method for ambulatory monitoring are that it is less susceptible to external noise (but not to low-frequency mechanical vibration), and that the cuff can be removed and replaced by the patient, for example to take a shower. The main disadvantage is that such recorders do not work well during physical activity, when there may be considerable movement artefact.

Ultrasound techniques

Devices incorporating this technique use an ultrasound transmitter and receiver placed over the brachial artery under a sphygmomanometer cuff. As the cuff is deflated the movement of the arterial wall at systolic pressure causes a Doppler phase shift in the reflected ultrasound, and diastolic pressure is recorded as the point at which diminution of arterial motion occurs [69]. Another vari-

---

[1]Etienne Marey, a French physiologist, has another claim to fame. In 1882 he invented the cine camera, which he called a photographic gun.

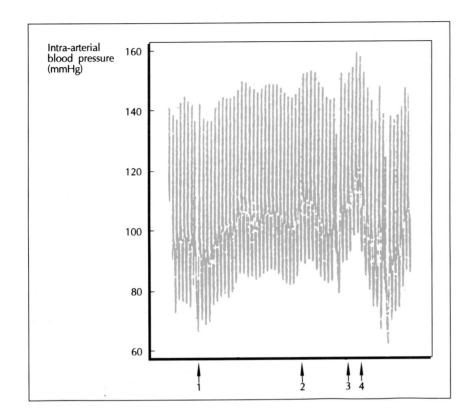

Fig. 2.10. An example of cuff-inflation hypertension, with intra-arterial recording. Arrow 1 indicates start of inflation, 2 the moment systolic pressure was recorded by the observer, 3 the moment diastolic pressure was recorded, and 4 the beginning of rapid cuff deflation. Reproduced with permission [57].

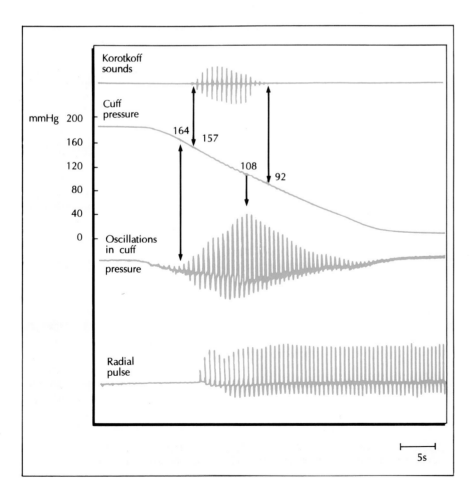

Fig. 2.11. The oscillometric technique of measuring blood pressure. Note that the cuff oscillations do not exactly correspond to the appearance and disappearance of Korotkoff sounds. Reproduced with permission [10].

Author	Systolic pressure	r	Diastolic pressure	r
Borow and Newburger [65]	−0.8 ± 3.5	0.984	−1.7 ± 2.3	0.969
Colan et al. [66]	+1.8 ± 4	0.979	+0.8 ± 4.2	0.941

Fig. 2.12. Average differences between direct and oscillometric measurements of blood pressure.

ation of this method detects the onset of blood flow at systolic pressure, which has been found to be of particular value for measuring pressure in infants and children [70,71]. Such devices compare favourably with those using other techniques [72], although their accuracy for measuring diastolic pressure in infants and children has been questioned [73].

Pulse transit time techniques

The velocity of the pulse wave along an artery is proportional to the arterial pressure. This principle has been used to evaluate changes in blood pressure by measuring changes in pulse wave velocity — by recording either the interval between the R wave of the electrocardiogram (ECG) and the radial pulse, or the interval between brachial and radial pulses. While this method has the advantages of not requiring a cuff and being theoretically suitable for beat-to-beat measurement of blood pressure, its accuracy has generally been found to be unacceptably low [74,75].

A commercial device has been developed recently (by Pulse Time Products Ltd, Chichester, UK), which is based on this method. It is a pocket-sized cuffless monitor which is held in one hand, with the ECG picked up from the palm and the thumb of the other hand placed on an electrode in the monitor. The arrival of the pulse wave at the wrist is detected by an optical transducer placed on the index finger. For reasons described above, the device has to be calibrated for each individual, but when this is done, it has been reported to give acceptably accurate measurements of both systolic and diastolic pressure [76].

Finger cuff method of Penàz

This interesting method was first developed by Penàz [77], and works on the principle of the 'unloaded arterial wall'. Arterial pulsation in a finger is detected by a photoplethysmograph under a pressure cuff. The output of the plethysmograph is used to drive a servo-loop which rapidly changes the cuff pressure to keep the output constant, so that the artery is held in a partially opened state. The oscillations of pressure in the cuff are measured, and have been found to resemble the intra-arterial pressure

wave in most subjects (see Fig. 2.9). This method gives an accurate estimate of systolic and diastolic pressure, although both may be underestimated (or overestimated in some subjects) when compared with brachial artery pressures [78]; the cuff can be kept inflated for up to 2 h. It is now commercially available as the Finapres recorder, and has been validated in several studies against intra-arterial pressures, mostly during anaesthesia for surgical operations [78–81]. These studies have shown that while there may be a sizeable systematic error in the recorded pressure (particularly in hypertensive patients), the device can accurately monitor changes in pressure. However, when there is intense peripheral vasoconstriction, the pressure recorded in the finger may be considerably lower than that in the systemic circulation [82]. During dynamic exercise systolic pressure is much higher when measured by the Finapres recorder than the corresponding intra-arterial (brachial artery) pressure, although the diastolic and mean pressures remain about the same [83]. Application of this device is likely to be greatest in situations where short-term blood pressure changes are being monitored, for example in tests of blood pressure reactivity or baroreflex sensitivity, for which it has been found to be quite accurate [81]. A prototype ambulatory monitor based on this principle has been developed, which has great promise, but is considerably more bulky than other monitors.

A variation of this method has been described by Aaslid and Brubakk [84], who measured flow with an ultrasound transducer placed over the brachial artery distal to a cuff. A servo-loop system operated to keep the artery partly compressed with a constant flow. This method also correlated well with intra-arterial pressures.

Oscillometric measurement in the finger

A recent development of the oscillometric technique has been to measure blood pressure in the finger, using a ring-shaped cuff which encircles it completely. The main advantage of this approach is that such recorders can be quite small. There are, however, several potential limitations. First, it is not clear to what extent the pressure in the finger resembles the pressure in the brachial or radial artery (direct recording from the finger is not feasible). This is not of great concern for a device such as the Finapres, whose main function is to monitor transient changes in pressure rather than its absolute level, but for self-monitoring or ambulatory monitoring it may pose a problem. According to one study the average difference between the pressure in the finger (measured oscillometrically) and the brachial artery (measured by the auscultatory technique) is only 1 mmHg for both systolic and diastolic pressure in normotensive subjects, but in hypertensive subjects the digital pressure may be as much as 19/13 mmHg lower [85].

The technique has also been developed for ambulatory monitoring [86]. Here the problems are related to movement. The effects of hydrostatic pressure differences between the finger and the heart are taken into account by measuring the pressure at heart level. Such recorders are, however, likely to be more susceptible to movement artefact than those which measure pressure from the upper arm.

Korotkoff signal (K₂) technique

We have recently described a technique of indirect blood pressure measurement which is based on waveform analysis of the Korotkoff signal [87,88]. This technique uses a specially designed transducer called a foil electret sensor (FES), which gives an accurate rendition of both the low-frequency and high-frequency components of the signal. With this technique, we have identified three components, which we have termed K_1, K_2 and K_3 (see Fig. 2.13). K_1 is a low-frequency, low-amplitude signal that can be detected at cuff pressures above systolic pressure (Fig. 2.13a). As cuff pressure

is reduced, a high-frequency component (K_2) develops (Fig. 2.13 b and c), the appearance of which corresponds precisely to systolic pressure. With further reduction of cuff pressure, a third component (K_3) appears, which resembles the arterial pressure waveform (Fig. 2.13 c and d). K_2 disappears at diastolic pressure, and therefore corresponds roughly to the audible Korotkoff sound.

The potential advantage of blood pressure measurement by the 'K₂ algorithm' is that it can be carried out on the basis of pattern recognition rather than by the absolute level of sound, which varies greatly from one individual to another. We suspect that K_2 originates from sudden movement of the arterial wall. We have shown that the K_2 method gives readings that are closer to true intra-arterial pressure than the auscultatory method. While this technique is not yet generally available, it can be replicated using any sensor–amplifier system that has an appropriately wide frequency response (including low frequencies).

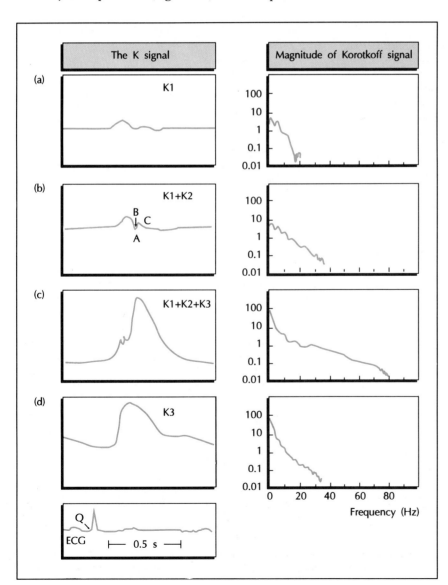

Fig. 2.13. Left-hand panels show waveform recorded with foil electret sensor from under the cuff during deflation from above systolic pressure to below diastolic pressure: (a) cuff pressure above systolic, K₁ is apparent; (b) at systolic pressure a high-frequency component (A,B,C) K₂ appears; (c) with cuff pressure between systolic and diastolic pressure a large low-frequency component (K₃) resembling the arterial pressure wave appears; (d) when cuff pressure is below diastolic, only K₃ remains. Right-hand panels show the corresponding spectral analysis. Reproduced with permission [87].

Measurement of blood pressure in special populations and circumstances

Infants and children

At the age of 4 days the median systolic pressure is only 75 mmHg, rising to 95 mmHg at 2 years. Up to the age of 14 years the blood pressure can be related to the height of the child, and nomograms have been published showing the normal range [89].

Conventional techniques, such as the auscultatory method, may give systematic errors in infants, where the true systolic pressure may be underestimated [70]. For indirect measurements the best technique is to use an ultrasonic flow detector (e.g. a Parks Doppler unit, GB Distributors, Instrumentarium Ltd, London, UK) coupled with an appropriately designed cuff (e.g. Pedisphyg, CAS Inc., Upper Montclair, New Jersey, USA) [70,71,73]. In children over the age of 12 years the auscultatory method may be used.

A particular problem associated with blood pressure measurement in children is knowing which sized cuff to select. Some authorities, such as the AHA [31], have recommended that the cuff size should be standardized to the circumference of the arm, while others have said that the length of the arm should also be taken into consideration [90]. Not surprisingly, there is a paucity of data based on intra-arterial measurements to resolve this issue. One of the most comprehensive studies was conducted by Whincup *et al.* [91], who compared the pressures obtained using three different cuff sizes (infant, child, and adult) in 838 children aged 5–7 years. Blood pressures were obtained with both the auscultatory and oscillometric techniques (using a Hawksley random-zero and Dinamap recorder). The findings with the two techniques were similar: the infant cuff gave readings that were about 6/2 mmHg higher than the child cuff, which in turn gave higher readings than the adult cuff, with a similar difference. These differences were about the same, whatever the arm circumference. The length of the arm had no influence on blood pressure independent of arm circumference. Thus, as shown in Fig. 2.14, if the conventional recommendations of choosing the cuff size according to the arm circumference are followed, there will be a stepwise change in the pressures recorded as arm circumference increases. On the basis of these findings, Whincup *et al.* recommended that a single cuff be used in such children. However, if more than one cuff size is used, the results can be corrected for a single cuff.

Pregnant women

In normal pregnancy there is a fall in blood pressure, together with an increase in cardiac output and a large decrease in peripheral resistance. As a result of this hyperkinetic state, Korotkoff-like sounds may be heard over the brachial artery without any pressure being applied to the cuff. These sounds are most probably due to turbulent flow in the artery — the compression murmur component described by McCutcheon and Rushmer [15] — and should be distinguished from the other component of the Korotkoff sounds, which is attributed to tautening of the arterial wall (see above). It is this latter component which is probably most closely related to diastolic pressure. In practice this distinction may be quite difficult. As a result of this, the use of phase 4 is generally recommended for registering diastolic pressure in pregnant women [92], which may be 12 mmHg higher than phase 5 [42]. However, while most European studies of hypertension in pregnancy have used phase 4, many American studies have used phase 5 [93].

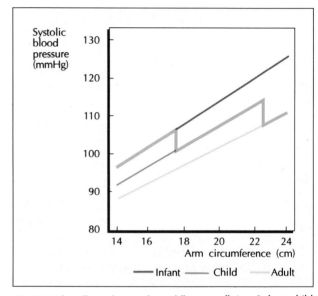

Fig. 2.14. The effect of using three different cuff sizes (infant, child, and adult) on the measurement of systolic pressure in children. The heavy blue line shows the consequences of following the AHA recommendations [91].

When the auscultatory method is compared with intra-arterial measurements during pregnancy there are considerable discrepancies between different studies, as shown in Fig. 2.3. These findings, however, do not provide any clear justification for recommending the use of phase 4 rather than phase 5 for measuring diastolic pressure in pregnant women.

Elderly subjects

In some older people there is an increase in systolic pressure without a corresponding increase in diastolic pressure (systolic hypertension), which has been attributed to a diminished distensibility of the arteries with increasing age. In extreme cases this may result in a diminished compressibility of the artery by the sphygmomanometer cuff, so that falsely high readings may be recorded. This condition is often referred to as pseudo-hypertension of the elderly [94]. In such patients vascular calcification may be seen on a plain radiograph [95]. It is important to emphasize that in this situation it may only be the diastolic pressure that is falsely elevated by the cuff method; systolic pressure may even be under-estimated [94]. In one study [28] which compared direct and indirect measurements of blood pressure in elderly subjects with systolic hypertension, it was found that the cuff method gave quite accurate readings for systolic pressure, but overestimated diastolic pressure by 18 mmHg (see Fig. 2.3). In another study [97] both systolic and diastolic pressure were overestimated by the cuff method. Therefore, in such individuals the only accurate method of measuring the arterial pressure is with direct intra-arterial recordings, which may reveal diastolic and systolic pressures 30 mmHg lower than non-invasive techniques. These patients represent the exception rather than the rule, however, because studies in healthy elderly subjects have not shown any greater discrepancy between direct and indirect measurements of pressure than in younger subjects [26,27,35].

The Osler manoeuvre

What is required for the detection of patients with pseudo-hypertension is a non-invasive test. Messerli *et al.* [96] evaluated a manoeuvre that was originally described by Osler in his textbook of medicine [96]. It is performed by inflating a sphygmomanometer cuff to above systolic pressure: if the brachial or radial artery is still palpable the manoeuvre is said to be positive. Messerli *et al.* confirmed that in patients who are 'Osler-positive' pseudo-hypertension is commonly present, with a false elevation of the non-invasively determined systolic and diastolic pressure of 10–54 mmHg, when compared with directly recorded pressure. Osler-negative patients have a much smaller discrepancy between non-invasive and invasive measurements of pressure.

Obese subjects

It is well known that the accurate estimation of blood pressure using the auscultatory method requires an appropriate match between cuff size and arm diameter. In obese subjects the regular adult cuff (12 × 23 cm) may seriously overestimate blood pressure [98]. The effects of arm circumference on the cuff method of measuring blood pressure were studied systematically by King [33]. Obesity was simulated by inserting sponge rubber between the arm and the cuff. The crucial finding was that the blood pressure obtained was independent of arm diameter as long as the cuff was of a sufficient size to encircle the arm. With inadequate cuff sizes he showed that the cuff pressure was not adequately transmitted to the arm, leading to serious overestimation of the blood pressure. Maxwell *et al.* [32] compared readings in obese subjects taken with the three available cuff sizes for adults, and recommended that the appropriate cuff size be selected according to the arm circumference, using somewhat different criteria than the recommendations of the AHA, which are shown in Fig. 2.5 . Van Montfrans [34] found arm circumference to be an unreliable guide to the difference between direct and indirect measurement of blood pressure and that a large cuff of 14 × 38 cm gave equally accurate results in both obese and non-obese subjects. The BHS recommend a 42 cm long cuff for obese arms [37].

Exercise

During dynamic exercise the auscultatory method may under-estimate systolic pressure by up to 15 mmHg, while during recovery it may be over-estimated by 30 mmHg [99,100]. Errors in diastolic pressure are unlikely to be as large, except during the recovery period, when falsely low readings may be recorded [100]. This is the reason why the AHA recommends taking the fourth phase of the Korotkoff sound after exercise.

Summary and conclusions

Blood pressure is not the same throughout the arterial bed, and the pressure wave becomes more peaked towards the periphery. This change occurs largely as a result of wave reflection, which will be affected both by vascular tone and stiffness. The gold standard for arterial blood pressure measurement continues to be intra-arterial recording, against which all other methods should ultimately be compared. The accuracy of this, however, is often suboptimal when under-damped fluid-filled recording systems are used.

For clinical purposes, non-invasive measurement is used almost exclusively. The Korotkoff sound technique is the most widely used method, and virtually all our clinical and epidemiological knowledge relating to blood pressure is based on its use. Although the overall agreement with intra-arterial pressure is reasonably close, there may be marked discrepancies between the two in some subjects. The fifth phase of the Korotkoff sounds is preferred for measuring diastolic pressure. Although traditionally it has been recommended to select the size of the sphygmomanometer cuff according to the circumference of the arm, it may be more reliable to use a large adult cuff for the majority of adults, and a single (child size) cuff for children. Many of the commercially available cuffs are too short. Observer error and observer bias are important sources of error with the Korotkoff sound technique, some of which may be reduced by using devices such as the Hawksley random-zero sphygmomanometer.

The next most widely used non-invasive technique is the oscillometric method, which is based on the observation that the maximal oscillation of pressure in a sphygmomanometer cuff occurs at mean arterial pressure, from which systolic and diastolic pressure can be detected indirectly. This method also has an acceptable accuracy.

Other non-invasive techniques include the use of ultrasound (reliable), pulse transit time (unreliable), and the finger cuff method of Penàz, which gives a reliable non-invasive estimate of beat-to-beat changes of pressure, although the absolute level may not be very accurate.

A more accurate version of the Korotkoff sound method uses a wideband frequency recording technique to detect both low- and high-frequency components. With this technique three distinct waveforms can be detected, one of which (K_2) corresponds to the audible Korotkoff sound. Visual detection of the appearance and disappearance of K$_2$ gives a more accurate measure of intra-arterial pressure than the auscultatory method.

Modification of the general recommendations for blood pressure measurement are appropriate in certain cases. In small children the auscultatory method does not work, and an ultrasound method may be used instead. In pregnant women there is debate about whether phase 4 or 5 should be used for recording diastolic pressure. In some elderly individuals, all non-invasive methods may be inaccurate because of incompressibility of the arteries, leading to the phenomenon of pseudo-hypertension.

References

1. McKay DW, Campbell NRC, Parab LS, Chockalingam G, Fodor JG: Clinical assessment of blood pressure. *J Human Hypertens* (in press).

2. Kroeker EJ, Wood EH: Beat-to-beat alterations in relationship to simultaneously recorded central and peripheral arterial pressure pulses during Valsalva maneuver and prolonged expiration in man. *J Appl Physiol* 1956, 8:483–494.

3. Kroeker EJ, Wood EH: Comparison of simultaneously recorded central and peripheral arterial pressure pulses during rest, exercise, and tilted position in man. *Circ Res* 1955, 3:623–632.

4. O'Rourke M: Basic concepts for the understanding of large arteries in hypertension. *J Cardiovasc Pharmacol* 1985, 7 (suppl): S14–S21.

5. O'Rourke M: Arterial stiffness, systolic blood pressure and logical treatment of hypertension. *Hypertension* 1990, 15:339–347.

6. Rowell LB, Brengleman GL, Blackman J, Murray JA: Disparities between aortic and peripheral pulse pressures recorded by upright exercise and vasomotor changes in man. *Circulation* 1968, 37:954–964.

7. Ting CT, Brin KP, Wang MS, Change MS, Chiang BM, Yin FCP: Arterial hemodynamics in human hypertension. *J Clin Invest* 1986, 78:1452–1471.

8. Nichols WW, O'Rourke MF, Avolio AP, *et al.*: Effects of age on ventricular/vascular coupling. *Am J Cardiol* 1985, 55:1179–1184.

9. Kelly R, Gibbs H, Morgan J, *et al.*: Brachial artery pressure measurements underestimate beneficial effects of nitroglycerin on left ventricular afterload. *J Am Coll Cardiol* 1989, 13:231A.

10. Geddes LA: *Cardiovascular Devices and their Applications.* New York: Wiley, 1984.

11. Bruner JMR, Krenis LJ, Kunsman JM, Sherman AP: Comparison of direct and indirect methods of measuring blood pressure. *Medical Instr* 1981, 15:11–21.

12. Kravetz LJ, Jennings RB, Goldbloom SD: Limitation of correction of frequency dependent artifact in pressure recordings using harmonic analysis. *Circulation* 1974, 50:992–997.

13. Korotkoff NS: On the subject of methods of measuring blood pressure. *Bull Imperial Military Med Acad St Petersburg* 1905, 11:365. Translated in *Classics in Arterial Hypertension* edited by Ruskin A. Springfield: Charles C. Thomas, 1956, pp 127–133.

14. Ettinger W: Auskultatorisch Methode der Blutdruck Bestimmung und ihr praktischer Wert. *Wien Klin Wochenschr* 1907, 20:992–996.

15. McCutcheon EP, Rushmer RF: Korotkoff sounds. An experimental critique. *Circ Res* 1967, 20:149–161.

16. Dock W: Occasional notes — Korotkoff sounds. *N Engl J Med* 1980, 302:1264–1267.

17. Ragan C, Bordley J: The accuracy of clinical measurements of arterial blood pressure, with a note on the auscultatory gap. *Bull Johns Hopkins Hosp* 1941, 69:504–528.

18. Kotte JH, Iglauer A, McGuire J: Measurements of arterial blood pressure in the arm and the leg: comparison of sphygmomanometric and direct intra-arterial pressures, with special attention to their relationship in aortic regurgitation. *Am Heart J* 1944, 28:476–490.

19. Roberts LN, Smiley JR, Manning GW: A comparison of direct and indirect blood-pressure determinations. *Circulation* 1953, 8:232–242.

20. Holland WW, Humerfelt S: Measurement of blood pressure: comparison of intra-arterial and cuff values. *Br Med J* 1964, 2:1241–1243.

21. Breit SN, O'Rourke MF: Comparison of direct and indirect arterial pressure measurements in hospitalized patients. *Aust N Z Med J* 1974, 4:485–491.

22. Hunyor SN, Flynn JM, Cochineas C: Comparison of performance of various sphygmomanometers with intra-arterial blood-pressure readings. *Br Med J* 1978, 2:159–162.

23. Gould BA, Hornung RS, Altman DG, Cashman PMM, Raftery EB: Indirect measurement of blood pressure during exercise testing can be misleading. *Br Heart J* 1985, 53:611–615.

24. Raftery EB, Ward AP: The indirect method of recording blood pressure. *Cardiovasc Res* 1968, 2:210–218.

25. Ginsburg J, Duncan S: Direct and indirect blood pressure measurements in pregnancy. *J Obstet Gynaecol Br Commonwealth* 1969, 76:705–710.

26. Finnegan TP, Spence JD, Wong DG, Wells GA: Blood pressure measurements in the elderly: correlation of arterial stiffness with differences between intra-arterial and cuff pressures. *J Hypertens* 1985, 3:231–235.

27. O'Callaghan W, Fitzgerald DJ, O'Malley K, O'Brien E: Accuracy of indirect blood pressure measurements in the elderly. *Br Med J* 1983, 286:1545–1546.

28. Vardan S, Mookherjee S, Warner R, Smulyan H: Systolic hypertension. Direct and indirect BP measurements. *Arch Intern Med* 1983, 143:935–938.

29. Thomson AE, Doupe J: Some factors affecting the auscultatory measurement of arterial blood pressure. *Can J Res* 1949, 27:72–80.

30. Kirkendall WM, Burton AC, Epstein FH, Fries ED: American Heart Association recommendations for human blood pressure determinations by sphygmomanometers. *Circulation* 1967, 36:980–987.

31. Frohlich ED, Grim C, Labarthe DR, Maxwell MH, Perloff D, Weidman WH: Recommendations for human blood pressure determination by sphygmomanometers. *Hypertension* 1988, 11:210A–222A.

32. Maxwell MH, Waks AV, Schroth PC, Karam M, Dornfeld L: Error in blood pressure measurement due to incorrect cuff size in obese patients. *Lancet* 1982, ii:33–35.

33. King GE: Errors in clinical measurement of blood pressure in obesity. *Clin Sci* 1967, 32:223–237.

34. van Montfrans GA, van der Hoeven GMA, Karemaker JM, Wieling W, Dunning AJ: Accuracy of auscultatory blood pressure measurement with a long cuff. *Br Med J* 1987, 295:354–355.

35. Russell AE, Wing LHM, Smith SA, *et al.*: Optimal size of cuff bladder for indirect measurement of arterial pressure in adults. *J Hypertens* 1989, 7:607–613.

36. Linfors EW, Feussner JR, Blessing CL, Starmer F, Neelon FA, McKee PA: Spurious hypertension in the obese patient. Effect of sphygmomanometer cuff size on prevalence of hypertension. *Arch Intern Med* 1984, 144:1482–1485.

37. Petrie JC, O'Brien ET, Littler WA, de Swiet M: British Hypertension Society recommendations on blood pressure measurement. *Br Med J* 1986, 293:611–615.

38. Mitchell PL, Parlin RW, Blackburn H: Effect of vertical displacement of the arm on indirect blood-pressure measurement. *N Engl J Med* 1964, 271:72–74.

39. WEBSTER J, NEWNHAM D, PETRIE JC, LOVELL HG: Influence of arm position on measurement of blood pressure. *Br Med J* 1984, 228:1574–1575.

40. SCHWAN A, PAVEK K: Change in posture during sleep causes errors in non-invasive automatic blood pressure recordings. *J Hypertens* 1989, 7 (suppl 6):62–63.

41. PICKERING GW: *High Blood Pressure.* London: Churchill, 1968.

42. VILLAR J, REPKE J, MARKUSH L, CALVERT W, RHOADS G. The measuring of blood pressure during pregnancy. *Am J Obstet Gynecol* 1989, 161:1019–1024.

43. EILERSTEN E, HUMERFELT S: The observer variation in the measurement of arterial blood pressure. *Acta Med Scand* 1968, 184:145–157.

44. AYMAN P, GOLDSHINE AD: Blood pressure determinations by patients with essential hypertension. I. The difference between clinic and home readings before treatment. *Am J Med Sci* 1940, 200:465–474.

45. MANCIA G, BERTINI G, GRASSI G, ET AL. Effects of blood pressure measurement by the doctor on patients' blood pressure and heart rate. *Lancet* 1983, ii:695–697.

46. PICKERING TG, JAMES GD, BODDIE C, HARSHFIELD GA, BLANK S, LARAGH JH: How common is white coat hypertension? *JAMA* 1988, 259:225–228.

47. COMSTOCK GW: An epidemiologic study of blood pressure levels in a biracial community in the southern United States. *Am J Hygiene* 1957, 65:271–315.

48. MCCUBBIN JA, WILSON JF, BRUEHL S, BRADY M, CLARK K, KORT E: Gender effects on blood pressures obtained during an on-campus screening. *Psychosom Med* (in press).

49. MURPHY JK, ALPERT BS, MOES DM, SOMES GW: Race and cardiovascular reactivity. A neglected relationship. *Hypertension* 1986, 3:1075–1083.

50. KING GE: Influence of rate of cuff inflation and deflation on observed blood pressure by sphygmomanometry. *Am Heart J* 1963, 65:303–306.

51. WILKINS R, BRADLY SE: Changes in arterial and venous blood pressure and flow distal to a cuff inflated on a human arm. *Am J Physiol* 1946, 147:260–269.

52. VEERMAN DP, VAN MONTFRANS GA, WIELING W: Effects of cuff inflation on self-recorded blood pressure. *Lancet* 1990, 335:451–453.

53. KRYLOV DO: The determination of the blood pressure by the acoustical means of N.S. Korotkov. *Izv Ven Med Akad* 1906, 13:113.

54. BLANK SG, WEST JE, MULLER FB, PECKER MS, LARAGH JH, PICKERING TG: The characterization of auscultatory gaps using wideband external pulse recording. *Hypertension* (in press).

55. IMAI Y, ABE K, SASAKI S, ET AL. Clinical evaluation of semi-automatic and automatic devices for home blood pressure measurement: comparison between cuff-oscillometric and microphone methods. *J Hypertens* 1989, 7:983–990.

56. PARATI G, POMIDOSSI G, CASADEI R, MANCIA G: Lack of alerting reactions to intermittent cuff inflations during noninvasive blood pressure monitoring. *Hypertension* 1985, 7:597–601.

57. MEJIA AD, EGAN BM, SCHORK NJ, ZEWIFLER AJ: Artefacts in measurement of blood pressure and lack of target organ involvement in the assessment of patients with treatment-resistant hypertension. *Ann Intern Med* 1990, 112:270–277.

58. BURKE MJ, TOWERS HM, O'MALLEY K, FITZGERALD DJ, O'BRIEN ET: Sphygmomanometers in hospital and family practice: problems and recommendations. *Br Med J* 1982, 285:469–471.

59. WRIGHT BM, DORE CF: A random-zero sphygmomanometer. *Lancet* 1970, i:337–338.

60. DE GAUDEMARIS R, FOLSOM AR, PRINEAS RJ, LUEPKER RV: The random-zero versus the standard mercury sphygmomanometer: a systematic blood pressure difference. *Am J Epidemiol* 1985, 121:282–290.

61. PARKER D, LIU K, DYER AR, GIUMETTI D, LIAO Y, STAMLER J: A comparison of the random-zero and standard mercury sphygmomanometers. *Hypertension* 1988, 11:269–272.

62. MAREY EJ: In *Pression et Vitesse du Sang. Physiologie Expérimentale. Travaux du Laboratoire de M. Marey.* Paris: Masson, 1875, **388**, pp 340–344. Translated in *Classics in Arterial Hypertension* edited by Ruskin A. Springfield: Charles C. Thomas, 1956.

63. MAUCK GB, SMITH CR, GEDDES LR, BOURLAND JD: The meaning of the point of maximum oscillations in cuff pressure in the indirect measurement of blood pressure. II. *J Biomech Eng* 1980, 102:28–33.

64. RAMSEY M: Noninvasive automatic determination of mean arterial pressure. *Med Biol Eng Comput* 1979, 17:11–18.

65. BOROW KM, NEWBURGER JW: Noninvasive measurement of central aortic pressure using the oscillometric method for analyzing systemic artery pulsatile blood flow: comparative study of indirect systolic, diastolic, and mean brachial artery pressure with simultaneous direct ascending aortic pressure measurements. *Am Heart J* 1982, 103:879–886.

66. COLAN SD, FUJI A, BOROW KM, MACPHERSON D, SANDERS SP: Noninvasive determination of systolic, diastolic, and end-systolic blood pressure in neonates, infants and young children: comparison with central aortic measurements. *Am J Cardiol* 1983, 52:867–870.

67. WIINBERG N, WALTHER-LARSEN S, ERIKSEN C, NIELSEN PE: An evaluation of semi-automatic blood-pressure monitors against intra-arterial blood pressure. *J Amb Mon* 1988, 1:303–309.

68. YELDERMAN M, REAM AK: Indirect measurement of mean blood pressure in the anesthetized patient. *Anesthesiology* 1979, 50:253–256.

69. WARE RW, LAENGER CJ: Indirect blood pressure measurement by Doppler ultrasonic kinetoarteriography. *Proc 20th Ann Conf Eng Med Biol* 1967, 9:27–30.

70. ELSEED AM, SHINEBOURNE EA, JOSEPH MC: Assessment of techniques for measurement of blood pressure in infants and children. *Arch Dis Child* 1973, 48:932–936.

71. STEINFELD L, DIMICH I, REDER R, COHEN M, ALEXANDER H: Sphygmomanometry in the pediatric patients. *J Pediatr* 1978, 92:934–938.

72. HOCHBERG HM, SOLOMON H: Accuracy of an automated ultrasound blood pressure monitor. *Curr Ther Res* 1971, 13:129–138.

73. REDER RF, DIMICH I, COHEN ML, STEINFELD L: Evaluating indirect blood pressure measurement techniques: a comparison of three systems in infants and children. *Pediatrics* 1978, 62:326–330.

74. POLLACK MH, OBRIST PA: Aortic-radial pulse transit time and ECG Q-wave to radial pulse wave interval as indices of beat-to-beat blood pressure change. *Psychophysiology* 1983, 20:21–28.

75. STEPTOE A, SMULYAN H, GRIBBIN B: Pulse wave velocity and blood pressure change: calibration and applications. *Psychophysiology* 1976, 13:488–493.

76. CARRUTHERS M, TAGGART P: Validation of a new, inexpensive, non-invasive miniaturized blood pressure monitor. *J Amb Mon* 1988, 1:163–170.

77. PENÀZ J: Photo-electric measurement of blood pressure, volume and flow in the finger. *Digest Tenth Int Conf Med Biol Eng*, Dresden, 1973, p. 104.

78. WESSELING KH, DE WIT B, SETTELS JJ, KLAWER WH: On the indirect registration of finger blood pressure after Penàz. *Funkt Biol Med J* 1982, 245:245–250.

79. TY SMITH N, WESSELING KH, DE WIT B: Evaluation of two prototype devices producing noninvasive, pulsatile, calibrated blood pressure measurement from a finger. *J Clin Monit* 1985, 1:17–29.

80. VAN EGMOND J, HASENBOS M, CRUL JF: Invasive versus non-invasive measurement of arterial pressure. Comparison of two automatic methods and simultaneously measured direct intra-arterial pressure. *Br J Anaesth* 1985, 57:434–444.

81. PARATI G, CASADEI R, GROPPELLI A, DI RIENZO M, MANCIA G: Continuous non-invasive finger blood pressure monitoring at rest and during laboratory testing: evaluation by intra-arterial recording. *J Hypertens* 1989, 13:647–655.

82. KURKI T, TY SMITH N, HEAD N, DEC-SILVER H, QUINN A: Non-invasive continuous blood pressure measurement from the finger: optimal measurement conditions and factors affecting reliability. *J Clin Mon* 1987, 3:6–13.

83.   KIDEMA RN, VAN DEN MEIRACKER AH, IMHOLZ BPM, *ET AL*: Comparison of Finapres non-invasive beat-to-beat finger blood pressure with intrabrachial artery pressure during and after bicycle ergometry. *J Hypertens* 1989, 7 (suppl 6):58–59.

84.   AASLID R, BRUBAKK AO: Accuracy of an ultrasound Doppler servo method for noninvasive determination of instantaneous and mean arterial blood pressure. *Circulation* 1981, 64:753–759.

85.   TAKAHASHI H, MATSUSUMA M, NISHIMURA M, *ET AL*: Usefulness of measurement of the digital blood pressure in patients with essential hypertension. *J Clin Exp Med* 1988, 146–154.

86.   IMAI Y, NIHEI M, ABE K, *ET AL*: A finger volume oscillometric device for monitoring ambulatory blood pressure: laboratory and clinical evaluations. *Clin Exp Hypertens* [A] 1987, 9:2001–2025.

87.   BLANK S, WEST JE, MULLER FB, *ET AL*: Wideband external pulse recording during cuff deflation: a new technique for evaluation of the arterial pressure pulse and measurement of blood pressure. *Circulation* 1988, 77:1297–1305.

88.   WEST JE, BUSCH-VISHNIAC IJ, HARSHFIELD GA, PICKERING TG: Foil electret transducer for blood pressure monitoring. *J Acoust Soc Am* 1983, 74:680–686.

89.   DE SWIET M, DILLON MJ, LITTLER W, O'BRIEN F, PADFIELD PL, PETRIE JC: Measurement of blood pressure in children. Recommendations of a working party of the British Hypertension Society. *Br Med J* 1989, 229:497.

90.   TASK FORCE ON BLOOD PRESSURE CONTROL IN CHILDREN: Report of the second task force on blood pressure control in children — 1987. *Pediatrics* 1987, 79:1–25.

91.   WHINCUP PH, COOK DG, SHAPER AG: Blood pressure measurement in children: the importance of cuff bladder size. *J Hypertens* 1989, 7:845–850.

92.   DE SWIET M: The physiology of normal pregnancy. In *Handbook of Hypertension. Vol 10. Hypertension in Pregnancy* edited by Rubin PC. Amsterdam: Elsevier, 1988, pp 1–15.

93.   TAYLOR DJ: The epidemiology of hypertension during pregnancy. *Handbook of Hypertension. Vol 10. Hypertension in Pregnancy* edited by Rubin PC. Amsterdam: Elsevier, 1988, pp. 223–240.

94.   SPENCE JD, SIBBALD WJ, CAPE RD: Direct, indirect and mean blood pressures in hypertensive patients: the problem of cuff artifact due to arterial wall stiffness, and a partial solution. *Clin Invest Med* 1980, 2:165–173.

95.   LITTENBERG B, WOLFBERG C: Pseudohypertension masquerading as malignant hypertension. Case report and review of the literature. *Am J Med* 1988, 64:539–542.

96.   MESSERLI FH, VENTURA HO, AMODEO C: Osler's maneuver and pseudohypertension. *N Engl J Med* 1985, 312:1548–1551.

97.   OSLER W: *Principles and Practice of Medicine.* New York: Appleton-Century, 1892.

98.   NIELSEN PE, JANNICHE H: The accuracy of auscultatory measurement of arm blood pressure in very obese subjects. *Acta Med Scand* 1974, 195:403–409.

99.   HENSCHEL A, DE LA VEGA F, TAYLOR HL: Simultaneous direct and indirect blood pressure measurements in man at rest and work. *J Appl Physiol* 1954, 5:506–508.

100. GOULD BA, HORNUNG RS, ALTMAN DG, CASHMAN PMM, RAFTERY EB: Indirect measurement of blood pressure during exercise testing can be misleading. *Br Heart J* 1985, 53:611–615.

3

Blood pressure monitors and their evaluation

Every new automatic or semi-automatic monitor which is developed uses a slightly different procedure for measuring blood pressure. Consequently, a new monitor must be tested for accuracy before it can be recommended for general use. While it is generally accepted that extensive testing should be done on at least one recorder of each type, it could also be argued that testing should be carried out on all of them, since it cannot be assumed that all units are identical. In practice this is inconvenient, but it is essential to check each recorder on each patient before a recording is started.

Recommendations for evaluation of non-invasive blood pressure monitors and observers

There are no generally agreed criteria for evaluating non-invasive blood pressure monitors. The most widely used technique has been to compare the readings obtained by the automatic recorder with simultaneously determined auscultatory readings, using either one or two observers. The Association for the Advancement of Medical Instrumentation (AAMI) and the BHS have published recommendations [1,2], both of which are described below. Ideally, intra-arterial pressures should be used as a reference, but this is often not feasible or ethical in practice. Furthermore, as we have seen in Chapter 2, there may be quite large differences between the intra-arterial and auscultatory measurments of blood pressure, which in some individuals may be as much as 25 mmHg. Such differences may be due to inaccuracies in both the direct and indirect measurements. It has been argued that, since all the information relating to the risks of hypertension and the benefits of treatment is based on readings taken with a mercury manometer, this should be the reference standard for automatic devices [3]. Most of the non-invasive methods cannot be expected to give readings that are any more accurate than the auscultatory method, which remains the usual method for comparison. At present, there is no automatic or semi-automatic recorder that is universally reliable, and so we would strongly recommend that every time such a device is used, it is calibrated against a standard method, which for practical reasons means a mercury sphygmomanometer and a trained observer. It is possible that, in the future, the K_2 method may be used rather than the auscultatory method.

Ideally, testing should be carried out in two situations: first, in controlled laboratory conditions, during which the accuracy can be evaluated; and second, with field testing, where factors such as convenience and reliability can be tested. This applies to both home and ambulatory monitors.

Evaluation of observers

Validation of each observer's technique is necessary before testing the recorders. For this purpose, training videotapes are available, and a double-headed stethoscope is advisable, so that two observers may listen to the same Korotkoff sounds. With this technique, differences in auditory acuity can be evaluated; under ideal circumstances more than 90% of readings taken by the two observers should be within 5 mmHg of each other.

Laboratory testing

Calibration against a mercury column is best performed using readings taken simultaneously from the same arm by the device being tested, and by one or two observers with a stethoscope placed just distal to the cuff, reading a mercury column connected to the cuff (Fig. 3.1). With devices which deflate the cuff automatically, there may be problems if large deflation steps are used (an example is the Spacelabs ambulatory recorder, which uses 8 mmHg steps), or if the cuff is deflated completely as

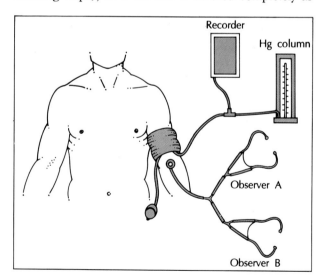

Fig. 3.1. Ideal situation for testing a non-invasive recorder against two trained observers, with the recorder connected to a mercury column via a T-piece. This enables simultaneous readings to be taken by the observers and the recorders.

soon as the recorder has registered diastolic pressure. An alternative (which may not always be possible) is to use manual deflation, which makes it easier for the observers but does not simulate the true operative conditions of the recorder. With this technique, a satisfactory device should give readings that are within 5 mmHg of the observers'.

If this technique is not practical, the observer can take auscultatory readings from the opposite arm. It is first necessary to check whether the pressure is the same in both arms, which can most easily be done by deflating two cuffs simultaneously, as shown in Fig. 3.2. This is less satisfactory for two reasons: there may be differences between the two arms; and it may be difficult to obtain the two sets of readings simultaneously. We have found that with the non-simultaneous technique two observers with a mercury sphygmomanometer can obtain correlation coefficients for paired readings of 0.98 for systolic pressure and 0.94 for diastolic pressure; 70% of readings should be within 5 mmHg of each other [4].

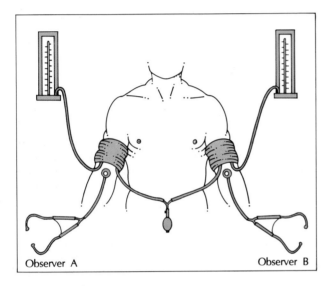

Fig. 3.2. Technique for checking whether the blood pressure is the same in the two arms.

The usual method of comparison is to take a relatively small number of paired readings, using the device being tested and the reference method, with the subject in the seated position. This is certainly adequate for devices intended for self-monitoring of blood pressure, but for ambulatory monitors it may also be advisable to obtain readings in three different positions — lying, sitting, and standing.

Field testing

The main purpose of field testing for the evaluation of home monitors is to check that the device is easy to use and robust. In most cases, home monitoring is performed by the patient alone, so that the ease with which the cuff can be applied single-handed is of importance. With ambulatory monitors an assessment of their performance in the more rigorous conditions of the field is also of interest. This would include both the acceptance by the patients, and the number of usable readings

obtained. It does not necessarily follow that differences between two sets of measurements made in the laboratory will remain the same throughout a 24-hour period. Two studies in which subjects wore a different monitor on each arm for 24 h showed that the discrepancies between the two may be different during the day and the night. In one study [5], subjects wore a Colin non-invasive monitor (Colin, Komaki-City, Japan) on one arm, and a finger-volume oscillometric device (BP-l00; ME Commercial Corp., Tokyo, Japan) on the other. During the day the systolic pressure readings were the same for the two recorders, but the diastolic pressure readings were consistently higher for the BP-100 device. However, during the night the systolic pressure readings were consistently higher for the Colin monitor, but the diastolic pressure readings were identical (Fig. 3.3). In the other study [6], the Spacelabs 5200 was compared with intra-arterial measurements: systolic pressures were closer during the night, and diastolic pressures were closer during the day.

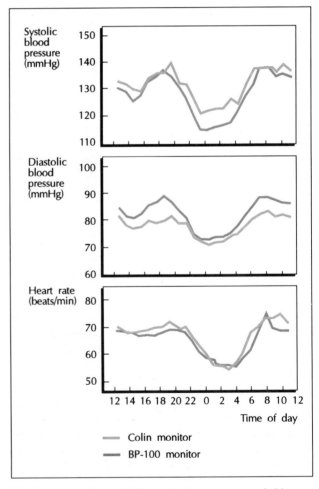

Fig. 3.3. Comparison of 24-hour blood pressure recorded by two different monitors, one on each arm, showing that the differences between the two may vary according to the time of day. Reproduced with permission [5].

Should more than one unit of each model be tested?

The vast majority of validation studies of blood pressure monitors have tested one unit of a particular model, with the implicit assumption that the unit tested is representative of all the units of that type. While this should certainly be true for some features of the recorder (such as the software design), for others (such as the sensitivity of the microphone) there could be significant variability. Relatively little attention has been given to the possibility that more than one unit of each type should be tested. One study, however, evaluated three Dinamap monitors of the same model and found virtually no difference between them, which is certainly reassuring [7]. Another study of 23 different home monitors carried out by Evans *et al.* [8], and described in the next section, found that 16 of the 23 brands showed no difference between two units of the same brand. Imai *et al.* [9] tested three units of eight different types of home monitor, and found minimal (less than 2 mmHg) inter-device variability. For testing oscillometric devices, they used an ingenious technique whereby a single cuff was linked via a four-way connector to three monitors and a stethoscope. This technique cannot, of course, be used with Korotkoff sound devices.

In contrast to these findings, O'Brien *et al.* [10] tested three units of each of six models, and found differences between individual units ranging from zero to 14 mmHg for systolic pressure, and from zero to 10 mmHg for diastolic pressure.

Procedures for comparing several recorders simultaneously

A few studies have compared several different monitors at one time. The usual set-up is shown in Fig. 3.4, where the recorder being tested is placed on one arm, and a standard or random-zero sphygmomanometer is placed on the other. Alternatively, two test recorders may be compared directly. We reported a study [4] in which a modified latin-square design was used to evaluate 11 brands of home blood pressure monitors. One of the most sophisticated studies to date was conducted by Evans *et al.* [8], who compared two units of each of 23 different home monitors. Each monitor was compared against readings taken by an observer using a Hawksley random-zero device on the other arm. To control for differences between observers, subjects, and arms they used a 'Youden square' design in a series of two-hourly sessions, during each of which four devices were tested on four subjects, with three pairs of observers (one of each pair operated the device). The testing was carried out in a series of 'rounds', with random allocation of observers, subjects, recorders, and starting arm. To begin with, each pair of observers was randomly allocated one subject and one recorder, and also which arm the recorder was put on. Three readings were taken, and then the observers switched over. Next, the recorder was switched to the other arm, and six more readings were taken. After this round of readings, the pair of observers tested another recorder on another subject, selected as shown in Fig. 3.5.

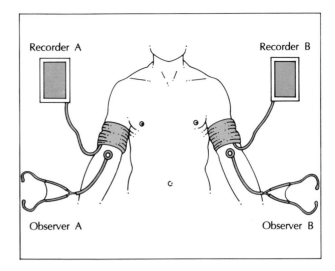

Fig. 3.4. Procedure for comparing two recorders using non-simultaneous readings on the two arms. One of the recorders may be a standard mercury sphygmomanometer.

Another study, conducted by O'Brien *et al.* [10], incorporated six phases of testing: observer training, observer assessment, before-use inter-device variability assessment, home use, after-use inter-device variability assessment, and device validation, in a sequence shown in Fig. 3.6. Observers were trained by an experienced physician using a multi-headed stethoscope, and with standard audiotapes and videotapes. Observers were accepted only if they obtained 85% of systolic and diastolic readings within 5 mmHg of readings obtained simultaneously by another observer. The before-use assessment of inter-device variability was carried out in a manner similar to Evans' Youden square design on 10 subjects with a rotation of three different units of each model, observers, and arms. One recorder was placed on each arm; devices that gave differences of more than 4 mmHg (systolic or diastolic pressure) were considered unacceptable. The 'home-use' phase was designed to assess the ease of use and reliability. The 'after-use' assessment was a repeat of the 'before-use' testing, to see whether the performance of the devices had changed. The final testing was the device validation, which was conducted only on the devices that had satisfied the criteria of the inital phases of testing, and followed the AAMI guidelines, described below. Each device was tested on 85 subjects using simultaneous testing with a double-headed stethoscope (as in Fig. 3.1), and three readings, giving a total of 255 readings per device.

While arduous and time consuming, this protocol had a number of exemplary features. First, observer reliability was checked before testing the devices. Second, the pre- and post-use testing served as as screening procedure for identifying grossly inaccurate or unreliable devices. Third, the criteria of acceptable accuracy were varied according to the level of blood pressure; 10 mmHg error at a sys-

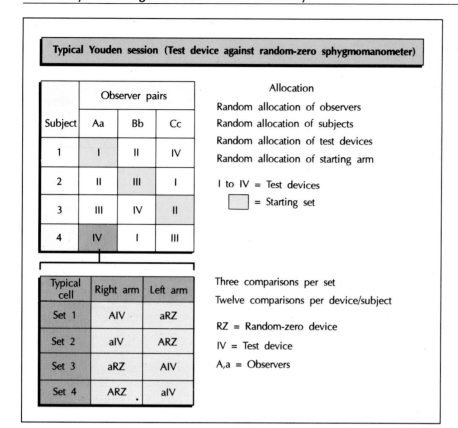

Fig. 3.5. Youden square design for testing several different recorders in one study. Reproduced with permission from Evans CE *et al.*, *J Hypertens* 1989, 7:133–142.

tolic pressure of 170 mmHg is unlikely to affect management very much, whereas at 90 mmHg it would make a big difference.

AAMI recommendations

The AAMI, based in the United States, has published[1] a series of recommendations for evaluating automated non-invasive blood pressure monitors for establishing acceptable criteria of accuracy [1]. These recommendations are summarized as follows:

(1)   The pressure transducer should be accurate to within ± 3 mmHg, over a range of 20–250 mmHg. The mean difference between paired measurements made by the device and the comparison system should be ± 5 mmHg or less, with a standard deviation of not more than 8 mmHg. Comparative measurements should be made with either auscultatory or intra-arterial readings.

(2)   For comparison of auscultatory monitors, at least 85 subjects should be studied, with systolic pressures ranging from 100 to 200 mmHg, and diastolic pressures ranging from 50 to 110 mmHg. The age range should be from 15 to 80 years, with the following distribution: less than 24 years, 6.5–13.5%; 25–44 years, 13–27%; 45–64 years, 19.5–40.5%; more than 64 years, 19.5–40.5%.

(3)   Two trained observers should take three sets of auscultatory blood pressure readings over a

10–30 min period in each subject, using the same arm as the recorder, unless the bleed rates of the device do not conform with the recommended rates [11]. In this case, simultaneous measurements may be performed in the two arms, provided that additional tests are carried out to check for blood pressure differences between them.

(4)   For intra-arterial comparisons 15 subjects should be studied with systolic pressures ranging from 90 to 190 mmHg, and diastolic pressures ranging from 60 to 100 mmHg. The age range should be 24–65 years. Between five and 10 paired measurements should be made on each subject.

(5)   The results should be reported as: (a) the means and standard deviation of the differences between the two methods for both systolic and diastolic pressures; (b) the correlation coefficients; (c) the regression equations; and (d) a scatter plot of the measurements, with lines showing the reliability of the estimated relationship (i.e. ± 1 and ± 2 standard errors).

Although these recommendations have been followed in a small number of studies, they were drawn up by equipment manufacturers, and have not so far been endorsed by any professional medical organizations. They were designed for electronic recorders in general, not just ambulatory monitors, and include no assessment of performance in the field, and no allowance for differences in

---

[1]This publication has not appeared in any medical journal, but can be obtained (for $55) from AAMI, 1901 North Fort Myer Drive, Suite 602, Arlington, VA 22209, USA.

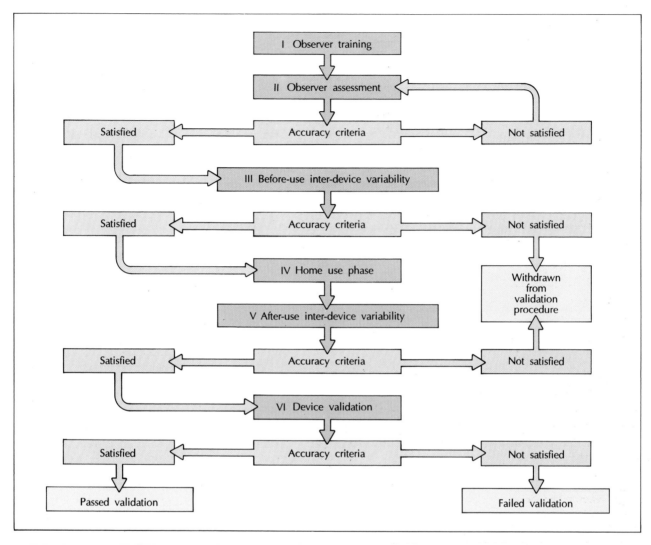

Fig. 3.6. Sequence of testing of home monitors used by O'Brien *et al.* Reproduced with permission [2].

arm size. The recommended method for data analysis is also no longer generally accepted as being optimal, as discussed below. These recommendations are currently being revised.

British Hypertension Society recommendations

The BHS has developed an elaborate protocol for evaluating ambulatory monitors, which was designed to overcome some of the shortcomings of the AAMI recommendations [2]. The procedure is outlined in Fig. 3.7. Two notable features are that it is based purely on non-invasive testing (for both practical and ethical reasons), and that most of the testing is carried out by a single observer.

Phase I consists of observer training and assessment, which includes a comparison with a trained observer with multi-headed stethoscopes, taking readings both from a videofilm and from normotensive and hypertensive subjects. Trainees should get 90% of systolic and diastolic readings within 5 mmHg of the expert's

readings, and 85% within 5 mmHg of another trainee's readings.

Phase II is a calibration test, and a test of inter-device variability. Three devices are selected, and each device's pressure transducer is calibrated against a mercury column. Ninety-five per cent of paired readings should be within 3 mmHg of each other.

Phase III involves field testing of the three devices, for each of which eight 24-hour recordings are obtained, in a total of 24 subjects. Readings are taken every 15 min during the day (9.00 a.m. to 10.00 p.m.) and every 30 min at night, giving a maximum of 75 readings per device. The performance is assessed both by the number of satisfactory readings, as judged by the system's own criteria (e.g. error codes, aborted readings), and by the acceptability to the subjects wearing them.

Phase IV is a repeat of inter-device variability (phase II), to see whether the performance has changed with use.

Phase V, the most intensive part of testing, is the laboratory validation similar to the AAMI procedure. It is carried out using one of the three devices, on 85 subjects

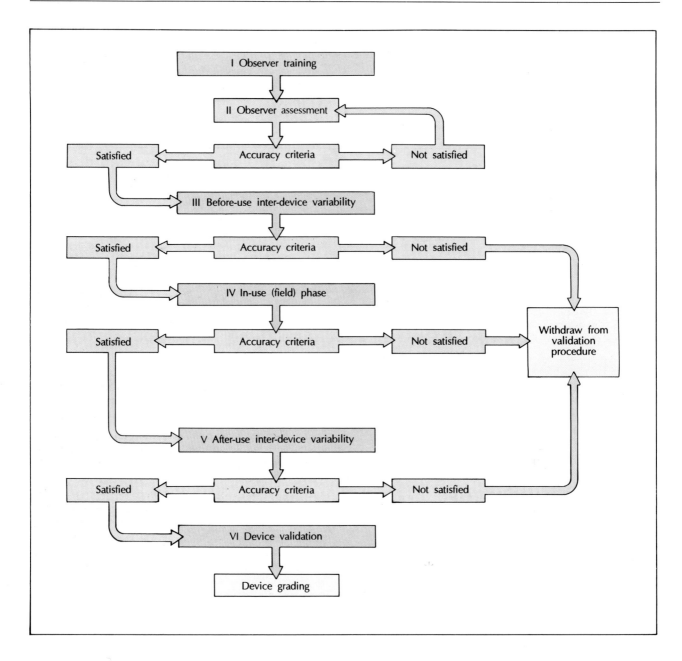

Fig. 3.7. Procedure recommended by the British Hypertension Society for the evaluation of non-invasive ambulatory recorders. Reproduced with permission [10].

(aged 15–80 years) whose blood pressures are evenly distributed over a systolic range of 100–240 mmHg, and a diastolic presure range of 60–120 mmHg. Two observers are used, each one testing half of the subjects, and taking three readings per subject. For devices with controllable deflation rates the simultaneous same-arm technique is used (Fig. 3.1). If the rate cannot be controlled manually, or is greater than 5 mmHg per second, sequential measurements are made on the same arm using a mercury sphygmomanometer and the device in alternation.

The results are analysed by the technique of Bland and Altman [12] (described below), and the devices are graded according to the percentage of readings within 5 mmHg of the mercury readings, as shown in Fig. 3.8.

While this procedure is certainly more appropriate for validating ambulatory monitors than the AAMI recommendations, one deficiency is that it does not require the devices to be tested in different postures.

How should the results be analysed?
The traditional method of analysing a comparison of two blood pressure recorders has been to use simple regression analysis, and to express the agreement between the

	Difference between observer and device readings (mmHg)*		
Grade	≤5	≤10	≤15
A	80	90	95
B	65	85	95
C	45	75	90
D		Worse than C	

*Values are cumulative % of readings.

Fig. 3.8. British Hypertension Society grading criteria for evaluation of ambulatory monitors.

two as the correlation coefficient, with graphical plots as in Fig. 3.9. In their influential and widely quoted paper [12], Bland and Altman have argued that this approach, although widely used, is inappropriate. There are three points to their argument. First, the correlation coefficient measures the strength of the relationship between the two measures, not the agreement between them. What we need to know is whether or not the two measures are the same, not whether or not they are related. Second, the correlation coefficient will depend on the range of pressures over which the measurements are made: in general the greater the range, the higher the correlation. Third, quite high correlations may be obtained when the agreement is poor.

Bland and Altman suggested that a better method of examining the data is to plot the average pressure measured by the two techniques against the difference between the two, as shown in Fig. 3.10. This gives a better idea of the extent of disagreement, which can be expressed numerically as the mean difference (d) and the standard

deviation of the differences (SDD). If the differences are normally distributed, as is likely to be the case, 95% of the readings will be between the limits d + 1.96 s and d − 1.96 s (approximately the mean ± 2 standard deviations). This range has been referred to as the limits of agreement.

While this method certainly has advantages over regression analysis, the means and standard deviations of the differences do not provide any information about the linearity of the agreement between the two measures. It is not uncommon, for example, for a recorder to overestimate blood pressure when it is low, and to underestimate it when it is high; this will be apparent from the regression equation, which in this case will have a slope of less than 1.0. For most clinical and research purposes, the accuracy of a recorder over the middle of the range is of greater concern than that at the two extremes; an error of 10 mmHg is of relatively little importance at 180 mmHg. A case could therefore be made for expressing the measurement errors over a variety of ranges (e.g. for systolic pressure, below 100 mmHg, between 100 and 150 mmHg, and above 160 mmHg).

Automatic and semi-automatic home blood pressure monitors

A large number of devices which monitor blood pressure automatically are now available. Virtually all use a sphygmomanometer cuff, and operate by Korotkoff sound detection, oscillometry, or ultrasound. Some of the devices are suitable for home monitoring of blood pressure, while others are better for laboratory studies. They have several obvious advantages: one is that they eliminate observer error and observer bias, and may print out the readings as well as displaying them. We have evaluated a number of such self-monitoring devices [4] using

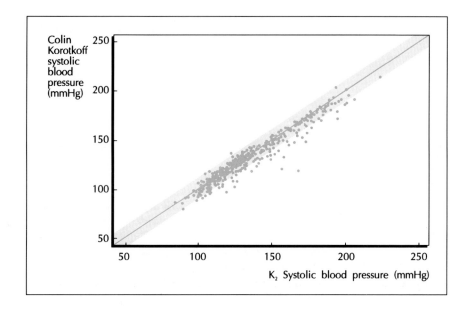

Fig. 3.9. The traditional way of plotting data obtained for the validation of a blood pressure monitor (the Colin ABPM 630) against a standard technique (the K_2 method), using linear regression analysis. The line is the line of identity bordered by ± 10 mmHg (courtesy of Dr S. Blank).

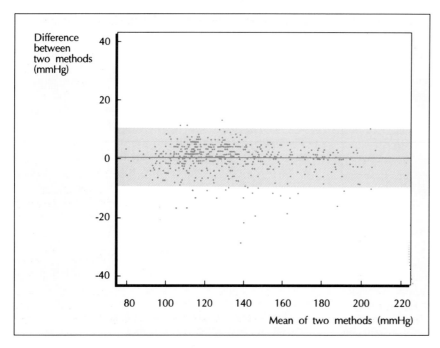

Fig. 3.10. The same data as in Fig. 3.9, plotted in the manner recommended by Bland and Altman. The line shows the mean difference bordered by ± 2 standard deviations (courtesy of Dr S. Blank).

the non-simultaneous two-arm technique (Fig. 3.4). From these evulations we have come to the following conclusions: first, many of the recorders are inaccurate, giving readings that are consistently more than 5 mmHg in error when compared with simultaneously determined auscultatory values (see Fig. 3.11); second, no single method recording, e.g. oscillometric or Korotkoff sound, is consistently superior; and third, there is no correlation between the price and the accuracy of the recorders.

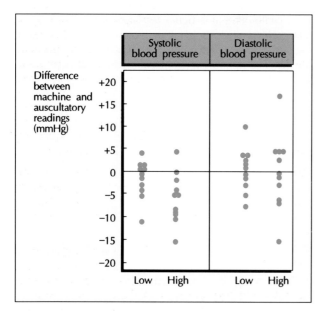

Fig. 3.11. Average differences between auscultatory and machine readings for 11 semi-automatic home monitors in normotensive (Low) and hypertensive (High) subjects. Data from [4].

It is essential that any automatic recorder be calibrated against auscultatory readings in each subject. Malatino and Brown [13] compared the Copal UA251 recorder

(Copal, Japan) with the Hawksley random-zero device and found excellent agreement, with a systematic difference of less than 1 mmHg and a standard deviation of less than 3 mmHg for both systolic and diastolic pressure readings.

In the study of O'Brien *et al.* [10] none of the six devices tested, which included five semi-automatic and an aneroid model, passed all the criteria, whereas a standard mercury sphygmomanometer tested in the same way did pass the criteria.

Telephonic transmission from home blood pressure monitors

Recently, a home blood pressure monitor (the Instromedix Barograf; Telelab, Hillsboro, Oregon, USA) has been developed which has the ability of not only storing the readings on a memory chip, but also transmitting them over a telephone via a modem to a personal computer, on which the data can be stored and analysed. This promising development is analogous to the technique of transmitting pacemaker signals over the telephone. It has great potential both for research purposes, and for monitoring patients' response to treatment. However, in its present form it is prohibitively expensive. We have validated it, and found it satisfactory [14].

The Vita-Stat automatic recorder

This device was first introduced in the United States in 1976, and was designed to be located in public places, such as supermarkets or pharmacies, to enable the general population to obtain a blood pressure reading either free of charge or at a nominal cost. There are now about 6500 such devices in use.

The subject places his or her arm in a looped cuff, which closes automatically over the upper arm. There is a microphone in the cuff which, when the arm is correctly placed, lies over the brachial artery. When the start button is pressed the cuff inflates automatically, and deflates at 4–6 mmHg per second. Readings are taken by Korotkoff sound detection and displayed on a screen. Such devices therefore, have the potential advantage of providing unbiased readings to large numbers of people who may have limited access to professional blood pressure measurements.

Vita-Stat automatic recorders have been evaluated in three studies [15–17], which examined nine, four and one recorder, respectively. Comparisons in each case were made with auscultatory readings taken by trained observers, using either a conventional mercury sphygmomanometer, or a random-zero machine. All three studies found better agreement for diastolic than systolic pressure, but it was not very good for either measurement. Furthermore, there were systematic errors for some of the devices, of up to 14 mmHg for systolic pressure and 7.5 mmHg for diastolic pressure [16]. Thus, these machines are not sufficiently accurate to be recommended for general use.

Ambulatory blood pressure monitors

Two types of ambulatory recorders have been developed — invasive and non-invasive. The former have the advantages of the greater accuracy of intra-arterial recording and of giving continuous beat-to-beat measurements, but are unsuitable for widespread clinical or epidemiological use. The non-invasive recorders are less accurate and give intermittent readings, but can be used for routine clinical evaluation. Both types are described below.

Invasive recorders

The most widely used invasive ambulatory recorder has been the Oxford Medilog device which records blood pressure continuously from a catheter in the brachial artery [18–20]. The central unit containing the transducer and tape recording system is worn in a harness on the chest, so that the transducer is always at the level of the heart. This technique ensures that errors in blood pressure measurement are not introduced as a result of changes in the position of the arm, but has the disadvantage of requiring a long connecting tube between the arterial cannula and the transducer, which severely limits the frequency response of the recording system [20]. Since every pressure wave is recorded, it is in theory possible to obtain a complete picture of blood pressure and heart rate changes over 24 h. In practice, however, there is some loss of data due to movement artefact and damping of the catheter, but at present this technique provides the only method for obtaining a true measure of the range of blood pressure and its variability in ambulatory patients. While this method is often regarded as the 'gold standard' for the validation of non-invasive recorders, its frequency response is flat to less than 8 Hz [6], which,

as discussed in Chapter 2, will result in significant underdamping of the pressure trace.

The technique has been used mainly in studies of blood pressure variability [21–23], and for documenting the effects of antihypertensive medications [24–27].

Non-invasive recorders

Several non-invasive ambulatory recorders have been developed, and more are likely to follow. Most of these have a conventional blood pressure cuff, and operate either on the Korotkoff sound technique or by oscillometry (see Fig. 3.12). One recorder (the Colin device) takes readings by both techniques, and gives simultaneous print-outs of both sets. This procedure has the theoretical advantage of enabling a check on the internal consistency of the readings. Recorders which operate on the Korotkoff sound principle typically have a piezo-electric microphone with a frequency response of about 15–30 Hz, which is positioned over the brachial artery. In some cases (e.g. the Suntech Accutracker II; Suntech, Raleigh, North Carolina, USA) R wave gating is used, so that only sounds detected at a certain interval after the R wave (150–300 ms) are accepted as Korotkoff sounds. This procedure is designed to minimize interference from artefactual sounds, for example from body movement. It does, however, require ECG electrodes for detecting the R waves, which is a slight added inconvenience.

Other techniques for eliminating artefactual sounds have been developed, such as the use of two microphones, one over the artery and one away from it, with subtraction of the two signals [28]. Ambulatory recorders using finger cuffs have also been developed [29], but may be susceptible to artefacts from movement and changes of environmental temperature. All monitors except the Remler M2000 are fully automatic, and most use a pump to inflate and deflate the cuff at pre-set intervals. The subject can also inflate the cuff on demand. The pumps on the earlier models tended to produce a visceral noise which might prove embarrassing to the subject, but the latest models are much quieter. The Colin recorder uses a CO_2 cylinder, which inflates the cuff noiselessly.

Such recorders typically give 50–100 readings over a 24-hour period. The blood pressure readings are stored in the memory of the recorder, and at the end of the 24-hour period can be downloaded onto a personal computer.

None of the currently available devices works in every patient, and problems are most pronounced in the elderly and the obese. It is important to calibrate the recorder against simultaneously determined auscultatory readings, which can be carried out using a mercury column. Some of the devices can be manually deflated during calibration (e.g. the Del Mar Avionics Pressurometer IV). Ideally, it should be possible to obtain paired readings that are within 5 mmHg of each other. It is helpful if the patient fills out a diary describing his or her activity, posture, and location, at the time of each reading, since these variables may have a substantial influence on blood pressure. The

Type of monitor	Mode of operation	Weight	Cuff inflation	Accuracy*	Author
Remler M2000	K sound	0.7 kg	Patient	0/−4	Pagny [37]
Physioport	K sound	1 kg	Pump	−2/−2	Langewitz [52]
Spacelabs 90202	Oscillometric	0.5 kg	Pump	1/−2.5	Santucci [46]
				1/−2.4	Von Pölnitz [47]
				0/−7	White [44] †
Spacelabs 90207	Oscillometric	0.3 kg	Pump	1/2	Cates [54]
Del Mar Avionics	K sound	0.8 kg	Pump	1/−2	Harshfield [42]
Pressurometer IV				−1/−1	Santucci [43]
				9/−6	White [44] †
Oxford Medilog	K sound	0.5 kg	Pump	2/−1	Hope [49]
Colin ABPM 630	Oscillometric	0.8 kg	CO_2	3/−12	White [44] †
				2/−7	White [50]
	K sound			−3/−12	White [44]
				0/−6	White [50]
Suntech Accutracker II	K sound	0.4 kg	Pump	3/−12	White [44] †
Takeda TM-2420	K sound	0.4 kg	Pump	−1/−3	Tochikubo [51]

*Accuracy: Mean difference between monitor and observer taking auscultatory readings for systolic and diastolic pressure. †In this study all four recorders tested gave lower diastolic readings than the observer's. However, intra-arterial readings were also lower (by 4 mmHg) than the observers' readings.

Fig. 3.12. Non-invasive ambulatory blood pressure monitors.

practical aspects of using these recorders are described in Chapter 9.

Few of the recorders so far evaluated give good readings during physical exercise, or in environments where there is a great deal of vibration. It is our policy to inform patients that they should keep their arm motionless by their side while a reading is being taken. Even with such precautions, there is still a proportion of readings that are artefactual, and must be edited out for the final analysis.

Accuracy of non-invasive ambulatory recorders

The accuracy of such recorders is limited by the inherent limitations of the non-invasive techniques used. Thus they are less accurate than direct intra-arterial recording. A large number of validation studies have been published in which readings taken by non-invasive recorders have been compared with simultaneously determined auscultatory readings taken with a mercury column. On the whole these reports have shown reasonably satisfactory correlations for the devices used most extensively — the Del Mar Avionics PIII [30–34], the Spacelabs 5200 [35–37], the Remler [38,39], and the Accutracker I [40,41]. There is now a second generation of ambulatory recorders, such as the Del Mar Avionics PIV [42–44], the Spacelabs 90202 and 90207 [43–48], the Oxford Medilog [49], the Suntech Accutracker II [44], the Colin APBM 630 [44,50], and the Takeda TM-2420 [51], all of which have been validated with generally satisfactory results. As with all non-invasive methods, systolic pressure is recorded more reliably than diastolic pressure. There does not appear to be any systematic difference between the accuracy of recorders which use the Korotkoff sound technique compared with the oscillometric technique.

Validation against intra-arterial measurements

Fewer studies have validated the non-invasive recorders against both auscultatory and intra-arterial readings. One of the problems with the comparison of direct and indirect measurements of pressure is that it is usually not possible to know exactly which pressure waves were taken by the non-invasive device to record systolic and diastolic pressure. It is therefore customary to take the average of several intra-arterial readings (e.g. for 15 s before and 15 s after the non-invasive measurement). While this should eliminate any systematic error between the two sets of readings, it will inevitably introduce some random scatter. White et al. [44] estimated the standard deviation of this to be about 3 mmHg for both systolic and diastolic pressure. The results of studies validating non-invasive monitors against intra-arterial studies are summarized in Fig. 3.13.

Graettinger et al. [48] evaluated the Spacelabs 5200 and 90202 devices. For systolic pressure the correlations with intra-arterial pressure were closer with the auscultatory readings than with the recorders' readings, while for diastolic pressure both recorders gave closer correlations than the auscultatory readings. The range of deviations between invasive and non-invasive measures of pressure was similar for all three methods. The Colin recorder has also been tested against intra-arterial pressures [50].

Baig et al. [53] found that the Accutracker I underestimated systolic pressure (by 7 mmHg), and overestimated diastolic pressure (by 6 mmHg). The relation-

Type of recorder	Accuracy*	Correlation	Author
Ambulatory			
Spacelabs 5200	5/−5	0.74/0.86	Graettinger et al. [48]
Spacelabs 90202	8/−8	0.89/0.81	Graettinger et al. [48]
(Auscultatory)†	8/−6	0.93/0.76	Graettinger et al. [48]
Spacelabs 90202	0.5/0.7	0.97/0.91	Von Pölnitz and Hifking [47]
	−2/3	–	White et al. [44]
(Auscultatory)†	−4/4	–	White et al. [44]
Colin ABPM 630			
Oscillometric	4.5/−1.2		White et al. [50]
	4/0	–	White et al. [44]
K sound	1.4/−0.1		White et al. [50]
	2/0	–	White et al. [44]
Del Mar PIV	6/2	–	White et al. [44]
Accutracker I	−6.7/6.2	0.92/0.89	Baig et al. [53]
Accutracker II	1/−3	–	White et al. [44]
Semi-automatic			
Takeda 751	3.5/5	0.84/0.89	Wiinberg et al. [55]
Copal 251	5/2	0.86/0.87	Wiinberg et al. [55]
(Auscultatory)†	4/7	0.91/0.91	Wiinberg et al. [55]

*Mean difference between monitor and intra-arterial pressure for systolic and diastolic pressure. †Comparisons made between auscultatory and intra-arterial pressure at time of testing the monitors.

Fig. 3.13. Comparisons of ambulatory and semi-automatic monitors with intra-arterial pressure.

ship between intra-arterial and machine systolic pressure was non-linear, such that the under-estimation by the machine was progressively greater at higher levels of pressure. Baig *et al.* commented that the 95% confidence limits (from +20 to −15 mmHg for systolic pressure, and from +6.5 to −19 mmHg for diastolic pressure) are considerably larger than for a standard mercury sphygmomanometer (for which the corresponding values would be +3.5 to −16.5 mmHg for systolic pressure and +19 to −3 mmHg for diastolic pressure). However, the much greater range for systolic pressure reflects this particular device's non-linearity at high systolic pressures.

The most extensive study to date was conducted by White *et al.* [44], who validated four monitors (the Colin ABPM 630, the Del Mar PIV, the Spacelabs 90202, and the Accutracker II) both at rest and during exercise (see below). As shown in Fig. 3.14, the agreement with intra-arterial pressure was in general no worse for the monitors than for observers taking auscultatory readings, and for two of them (the Colin and the Accutracker) was significantly better.

Relatively few comparisons of intra-arterial and non-invasive measurements of blood pressure measured over 24 h have been published. Casadei *et al.* [6] compared the Spacelabs 5200 with intra-arterial monitoring in eight hospitalized patients. For the group as a whole, the average 24-hour pressures were the same for the two techniques, but there were large individual differences of up to 25 mmHg. The authors concluded that such dis-

crepancies could not be attributed to the different sampling intervals (every beat for the intra-arterial measurements, but once every 15 min for the Spacelabs monitor), because they had previously shown that sampling at intervals of 5–30 min provides 24-hour average values that are virtually identical to beat-by-beat sampling [54]. Casadei *et al.* concluded that the Spacelabs device cannot accurately measure blood pressure throughout the 24-hour period. Rather than blaming this particular recorder, however, a more plausible explanation would be that this is another example of the generally poor correlation between direct and indirect methods of measurement. This conclusion is supported by the statement that the Spacelabs recorder agreed with auscultatory readings to within 5 mmHg.

Validation during exercise

The non-invasive measurement of blood pressure during dynamic exercise has always been unreliable, and this applies equally to the newer ambulatory monitors. White *et al.* [44] tested four monitors against intra-arterial pressure both at rest and during isometric and bicycle exercise. During isometric exercise the average errors and the limits of agreement were generally similar to auscultatory readings taken by trained observers, but during bicycle exercise two of the recorders (the Accutracker and Colin) performed reliably, while two others (the Spacelabs and the Del Mar) gave gross errors.

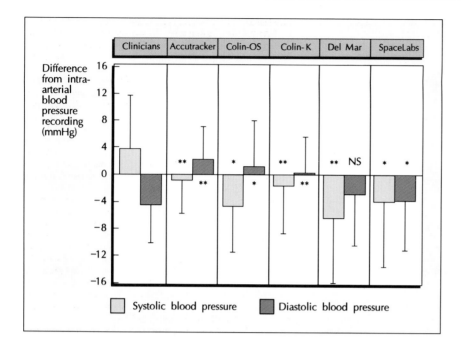

Fig. 3.14. Comparison of differences between intra-arterial and non-invasive measurements of blood pressure for clinicians (using the auscultatory method) and four ambulatory monitors – Accutracker II, Colin ABPM 560 (OS, oscillometric, K Korotkoff modes, Del Mar PIV, and Spacelabs 90202). Reproduced with permission from White et al., Am J Cardiol 1989, 65:60–66.

Summary and conclusions

The technology for non-invasive automatic monitoring of blood pressure is advancing at a rapid rate, and many recorders are now available which are sufficiently small and accurate to make ambulatory monitoring a practical and reliable procedure. They operate either by the Korotkoff sound technique or by the oscillometric technique, and there does not appear to be any consistent superiority of one over the other. All such monitors suffer from the inherent inaccuracies of the non-invasive methods, and are less reliable at the extremes of blood pressure, for example during vigorous exercise and sleep.

An even larger number of semi-automatic home monitors are available, which are mostly much less accurate, and in many cases unacceptably so.

Any new automatic or semi-automatic monitor must be subjected to a formal evaluation of its accuracy and reliability before it can be recommended for use. Although there is no universally agreed standard, some generally accepted guidelines are recommended. First, while comparisons against intra-arterial pressures are optimal, validation against the auscultatory method is generally acceptable, since this remains the 'gold standard' for clinical measurement. Second, two trained observers, whose technique has been previously validated, should take readings for comparison against the device being tested. This can be carried out either with the 'simultaneous — same arm' technique, or with the 'non-simultaneous — both arms' technique. While there should be no systematic error for either method, the scatter of readings will be higher with the latter. Third, the testing should be carried out in a variety of subjects with different ages, arm diameters, and blood pressures. Fourth, the circumstances of testing should, as closely as possible, simulate the circumstances in which the recorder will actually be used.

References

1. ASSOCIATION FOR THE ADVANCEMENT OF MEDICAL INSTRUMENTATION: *Proposed Standard for Electronic or Automated Sphygmomanometers.* Arlington, VA: AAMI, 1985.

2. O'BRIEN E, PETRIE J, LITLER WA, ET AL: **The British Hypertension Society protocol for the evaluation of automated and semi-automated blood pressure measuring devices with special reference to ambulatory systems.** *J Hypertens* 1990, 8:607–619.

3. SLOAN PJM, ZEZULKA A, DAVIES P, SANGAL A, BEEVERS M, BEEVERS DG: **Standardized methods for comparison of sphygmomanometers.** *J Hypertens* 1984, 2:547–551.

4. PICKERING TG, CVETKOVSKI B, JAMES GD: **An evaluation of electronic recorders for self monitoring of blood pressure.** *J Hypertens* 1986, 4 (suppl 5):S328–S330.

5. IMAI Y, SASAKI S, MINAMI N, ET AL: **Difference in the nocturnal behavior of blood pressure between monitoring with the arm-cuff method and with the finger-volume oscillometric method.** *J Hypertens* 1988, 6 (suppl 4):61–63.

6. CASADEI R, PARATI G, POMIDOSSI G, ET AL: **24-hour blood pressure monitoring: evaluation of Spacelabs 5300 monitor by comparison with intra-arterial blood pressure recordings in ambulant subjects.** *J Hypertens* 1988, 6:797–803.

7. SPYCHERELLE Y, GUEGUEN R, ANDRE JL, DESCHAMPS JP: **La mesure de la pression artérielle par méthode automatique.** *Arch Mal Coeur* 1988, 81:997–1000.

8. EVANS CE, HAYNES RB, GOLDSMITH CH, HEWSON SA: **Home blood pressure-measuring devices: a comparative study of accuracy.** *J Hypertens* 1989, 7:133–142.

9. IMAI Y, ABE K, SASAKI S, ET AL: **Clinical evaluation of semi-automatic and automatic devices for home blood pressure measurements: comparison between cuff-oscillometric and microphone methods.** *J Hypertens* 1989, 7:983–990.

10. O'BRIEN E, ATKINS N, MEE F, O'MALLEY K: **Inaccuracies of sphygmomanometers for home measurement of blood pressure.** *J Hypertens* 1990, 8:621–624.

11. ASSOCIATION FOR THE ADVANCEMENT OF MEDICAL INSTRUMENTATION: *American National Standards for Non-Automated Sphygmomanometers.* ANSI/AAMIU. SP9-1986, Arlington, VA, 1986.

12. BLAND JM, ALTMAN DG: **Statistical methods for assessing agreement between two methods of clinical measurements.** *Lancet* 1986, i:307–310.

13. MALATINO L, BROWN WCB: Comparison of a new portable electronic sphygmomanometer (Copal UA 251) with the Hawksley random zero machine. *Clin Exp Hypertens* [A] 1988, 10:589–596.

14. JAMES GD, YEE LS, CATES EM, SCHLUSSEL YR, PECKER MS, PICKERING TG: A validation study of the Instromedix Baro-Graf QD home blood pressure monitor. *Am J Hypertens* 1990, 3:717–720.

15. BERKSON DM, WHIPPLE IT, SHIREMAN L, BROWN MC, RAYNOR W, SHEKELLE RB: Evaluation of an automated blood pressure measuring device intended for general public use. *Am J Public Health* 1979, 69:473–479.

16. POLK FB, ROSNER B, FEUDO R, VANDENBURGH M: An evaluation of the Vita-Stat automatic blood pressure measuring device. *Hypertension* 1980, 2:221–227.

17. WHELTON PK, THOMPSON SG, BARNES GR, MIALL WE: Evaluation of the Vita-Stat automatic blood pressure recorder. A comparison with the random-zero sphygmomanometer. *Am J Epidemiol* 1983, 117:46–54.

18. BEVAN AT, HONOUR AJ, SCOTT FG: Direct arterial pressure recording in unrestricted man. *Clin Sci* 1969, 36:329–344.

19. STOTT FD, TERRY VG, HONOUR AJ: Factors determining the design and construction of a portable pressure transducer system. *Postgrad Med J* 1976, 52 (suppl 7):97–99.

20. GOLDBERG AD, RAFTERY EB, GREEN HL: The Oxford continuous blood pressure monitor: technical and clinical evaluation. *Postgrad Med J* 1976, 52 (suppl 7):104–109.

21. CONWAY J: Blood pressure and heart rate variability. *J Hypertens* 1986, 4:261–263.

22. WATSON RD, STALLARD TJ, FLINN RM, LITTLER WA: Factors determining direct arterial pressure and its variability in hypertensive man. *Hypertension* 1986, 2:333–341.

23. MANCIA G, FERRARI A, GREGORINI L, ET AL: Blood pressure variability in man: its relation to high blood pressure, age, and baroreflex sensitivity. *Clin Sci* 1980, 59:401s–404s.

24. MANN S, MILLAR-CRAIG MW, BALASUBRAMANIAN V, CASHMAN PMM, RAFTERY EB: Ambulant blood pressure: reproducibility and the assessment of interventions. *Clin Sci* 1980, 59:497–500.

25. GOULD BA, MANN S, DAVIES AB, ALTMAN DG, RAFTERY EB: Does placebo lower blood-pressure? *Lancet* 1981, ii:1377–1381.

26. GOLDBERG AD, RAFTERY EB: Patterns of blood-pressure during chronic administration of postganglionic sympathetic blocking drugs for hypertension. *Lancet* 1976, ii:1052–1054.

27. FLORAS JS, JONES JV, HASSAN MO, SLEIGHT P: Ambulatory pressure during once-daily randomized double-blind administration of atenolol, metoprolol, pindolol, and slow-release propranolol. *Br Med J* 1982, 285:1387–1392.

28. OGASAWARA S, FREEDMAN SB, RAM J, KELLY DT: Evaluation of a microprocessor-controlled sphygmomanometer for recording blood pressure during exercise. *Am J Cardiol* 1989, 64:806–808.

29. YAMAKOSHI K, KAWARADA A, KAMIYA A, SHIMAZU H, ITO H: Long-term ambulatory monitoring of indirect arterial blood pressure using a volume-oscillometric method. *Med Biol Eng Comput* 1985, 23:459–465.

30. HARSHFIELD GA, PICKERING TG, LARAGH JH: A validation study of the Del Mar Avionics ambulatory blood pressure system. *Ambulatory Electrocardiography* 1979, 1:7–12.

31. SHEPS SG, ELVEBACH LR, CLOSE EL, KLEVEN MK, BISSEN C: Evaluation of the Del Mar Avionics ambulatory blood pressure recording device. *Mayo Clin Proc* 1981, 56:740–743.

32. MESSERLI FH, GLADE LB, VENTURA HO, ET AL: Diurnal variations of cardiac rhythm, arterial pressure and urinary catecholamines in borderline and established essential hypertension. *Am Heart J* 1982, 104:109–114.

33. WARD A, HANSON P: Accuracy and reproducibility of ambulatory blood pressure recorder measurements during rest and exercise. In *Ambulatory Blood Pressure Monitoring* edited by Weber MA, Drayer JIM. Darmstadt: Steinkopff, 1984, pp 51–56.

34. GOULD BA, HORNING RS, CASHMAN PMM, RAFTERY EB: Ambulatory blood pressure: direct and indirect. In *Ambulatory Blood Pressure Monitoring* edited by Weber MA, Drayer JIM. Darmstadt: Steinkopff, 1984, pp 9–20.

35. HARSHFIELD GA, PICKERING TG, BLANK S, LINDAHL C, STROUD L, LARAGH JH: Ambulatory blood pressure monitoring: recorders, applications, and analysis. In *Ambulatory Blood Pressure Monitoring* edited by Weber MA, Drayer JIM. Darmstadt: Steinkopff, 1984, pp 1–8.

36. DEMBROSKI TM, MACDOUGALL TM: Validation of the Vita-Stat automated noninvasive blood pressure recording device. In *Cardiovascular Instrumentation: Applicability of New Technology to Biobehavioral Research* edited by Herd JA, Gotto AM, Kaufman PC, Weiss SM. Bethesda, MD: National Institutes of Health, 1984, pp 53–77.

37. PAGNY J-Y, CHATELLIER G, DEVRIES C, JANOD J-P, CORVOL P, MENARD J: Evaluation of the Spacelabs ambulatory blood pressure recorder: comparison with the Remler M2000. *Cardiovasc Rev Rep* 1987, 8:31–36.

38. HINMAN AT, ENGEL BT, BICKFORD AF: Portable blood pressure records: accuracy and preliminary use in evaluating intradaily variations in pressure. *Am Heart J* 1962, 64:663–668.

39. WAEBER B, JACOT DES GOMBES B, PORCHET M, BRUNNER HR: Accuracy, reproducibility and usefulness of ambulatory blood pressure recordings obtained with the Remler System. In *Ambulatory Blood Pressure Monitoring* ed d by Weber MA, Drayer JIM. Darmstadt: Steinkopff, 1984, p 65–70.

40. WHITE WB, SCHULMAN P, MCCABE EJ, NARDONE M: Clinical validation of the Accutracker ambulatory blood pressure monitor. *J Clin Hypertens* 1987, 3:500–509.

41. LIGHT KC, OBRIST PA, CUBEDDU LX: Evaluation of a new ambulatory blood pressure monitor (Accutracker 102): laboratory comparisons with direct arterial pressure, stethoscopic ausculatatory pressure, and readings from a similar monitor. (Spacelabs model 5200). *Psychophysiology* 1988, 25:107–116.

42. HARSHFIELD GA, HWANG C, GRIM CE: A validation study of the Del Mar Avionics Pressurometer IV according to AAMI guidelines. *J Hypertens* 1988, 6:913–918.

43. SANTUCCI S, CATES EM, JAMES GD, SCHLUSSEL YR, STEINER D, PICKERING TG: A comparison of two ambulatory blood pressure monitors, the Del Mar Avionics Pressurometer IV and the Spacelabs 90202. *Am J Hypertens* 1989, 2:797–799.

44. WHITE WB, LUND-JOHANSEN P, OMVIK P: Assessment of four ambulatory blood pressure monitors and measurements by clinicians versus intraarterial blood pressure at rest and during exercise. *Am J Cardiol* 1989, 65:60–66.

45. CATES EM, SCHLUSSEL YR, JAMES GD, PICKERING TG: A validation study of the Spacelabs 90207 ambulatory monitor *J Amb Mon* (in press).

46. SANTUCCI S, STEINER D, ZIMBLER M, JAMES GD, PICKERING TG: A validation study of the Spacelabs 90202 and 5200 ambulatory blood pressure monitors. *J Amb Mon* 1988, 1:211–216.

47. VON PÖLNITZ A, HÖFLING B: Validation of the Spacelabs Model 90202, a non-invasive, ambulatory blood-pressure monitoirng device: intra-arterial and mercury column comparison study. *J Amb Mon* 1989, 2:169–173.

48. GRAETTINGER WR, LIPSON HL, CHEUNG DG, WEBER MA: Validation of portable noninvasive blood pressure monitoring devices: comparisons with intra-arterial and sphygmomanometer measurements. *Am Heart J* 1988, 116:1155–1160.

49. HOPE SL, ALUN-JONES E, SLEIGHT P: Validation of the accuracy of the Medilog ABP noninvasive blood pressure monitor. *J Amb Mon* 1988, 1:39–51.

50. WHITE WB, LUND-JOHANSEN P, MCCABE EJ: Clinical evaluation of the Colin ABPM 630 at rest and during exercise: an ambulatory blood pressure monitor with gas-powered cuff inflation. *J Hypertens* 1989, 7:477–483.

51. TOCHIKUBO O, MINAMISAWA K, MIYAJIMA E, ISHII M, YAMAGA A, YUKINARI Y: A new compact 24-hour indirect blood-pressure recorder and its clinical application. *Jpn Heart J* 1988, 29:257–269.

52. LANGEWITZ W, DÄHNERT A, RÜDDEL H: Zur Validität der Blutdruckmessung eines neuen tragbaren automatischen Blutdruckmessgerätes (Physioport). *Medwelt* 1987, 38:816–821.

53. BAIG MW, WILSON J, WADE G, LONSDALE D, PERRINS EJ: Clinical evaluation of the Accutracker ambulatory blood-pressure monitoring system. *J Amb Mon* 1989, 2:175–182.

54. DiRIENZO M, GRASSI G, PEDOTTI A, MANCIA G: Continuous vs intermittent blood pressure measurements in estimating 24-hour average blood pressure. *Hypertension* 1983, 5:264–269.

55. WIINBERG N, WALTHER-LARSEN S, ERIKSEN C, NIELSEN PE: An evaluation of semi-automatic blood-pressure monitors against intra-arterial blood pressure. *J Amb Mon* 1988, 1:303–309.

4 Short-term variability of blood pressure, and the effects of physical and mental activity

Blood pressure variability is clearly a central theme of this book. It is, however, a term that is often used rather loosely, as if it were a single entity that could be adequately described by a single number. In fact, it encompasses a number of sources of variation with different time courses, ranging from a few seconds to a year, and with quite different origins (Fig. 4.1). In this chapter we will review the short-term variability of pressure, that is variability with a periodicity of less than 24 hours, and in the next chapter will review ultradian[1], diurnal and seasonal changes.

How should blood pressure variability be expressed?

Variability is a quantitative concept, and the way in which it is expressed has a major effect on the numbers that are obtained. The first consideration is the time span over which variability is measured: short-term variability, as measured over periods of up to half-an-hour or so, will be influenced largely by respiratory variations and Mayer waves, described below. Measurements made over longer periods will be influenced by changes in physical activity, location, and time of day, and yield a different set of numbers.

Another important consideration is the choice of an absolute, as opposed to a relative, measure of variability. The classic example of the former is the standard deviation (in this case expressed as mmHg) and of the latter the coefficient of variation (the standard deviation expressed as a percentage of the average level). Which is more appropriate has been the subject of considerable debate. The main question here is whether the variability of blood pressure normally changes in proportion to its absolute level. If this is the case, the standard deviation will change, but the coefficient of variation will not. This was addressed in a recent study by Jacob *et al.* [1], who examined the effects of systematically raising or lowering the blood pressure of rats with denervated carotid and aortic baroreceptors, a situation which results in an increase of variability without much influence on the absolute level. When variability was expressed as the standard deviation they found no consistent changes of variability either during spontaneous changes or when the absolute level of pressure was raised by pressor infusions. When pressure was lowered by vasodilators, two of them (adenosine and nitroprusside) had no effect on variability, while a third one (nisoldipine) reduced it. The authors concluded that variability does not necessarily change *pari passu* with the absolute level of pressure, and hence that absolute measures of variability are the more appropriate.

The third factor which will influence the estimate of variability is the set of circumstances in which the measurements were made. In the same subject, very different measures of variability will be obtained depending on whether the subject is resting quietly or physically active. An extreme example of this is patients with autonomic failure (see Chapter 5), whose blood pressure variability

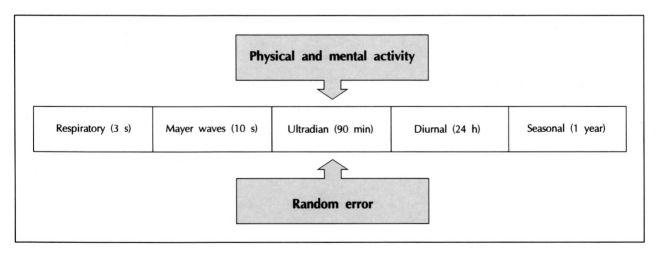

Fig. 4.1. The principal sources of blood pressure variability and their periodicities.

---

[1]Strictly speaking, the discussion of ultradian rhythms, which have a periodicity of 90 minutes, should be included in this chapter. Since, however, their existence in man has been demonstrated only during sleep, they are discussed in Chapter 5.

is greater than normal while they are active during the day, but whose nocturnal blood pressure fall is less than normal [2]. In active subjects, therefore, such as are commonly studied by ambulatory monitoring, a case can be made for normalizing the blood pressure variability to the activity of the subject. This relates to the concept of reactivity, which is reviewed extensively in Chapter 12.

Spontaneous short-term variability

As shown schematically in Fig. 4.1, a number of discrete sources of blood pressure variability can be identified. At the high frequency end of the spectrum are respiratory fluctuations, followed by Mayer waves. Ultradian variations, with a periodicity of 90 min, are not clearly established in man. These spontaneous variations can be masked by the effects of superimposed physical and mental activity, so that they are best studied in a steady-state condition.

Short-term blood pressure variability, of which respiratory fluctuation is the dominant cause, can only be assessed by beat-to-beat monitoring, for example using intra-arterial recording. Mancia et al. [3] studied blood pressure and heart rate variability in a series of normotensive and hypertensive individuals using intra-arterial ambulatory monitoring. Variability was expressed as the standard deviation (i.e. the absolute level) and variation coefficient (i.e. the percentage level), measured over two intervals: 30 min (short-term variability) and 24 h (long-term variability) calculated from the hourly averages. The short-term variability was about two-thirds of the magnitude of the long-term variability. One of their principal findings was that both the mean levels and the short-term variabilities of blood pressure and heart rate tend to change in parallel: thus during sleep there is a decrease not only of blood pressure and heart rate, but also of their variabilities. These within-subject changes of variability are shown in Fig. 4.2. With increasing age, there is

an increase in short-term blood pressure variability, but a decrease in heart rate variability [3].

An important consideration is the extent to which the variability of blood pressure is linked to heart rate. Parati et al. [4] analysed intra-arterial recordings of blood pressure and heart rate, and expressed the variability as the average of 1 min coefficients of variation. Atropine greatly reduced the heart rate variability, but had little effect on blood pressure variability, suggesting that the short-term variability of blood pressure is regulated by changes of vasomotor tone rather than of heart rate. Rawles et al. [5] measured cardiac output and blood pressure non-invasively in hypertensive subjects, and also concluded that blood pressure lability was mediated more by changes of peripheral resistance than cardiac output. However, Clement et al. [6,7] concluded that this variability may be partly under vagal control (presumably via the effect on heart rate), since it persists despite blockade of either the alpha- or beta-adrenergic system, but is attenuated by vagal blockade with atropine. Such variability is more pronounced in patients with higher pressures [8].

Respiration and blood pressure variability

The respiratory variations in blood pressure were studied by Dornhorst et al. [9], who established a number of important associations. At normal rates of breathing the pressure falls during most of inspiration, but at slower rates inspiration is associated with a rising pressure (Fig. 4.3). Sinus arrhythmia, that is the change of heart rate associated with respiration, does not contribute to the blood pressure change; this statement was based on the observation that the appearance and disappearance of sinus arrhythmia did not alter the rhythm of blood pressure. During periods of apnoea, rhythmical variations of blood pressure may still be apparent, at a rate of six per minute (0.1 Hz), which Dornhorst et al. referred to as Traube waves, but which are usually known

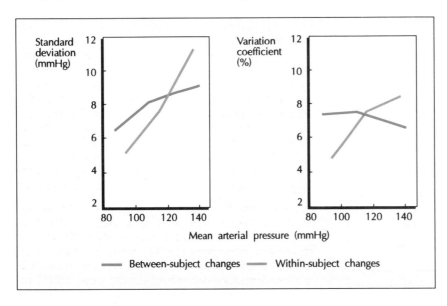

Fig. 4.2. Comparison of between- and within-subject changes of short-term blood pressure variability as a function of the average pressure. Data plotted by permission from [3].

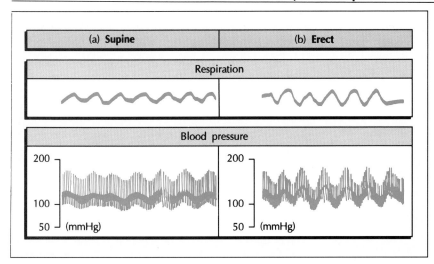

Fig. 4.3. Respiratory fluctuations of blood pressure, as described by Dornhorst *et al.* [9]: (a) subject supine; (b) subject erect. Upper trace is respiration, lower is blood pressure. Reproduced with permission [9].

as Mayer waves. Finally, the fluctuations of blood pressure are more marked when standing than when supine, as shown in Fig. 4.3. Some of the changes in blood pressure can be attributed to the mechanical effects of breathing on venous return and modulation of stroke volume, since they persist after ganglionic blockade. Dornhorst *et al.* concluded that changes in vascular tone were also important (as evidenced by the Traube waves seen during apnoea), but that changes of heart rate were not.

Mayer waves

There are also periodic waves of blood pressure which are slower than the respiratory oscillations. These are usually referred to as Mayer waves. In experimental animals they are most prominent in the presence of acidosis or cerebral ischaemia, particularly after bleeding [10,11]. It has been suggested that they may be mediated via the chemoreceptors [12]. They have a periodicity of three to five cycles/min in the dog (0.05–0.08 Hz), and somewhat shorter in man (0.07–0.12 Hz). They can be seen quite clearly during apnoeic episodes, as shown in Fig. 4.4, which is taken from the classic paper by Dornhorst *et al.* [9].

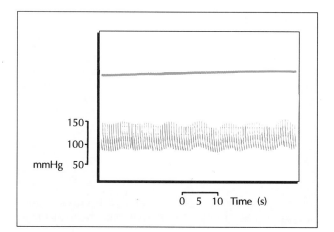

Fig. 4.4. Mayer waves occurring during apnoea. Reproduced with permission [9].

Power spectral analysis of blood pressure and heart rate variability

It has been known for many years that both heart rate and blood pressure exhibit rhythmical fluctuations, of which respiratory sinus arrhythmia and Mayer waves are examples. Using the techniques of power spectral analysis it has recently become possible to quantify these fluctuations, and relate them to the two limbs of the autonomic nervous system, the sympathetic and the vagus.

The technique was first developed for heart rate variability, and was based on analysis of the beat-to-beat variations occurring during steady-state conditions, with the respiration rate held constant. Two methods of analysis have been used: the first, described by workers in Boston, used fast Fourier transform to provide the power spectral analysis, and the second, described by workers in Milan, used autoregression techniques. The results are generally similar; both show the relative preponderance of different frequencies with either two or three distinct peaks. In the original description by the Boston group [13], who studied dogs, there were three peaks: a low-frequency peak at 0.04 Hz, which appeared to be dependent on the activity of the sympathetic nervous system and the renin–angiotensin system, a medium-frequency peak at 0.1 Hz, and a high-frequency peak at 0.4 Hz, the last two of which were due to vagal activity. The same group described two peaks in man, at 0.1 and 0.25 Hz [14]. Using the autoregression analysis technique the Milan group have described three peaks in man: P_1 at 0.07–0.1 Hz, reflecting sympathetic activity; P_2 at 0.12 Hz, and P_3 at 0.25–0.27 Hz, both reflecting vagal activity [15]. In our experience, these discrete peaks are often not discernible. Furthermore, the frequency of the 'vagal' peak is actually set by the frequency of breathing. If paced breathing is used, the height and position of this peak can be made to change.

The contributions of the sympathetic and parasympathetic systems to these peaks have been demonstrated with selective autonomic blockade, for example using atropine and propranolol [14,16]. Moving from the supine to the upright position causes a relative increase in the low-frequency/sympathetic-activity peak, and a relative decrease in the high-frequency/vagal-activity peak

[14,15]. It has long been suspected that sympathetic activity may be increased in hypertension, and it is of particular interest that, when compared with age-matched normotensive subjects, hypertensives show a greater low-frequency (0.1 Hz) component, and a smaller high-frequency (0.26 Hz) component, suggesting not only an increased level of sympathetic activity, but also a decreased level of vagal activity, which would be consistent with their slightly higher heart rates [17].

Relatively little work has so far been done on power spectral analysis of blood pressure variability. Pagani *et al.* [18] have analysed heart rate and systolic pressure variabilities in 24-hour recordings made with a catheter-tipped (and hence high-fidelity) transducer in ambulatory hypertensive patients. During the day there was a predominantly low-frequency (approximately 0.1 Hz) component, which was more evident in the pressure than in the heart rate spectrum. The high-frequency component (0.25 Hz) was detectable only at night, when it was present in both traces. In a study of hospitalized patients Furlan *et al.* [19] were able to demonstrate a diurnal rhythm of sympathetic activity (measured as the low-frequency blood pressure oscillations) which was maximal at about 9.00 a.m., and lowest during the night. Interestingly, the 0.1 Hz peak increased sharply at 6.00 a.m. when the patients were awakened, but the absolute level of blood pressure did not increase much until they got out of bed 3 h later. Mancia *et al.* [20] also found the 0.1 Hz band to be more prominent during the day than at night.

Two comments can be made about these findings: first, because the patients were ambulatory during the day and in bed at night, the absence of any clearly defined peaks in the heart rate spectrum during the day may have been because they were swamped by the effects of changing physical and mental activities on heart rate; at night there would be less interference. Second, they suggest that the sympathetic plays a greater role than the vagus in the modulation of systolic pressure variability, particularly during the day. Whether this would apply to normotensive individuals in whom vagal tone appears to be greater cannot be judged from these data.

Factors influencing individual differences in blood pressure variability

The idea that individual differences in blood pressure variability may play a role in the development of hypertension is not new [21], and led to the development of the 'reactivity hypothesis', which is reviewed in Chapter 12. As mentioned earlier, however, comparisons of blood pressure variability may depend on the circumstances in which variability is measured, and on how it is expressed. Situations in which it is commonly evaluated include reactivity testing (in which the response to a standardized stimulus is measured), ambulatory monitoring (which will include the response to non-standardized stimuli and spontaneous variability), and readings taken

during a period of quiet rest (when the influence of extraneous stimuli should be minimal).

The factors which influence blood pressure variability other than the level of the blood pressure and the role of the baroreceptors (see below) have received relatively little attention. There is general agreement that variability assessed by ambulatory monitoring increases with age [22,23], which may be partly accounted for by the diminished baroreflex sensitivity associated with ageing, although other factors may also be involved [23]. Ambulatory blood pressure variability has also been reported to be increased in high-renin patients [23].

In a study of blood pressure variability measured while resting, Puddey *et al.* took 10 readings at 2 min intervals on each of three consecutive days using a Dinamap recorder (Critikon, Tampa, Florida, USA) in 343 working men [24]. Variability was expressed as the average coefficient of variation for each of the 3 days. Systolic (but not diastolic) variability was higher in those who consumed more alcohol.

Personality variables may also be relevant. There is a large but conflicting literature on the association between increased blood pressure reactivity and the type A behaviour pattern [25]. Puddey *et al.* [24] found diastolic pressure variability to be greater in type A subjects. They also found that individuals who scored highly on verbal aggression and extraversion had higher variability.

The role of the baroreceptors

It has long been recognized that the aortic and carotid sinus baroreceptors play a buffering role in the regulation of blood pressure. Stimulation of the baroreceptors by an increase in pressure causes a reflex bradycardia and vasodilatation, and baroreflex sensitivity can be measured by increasing carotid sinus pressure (e.g. using vasoconstrictor agents to raise the systemic pressure, or by neck suction) and measuring the reflex response. Direct evidence for the tonic role of the baroreceptors in man comes from muscle sympathetic nerve recordings, which show a suppression of sympathetic activity during spontaneous increases in pressure [26]. A consistent finding from intra-arterial ambulatory monitoring studies has been that subjects with diminished baroreflex sensitivity show increased blood pressure variability, with a negative correlation between the two [27–29]. Indeed, when comparing the associations between age, mean arterial pressure, and baroreflex sensitivity with blood pressure variability, Floras *et al.* [29] found that only baroreflex sensitivity was a significant predictor. In this situation the heart rate changes are buffering rather than causing the variations in blood pressure. Conway *et al.* [30] found that subjects with high baroreflex sensitivity showed greater heart rate variability during ambulatory monitoring and a smaller fall in blood pressure during the night than subjects with lower reflex sensitivity. Mancia *et al.* [20] analysed 24-hour blood pressure and heart rate recordings to look for episodes in which there appeared to be a reflex modulation of blood pressure and heart rate, that is, where increasing pressure was associated with a decreasing rate, and *vice versa*. Such episodes accounted for 15% of the total heart beats, and were more common during the day, when the pressure was higher and more labile than during the night. They were less frequent in hypertensive than in normotensive individuals.

The baroreceptors may modulate the blood pressure changes occurring in response to physical or mental activity: Conway *et al.* [30] found that the increase in pressure during mental arithmetic was greatest in subjects with the lowest baroreflex sensitivity, and Floras *et al.* [31] showed the same during dynamic exercise.

The baroreflex does not operate as a fixed entity, but appears to be under central control. Stimulation of brainstem defence areas inhibits baroreflex responses [32], and the reflex bradycardia occurring in response to phenylephrine injections is impaired during mental arithmetic [33] or exercise [34].

When the baroreceptors are denervated there is a dramatic increase in blood pressure variability [35,36] as shown in Fig. 4.5. Earlier studies indicated that this procedure also produced sustained hypertension, but this may be another example of the importance of the circumstances of measurement, since continuous 24-hour recordings have, for the most part, shown that while variability is dramatically increased, the level of mean pressure is not [35,37]. The increased lability of pressure is mediated by the sympathetic nervous system, since plasma noradrenaline levels are increased [37], and the variability can be normalized by ganglionic blockade [38], as shown in Fig. 4.6.

A few isolated case reports have appeared of the consequences of baroreceptor denervation in man. The best studied case was described by Aksamit *et al.* [39] of a man who developed paroxysmal hypertension following bilateral carotid bypass surgery. Between paroxysms his pressure was normal. The increases in pressure were accompanied by an increase in heart rate and plasma noradrenaline. Reflex changes in heart rate and muscle sympathetic nerve activity occurring in response to drug-induced changes of pressure were absent. Another illustrative case was described by Kuchel *et al.* [40] of a woman with a 30-year history of paroxysms of hypertension induced by emotion or postural change, alternating with orthostatic hypotension. The hypertensive episodes were associated with an increase in heart rate and plasma catecholamines. Baroreflex sensitivity was impaired, and the blood pressure increase during a cold pressor test was greatly enhanced (from 130/88 mmHg at rest to 180/130 mmHg).

In hypertensive patients the reflex is reset to maintain the pressure at the higher level. The reflex regulation of heart rate is impaired [41], as has been shown repeatedly by the phenylephrine method. However, the reflex blood pressure response to neck suction is the same in normotensive and hypertensive individuals, which suggests that there is no impairment in the control of the peripheral circulation [42]. This somewhat paradoxical finding may be explained by the hypertrophy of the peripheral arteries, which would result in an exaggerated vasoconstrictor response to a given level of sympathetic nerve activity. In any event, the fact that the decreased reflex heart rate response can be directly correlated with increased blood pressure variability [27,28] suggests that the baroreflex is indeed less effective in regulating blood pressure in hypertensive patients. This impairment is most probably a consequence rather than a cause of the hypertension,

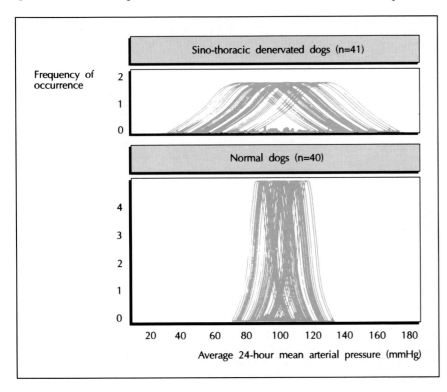

Fig. 4.5. Effects of baroreceptor denervation on blood pressure level and variability in dogs. Reproduced with permission from [35].

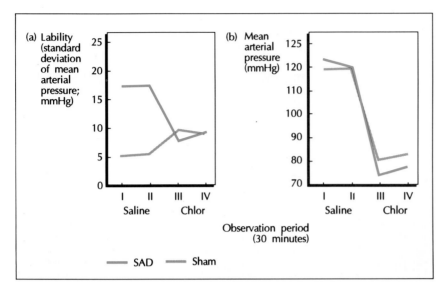

Fig. 4.6. Effects of ganglionic blockade on blood pressure variability in rats with sinoaortic denervation (SAD) and sham-operated control rats (Sham). Arterial pressure was measured for two 30 min periods (I and II) during saline infusions, and for two more periods (III and IV) following chlorisondamine (Chlor, a ganglionic blocking agent): (a) blood pressure variability (standard deviation of mean arterial pressure); (b) the average level of blood pressure. Reproduced with permission [38].

since it is not present in 'prehypertensive' young adults [43].

The role of the central nervous system

A characteristic finding of baroreceptor modulation of blood pressure variability is that when blood pressure is increasing, heart rate (or muscle sympathetic nerve activity) is decreasing, and *vice versa*. While this certainly occurs, the correlation between blood pressure variability and baroreflex sensitivity is relatively weak (around −0.3 to −0.5), and for much of the time heart rate and blood pressure rise and fall together. In such situations, the central nervous system can be assumed to be playing the primary role in regulating blood pressure.

The autonomic nervous system is thought to play the dominant role in regulating blood pressure changes during normal activities, including the diurnal or circadian changes. In the rat, much of the apparently spontaneous variability of blood pressure can be attributed to activities such as eating, drinking, grooming and exploring [44]. The effects of these activities on pressure are greatly attenuated by chemosympathectomy. Sympathetic blockade does not invariably lead to a decreased blood pressure lability, however. In rats monitored in their home cage for an hour, Alper *et al.* [38] observed that ganglionic blockade resulted in an increased lability (Fig. 4.5). Thus, it appears that the autonomic nervous system can have both a buffering and a mediating role. In man, blood pressure varies over 24 hours in parallel with changes in plasma catecholamines [45], although individual differences in resting plasma catecholamine levels are not correlated with differences in blood pressure variability [22].

Reis and LeDoux [46] have pointed out that separate neural mechanisms may regulate the tonic and phasic components of blood pressure. Tonic control is regulated by the adrenaline-containing Cl neurons in the medulla, while the phasic changes occurring in response to

behavioural stimuli are influenced by the hypothalamus, limbic system, and basal forebrain.

Effects of physical and mental activity on blood pressure variability

If the effects of environmental stimuli and changes in physical activity are minimized, the profile of blood pressure during the day becomes relatively flat, with a fall of about 20% during sleep [47,48]. It has also been shown that diurnal blood pressure changes are less pronounced in hospitalized patients than in patients studied in their natural environment [49]. Both the average level of blood pressure and its variability are reduced during periods of bed rest compared with periods of physical activity [50].

It is possible to monitor physical activity by an electronic device known as an actigraph, which is worn on the wrist or waist, and which can register body movement in 1 min epochs over periods of 24 hours. Van Egeren has pioneered the use of this device in conjunction with ambulatory blood pressure monitoring, and, as shown in Fig. 4.7, has found a close parallelism between changes in physical activity and blood pressure [51]. Some of the more relevant activities influencing the changes of blood pressure and other variables that might be detected by ambulatory monitoring are briefly reviewed below; they are divided into physical and mental activities, although obviously there is considerable overlap.

Posture

Posture is an important source of blood pressure variance, particularly in ambulatory monitoring studies. Changing from the supine to the upright position causes an increase in diastolic pressure with little or no change in systolic pressure. This occurs because venous return, and hence also stroke volume, is decreased with a compensatory increase in heart rate to maintain cardiac output. In ambulatory monitoring studies Gellman *et al.* [52]

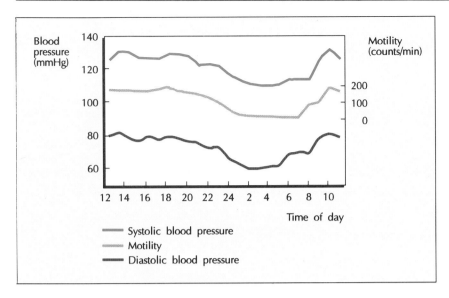

Fig. 4.7. Twenty-four-hour systolic blood pressure, diastolic blood pressure, and motility measured by an actigraph. Values are the means of 47 subjects. Reproduced with permission [51].

have claimed that changes in posture account for a major portion of overall blood variance (33% of systolic, and 47% of diastolic). However, their analysis included walking as a postural component, as well as standing. It is our belief that their findings can largely be explained by the effects of the activities associated with different postures rather than the posture themselves; as shown in Fig. 4.8, the changes in blood pressure occurring simply as the result of changing posture are rather modest.

	Average blood pressure (systolic/diastolic, mmHg)
Supine	137.1 ± 27.4/76.1 ± 13.6
Sitting	139.0 ± 28.8/83.8 ± 15.2
Standing	133.3 ± 27.0/85.6 ± 14.5

Fig. 4.8. Effects of postural change on blood pressure, measured by a Colin ABPM 630 ambulatory monitor during a validation study performed in 61 subjects (unpublished data).

Dynamic exercise

Dynamic exercise raises systolic pressure and heart rate, with little effect on diastolic pressure. In normotensive subjects systolic pressure during intense exercise may reach 200 mmHg or more.

Intra-arterial recordings made during running [53] may indicate a periodic fluctuation of pulse pressure, with oscillations of between 30 and 100 mmHg. This phenomenon appears to be the result of a beat phenomenon, where the normal variations in pressure are amplified by pressure waves induced by the rhythmic pounding of the feet. The phenomenon does not occur during cycling.

Static (isometric) exercise

Static (isometric) exercise, such as occurs during weight-lifting, produces a very different blood pressure response, with a marked increase in both systolic and diastolic pressure. The extent of this increase is a function of the intensity of contraction rather than of the bulk of muscle being used: at 50% of maximal voluntary contraction mean arterial pressure may increase by 40 mmHg within 1 min [54].

During isometric exercise such as lifting barbells, huge increases in intra-arterial pressure may occur, with levels as high as 345/245 mmHg having been recorded [55], as shown in Fig. 4.9. These are partly the result of the associated Valsalva manoeuvres, since they are accompanied by sudden increases in intra-thoracic and intra-abdominal pressure.

Sexual intercourse

Sexual intercourse, another form of exercise, can produce a dramatic transient rise in pressure, ranging from 25 to 120 mmHg in systolic, and 24 to 48 mmHg in diastolic pressure [56]. These changes are reversed within a few minutes after orgasm.

Micturition and defaecation

Micturition and defaecation produce transient changes that resemble a Valsalva manoeuvre, with a brief rise in pressure followed by a precipitous fall, and then a marked rise corresponding to the overshoot phase of the Valsalva [57].

Ingestion of food and drink

Most of the studies investigating the effects of ingested substances have been carried out in the laboratory, but their results may in most cases be extrapolated to the

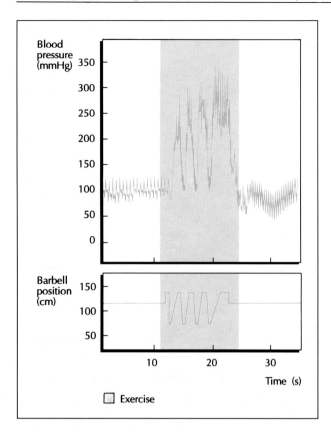

Fig. 4.9. Intra-arterial blood pressure changes during weight-lifting with barbells. Four repetitions to exhaustion were performed. Reproduced with permission [55].

field. In younger subjects there is an increase in heart rate and cardiac output, a decrease in diastolic pressure, and little change in systolic pressure 3 h after a meal [58,59]. In older subjects there may be a pronounced fall in both systolic and diastolic pressure after food [60]. Peitzman and Berger [61] compared the effects of a breakfast of two eggs, two slices of toast, and orange juice in healthy elderly subjects (mean age 82 years) and controls (aged 35 years). The average fall in blood pressure between 30 and 60 min after the meal was 16/10 mmHg in the elderly, but only 4/3 mmHg (not significant) in the young [61].

Smoking

Smoking a cigarette raises both heart rate and blood pressure. In a laboratory study of healthy young men Thomas and Murphy [62] found that smoking a single cigarette raised systolic pressure by about 3 mmHg and diastolic by about 4 mmHg. These increases were similar in smokers and non-smokers, but were more marked in subjects with a family history of hypertension than in those without. Roth *et al.* [63] reported much bigger changes (19/14 mmHg), but this may have been because their subjects smoked two cigarettes. In patients who were studied smoking in their natural environment during intra-arterial ambulatory blood pressure monitoring, Cellina *et al.* [64] found increases of about 11/5 mmHg, sometimes preceded by a transient fall in pressure; changes were quantitatively similar in normo-

tensive and hypertensive subjects. The effect on blood pressure was seen within a few minutes, and lasted about 15 min.

Alcohol

Alcohol may increase heart rate, with small but variable effects on blood pressure in normal subjects, ranging from no significant change to an increase of 5/7 mmHg 1 h after ingestion of 0.75–1.3 g alcohol per kg body weight, equivalent to social drinking [65–69]. In hypertensive people blood pressure has been reported to increase within 1 h of drinking alcohol in moderate drinkers (by about 10/4 mmHg), but not in light drinkers [70]. Studies of more prolonged drinking (over several days) have also shown variable effects in normotensive people, with more consistent increases in hypertensive people [71,72].

A large number of epidemiological surveys have shown a strong association between alcohol intake and hypertension; these have been reviewed by MacMahon [73].

Caffeine

Caffeine increases blood pressure, plasma catecholamines, and renin, but not heart rate [74]. The increase in blood pressure begins within 15 min of drinking coffee, is maximal in about 1 h, and may last for as long as 3 h. Typical increases are between 5/9 mmHg [67] and 14/10 mmHg [75]. Drinking decaffeinated coffee produces little or no change [74]. These changes are dependent on the level of habitual caffeine intake [76]: in people who do not use it regularly they are much larger than in habitual users (12/10 and 4/2 mmHg, respectively). Older subjects show bigger increases in pressure than younger ones [76]. Caffeine also has an additive effect on the blood pressure response to mental stress: higher absolute levels of pressure are achieved after caffeine, but the rise in pressure during the stressor is not affected [77,78].

Increased caffeine intake is not associated with sustained hypertension, however. Switching from caffeinated to decaffeinated coffee has been shown to lower casual blood pressure by only 1 mmHg [79]. If anything, coffee drinkers tend to have lower blood pressures than non-drinkers [80]. Coffee and cigarettes are often taken together, and a study by Freestone and Ramsay showed that they may have an interactive effect [81]. As shown in Fig. 4.10, smoking a cigarette elevated blood pressure for 15 min, whereas drinking coffee had no effect for an hour, when there was a significant increase. When the cigarette and coffee were taken together, however, there was a significant increase in pressure of about 10 mmHg, which was seen within 5 min, and was still present 2 h later.

Salt

In a study of the effects of varying sodium intake on blood pressure, we observed [82] that the effects of

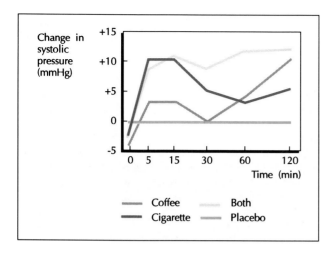

Fig. 4.10. Effects of smoking a cigarette and drinking coffee, alone and in combination, on blood pressure. Data plotted with permission [81].

physical activity and posture on blood pressure were generally similar on the high and low sodium diet.

Talking

Talking is a potent pressor stimulus that has both physical and psychological components. These have been extensively investigated by Lynch [83–88]. Reading aloud produces an immediate increase in both systolic and diastolic pressure (by about 10/7 mmHg in normotensive individuals) and in heart rate, with an immediate return to baseline levels once silence is resumed [83]. Reading silently, however, does not affect the pressure [86]. Speaking fast produces a bigger increase than speaking slowly [86]. The role of psychological factors is shown by the finding that talking in front of a group produces a bigger increase than reading aloud while alone [83]. Of particular relevance to the clinical measurement of blood pressure (see Chapter 7) is the perceived status of the person being spoken to: an experimenter posing as a physician will evoke higher pressures than one posing as an experimenter with equal status to the subject [84]. The size of the audience is also a factor [87]. Similar increases in pressure are seen in deaf-mutes when they are communicating by sign language, suggesting that the act of communicating *per se* may be partly responsible for the increased pressure [85].

Linden [89] also came to the conclusion that the blood pressure changes accompanying speech are determined to a much greater extent by the emotional content of speech than by the physical efforts required.

Mental activity and emotion

At least two studies have reported some correlation between self-rated mental 'stress' or 'arousal' and blood pressure during non-invasive ambulatory monitoring [90,91]. We have reported higher levels of blood pressure when people are at work than when they are at

home, which we have attributed to mental rather than physical factors, because most of our subjects had sedentary jobs [92,93].

Mood has also been reported to be a potent determinant of blood pressure during ambulatory monitoring. We have found that self-reported levels of anger, anxiety, and happiness are correlated with blood pressure: systolic pressure decreased as the intensity of happiness increased, and diastolic pressure increased with the intensity of anxiety [94]. There appear to be significant gender differences in the effects of physical and mental activities on blood pressure. In a study of 137 men and 67 women who wore an ambulatory blood pressure monitor, we found that mood had a greater effect on systolic pressure in men, while posture had a greater effect in women [95]. In addition, men showed the biggest mood-related blood pressure change during anger, while women showed the biggest change during anxiety.

How much of the variability of blood pressure measured during ambulatory monitoring can be explained by differences in physical and mental activity?

In the past, analyses of ambulatory recordings of heart rate and blood pressure have typically expressed the data in terms of the mean level plus an overall measure of variability. While this approach provides much useful information, students of behaviour want to quantify the effects of specific activities or moods on such variables. In the case of blood pressure, we were interested to see how much of the overall variance could be accounted for by changes in activity [96]. We found that coding for the average effect of 15 commonly occurring activities (including sleep) on blood pressure (using the patient's clinic pressure as a covariate) accounted for 41% of systolic and 36% of diastolic variance. Time of day was a less important determinant of blood pressure. The average effects of these activities on blood pressure are shown in Fig. 4.11.

In a subsequent analysis [97] we compared the relative effects of three major determinants of daytime blood pressure variance: activity (including postural effects), mood, and the place of measurement. Of these, activity was by far the most important, with mood coming next, and place of measurement having a lesser influence (being significant for systolic but not diastolic pressure). The most significant finding of this study was that the effects of activity and mood on blood pressure were additive.

Although these modelling techniques can account for a sizeable portion of the overall variation in blood pressure or other variables, it is only a first approximation. Thus, the idea that the effects of each activity can be represented by a single coefficient is an oversimplification, because the intensity of any activity may vary, and individual subjects will have different pressure responses to the same activity, for example from differences in barore-

	Systolic pressure (mmHg)	Diastolic pressure (mmHg)
Meetings	+ 20.2	+ 15.0
Work	+ 16.0	+ 13.0
Transportation	+ 14.0	+ 9.2
Walking	+ 12.0	+ 5.5
Dressing	+ 11.5	+ 9.7
Chores	+ 10.7	+ 6.7
Telephone	+ 9.5	+ 7.2
Eating	+ 8.8	+ 9.6
Talking	+ 6.7	+ 6.7
Desk work	+ 5.9	+ 5.3
Reading	+ 1.9	+ 2.2
Business (at home)	+ 1.6	+ 3.2
Television	+ 0.3	+ 1.1
Relaxing	0	0
Sleeping	− 10.0	− 7.6

Changes are shown relative to blood pressure while relaxing.

Fig. 4.11. Average changes of blood pressure associated with 15 commonly occurring activities.

flex sensitivity. Furthermore, we have evidence (Pieper *et al.*, in preparation) that there may be a 'carry-over' effect, such that the effects of a particular activity (e.g. being at work) on blood pressure may still be detectable after the activity has ceased (e.g. after returning home).

Comparison of blood pressure variability in normotensive and hypertensive subjects

Several studies using intra-arterial ambulatory monitoring have shown that blood pressure variability, usually measured as the standard deviation of the daytime pressure, tends to be higher in hypertensive than in normotensive people [22,36,98]. However, if variability is normalized by calculating the variation coefficient, there is no longer any difference between normotensive and hypertensive people [22]. Mann *et al.* [2] expressed variability as the 'average hourly change' (the mean absolute difference between consecutive hours), and found that while simple regression analysis was related to both age and mean pressure, with multiple regression analysis only age remained a significant predictor. This is in contrast to the within-subject relationship between the level of blood pressure and its variability, where there is an increase in both the absolute and the percentage variability with increasing pressure (Fig. 4.2). Floras *et al.* [98] found that increased blood pressure variability was related not only to higher mean pressures, but also to increased age and diminished baroreflex sensitivity. Multiple regression analysis showed that the only independent predictor of variability was baroreflex sensitivity. Heart rate variability is similar in normotensive and hypertensive subjects [3].

We compared four measures of blood pressure variability or reactivity in three groups of subjects (58 normotensive subjects [99], 578 mild hypertensive subjects with clinic blood pressures below 160/106 mmHg, and 66 established hypertensives with clinic pressures above 160/105 mmHg), all of whom wore a non-invasive blood pressure monitor for 24 h. The first measure was the change in pressure from work to home, which was found to be greater in the hypertensives than in the normotensive subjects (for systolic pressure, the changes were 3, 8, and 7 mmHg, respectively, for the three groups), and the change between home and sleep, which showed no difference (12, 14, and 13 mmHg, respectively). The second measure was blood pressure variance, which showed a progressive increase with the level of pressure (the average daytime systolic pressure variances being 130, 145, and 244 mmHg for the three groups, respectively), as shown in Fig. 4.12. The third measure was the range (defined as the difference between the upper and lower 5% of readings). This was also greater in the hypertensive groups. Finally, the blood pressure response to specific activities (both physical and mental) was greater in the hypertensive groups.

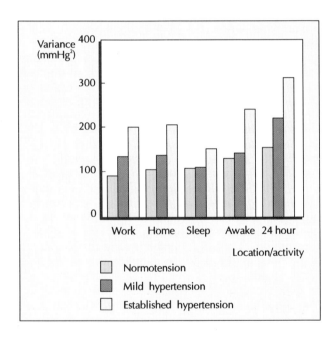

Fig. 4.12. Blood pressure variance measured by non-invasive ambulatory monitoring in different situations in three groups of subjects, with normal blood pressure, mild hypertension, or established hypertension. Reproduced with permission [99].

Other studies comparing blood pressure changes during physical or mental activity have given a less clear-cut picture. The increase in systolic pressure during dynamic exercise is normal in patients with borderline hypertension, but exaggerated in those with more severe disease [100,101]. However, the maximal exercise capacity may be reduced in hypertension [102]. Elderly hypertensives show similar blood pressure responses to age-matched normotensive subjects [103].

There is a tendency for hypertensives to show greater absolute increases in blood pressure during mental reactivity tasks, such as mental arithmetic or reaction time tasks. In a review of such studies, we found that 11 out of 22 (50%) studies which used active coping tasks (mental tasks requiring a specific response from the subjects) reported increased reactivity in systolic pressure in borderline hypertensive subjects, and seven out of 10 (70%) studies found increased reactivity in established hypertensive subjects [104]. It is likely that these differences would be less marked if reactivity was expressed in terms of the percentage change from the baseline level rather than the absolute change. Lynch *et al* [105] have claimed that hypertensive subjects tend to show greater increases in blood pressure during talking than normotensive subjects, on which they have based a somewhat rickety theory that hypertension may be related to problems with communication. In fact, their data [88] show no consistent differences between the effect of talking in normotensive subjects (an increase of 8/10 mmHg) and hypertensives (an increase of 8/9 mmHg).

Effects of antihypertensive treatment on blood pressure variability and reactivity

These subjects are reviewed in Chapters 10 and 12.

Can blood pressure variability change independently of the average level?

It has been clear for many years that blood pressure variability is closely related to the average level of pressure, being greatest when the pressure is high, such as during vigorous exercise, and at its minimum during sleep. This relationship has been quantified by Mancia's group (see Fig. 4.2) and shown to apply for both absolute and relative measures of variability.

That this relationship is not invariable has been demonstrated in a study by van der Meiracker *et al* [106]. Patients with mild, untreated hypertension were studied in hospital with intra-arterial 24-hour monitoring. Half the subjects were ambulatory during the day while the others remained in bed for the entire 24 h. The ambulatory subjects had higher average levels of pressure during the day than the subjects in bed, but their variability (measured as the standard deviation) was not significantly higher, as shown in Fig. 4.7. Furthermore, 'sensory deprivation' (resting quietly with the eyes open) did not affect the mean blood pressure in comparison with simple bed rest, but did result in a marked reduction in blood pressure variability (Fig. 4.13). These results suggest that the effects of physical and mental activity on the blood pressure level and its variability can be dissociated from each other.

An analogous dissociation between these two components of blood pressure has been described in experi-

mental animal studies which have shown that selective interruption of baroreceptor reflexes can increase the variability of blood pressure without affecting its tonic level [107,108].

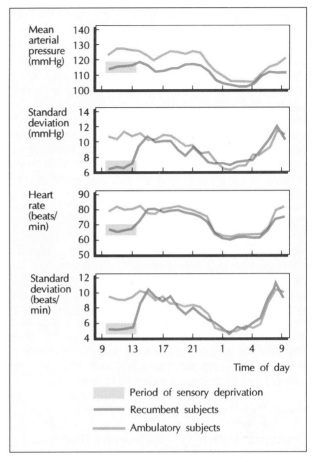

Fig. 4.13. Hourly changes in blood pressure and heart rate in subjects who were either ambulatory during the day or recumbent for 24 hours. Reproduced with permission [106].

The primacy of blood pressure as the regulated haemodynamic variable, and the separate regulation of short- and long-term variation

One of the most striking findings to emerge from studies of blood pressure variability is that the short-term fluctuations in blood pressure are remarkably similar in normotensive and hypertensive individuals, both qualitatively and quantitatively. Even more remarkably, antihypertensive treatment often has little effect on the blood pressure changes accompanying physical and mental activity, although it may have profound effects on the overall level of pressure. Thus, as Julius [109] has stated:

'...hypertension is not a disease of blood pressure regulation. The pressure is set at a higher level and around that setting it is regulated in a normal fashion'.

A recent study by Ravogli *et al* [110] of genetic factors in hypertension provides strong evidence in support of this view. They found that normotensive young adults with a positive family history of hypertension showed a slight, but significant, elevation in blood pressure measured casually, during prolonged rest, and during ambulatory monitoring, in comparison with subjects who had a negative family history of hypertension. There were, however, no differences in either the variability of blood pressure or the reactivity to pressor stimuli.

Blood pressure is the product of peripheral resistance and cardiac output, and it is these two variables which are under direct physiological control, by the tone of the arterioles, and by the pumping action of the heart. Of the three, it is only blood pressure that is monitored directly by the central nervous system, and it appears to be blood pressure which is the primary regulated variable during acute changes in autonomic activity. This point has been argued by Julius [109], in his editorial entitled 'The blood pressure seeking properties of the central nervous system'. The importance of pressure over peripheral resistance and cardiac output is best illustrated by haemodynamic studies of the effects of autonomic blocking drugs on the pressor responses to acute mental or physical challenge. An example of this is provided by a study of the haemodynamic effects of quiet speaking carried out by Ulrych [111]. In the untreated state, blood pressure rose predominantly as a result of increased in cardiac output. The salient finding of this study was that administration of a beta blocker (oxprenolol) blocked the increase in cardiac output, but not blood pressure, which still increased by the same amount, being now mediated by vasoconstriction. The same occurs during isometric exercise, where treatment with a beta blocker again has no effect on the pressor response, but radically alters the haemodynamic pattern by which this occurs [112], as shown in Fig. 4.9. Similar observations have been made with stimuli (such as noise) which elevate pressure primarily by vasoconstriction; in this situation administration of an alpha blocker has little effect on the increase in pressure, but shifts the haemodynamic response from vasoconstriction to increased cardiac output [113].

An important point is the time course of the different regulatory processes. The traditional view of blood pressure regulation, as expounded by Guyton [114], is that the central nervous system is predominantly responsible for regulating the short-term changes in blood pressure (which includes the situations discussed in this chapter) but that it is relatively unimportant in controlling longer term changes (over days or weeks), when other factors such as the regulation of fluid balance by the kidney and structural changes in resistance vessels assume a greater role. A sustained neurogenic increase in blood pressure has been achieved for up to 7 days in a study by Liard *et al.* [115] using electrical stimulation of the stellate ganglion in dogs. Interestingly, the increased pressure was mediated by an increase in cardiac output at first, but subsequently by an increase in peripheral resistance. The blood pressure returned to normal immediately after the stimulation was stopped.

One mechanism by which normal short-term regulation of blood pressure can be maintained by the central nervous system in the face of an altered basal level is by

resetting the baroreceptors, which can take place quite rapidly, and is complete within 48 h [116]. Nevertheless, it should be pointed out that the baroreflex plays only a minor role in regulating the acute blood pressure changes during physical and mental activity (since the increases in pressure are typically accompanied by increases in heart rate, while the baroreflex acts to decrease heart rate), although the baroreceptors presumably provide the necessary afferent input to the brain.

Clinical conditions in which blood pressure variability is increased

Individual patients are commonly given the diagnosis of 'labile' hypertension. At one time this was used to describe patients with borderline hypertension whose pressure was at times above, and at times below, an arbitrary dividing line. Patients with more severe hypertension, whose pressure was always above this point, were regarded as having 'fixed' hypertension. It is now quite clear that hypertension does not go through a transient phase of increased variability, and that the trend is for variability to continue to increase with the patient's age and blood pressure.

Nevertheless, there are patients whose blood pressure does show an increased variability. Some of these will, of course, merely represent the upper end of the distribution curve of blood pressure variability. Others, less commonly, may have a discrete lesion of their central or peripheral nervous system which impairs the normal blood pressure homeostasis. These are reviewed below, and summarized in Fig. 4.14.

● Phaeochromocytoma
● Autonomic neuropathies
● Baroreceptor denervation
● High spinal cord lesions
● Hypersomnia/sleeplessness syndrome

Fig. 4.14. Clinical conditions associated with increased blood pressure variability.

Phaeochromocytoma
This is the archetypal paroxysmal hypertension, where the surges in blood pressure may be related to catecholamine release. The nocturnal fall in blood pressure may be absent, as reviewed in Chapter 5. Periods of hypotension are usually not seen.

Autonomic neuropathies
Degeneration of the efferent autonomic nerves, which may involve both sympathetic and parasympathetic components, typically leads to increased blood pressure vari-

ability characterized by episodes of both hypo- and hypertension. The neuropathy may be idiopathic, a part of the Shy-Drager syndrome, or associated with diabetes mellitus. As described above, all these conditions are characterized by an absence of the nocturnal blood pressure fall (see Chapter 5). The hypotensive episodes occur with the upright position, or after meals.

Baroreceptor denervation

In this situation, which may result from bilateral carotid artery surgery, the lesion is on the afferent side of the reflex arc and the efferent sympathetic nerves are intact. Blood pressure variability is increased, with episodes of both hypo- and hypertension. What happens to the pressure at night is unclear.

Spinal cord lesions

In patients with high spinal cord lesions which result in tetraplegia or paraplegia, the connections between the central and peripheral components of the sympathetic nervous system are interrupted. This results in a disinhibition of visceral cardiovascular reflexes, causing situations such as bladder distension or muscle spasm which produce paroxysmal hypertension. A unique feature of this condition is that these episodes are associated with a reflex bradycardia, mediated via the vagus nerves [117].

Hypersomnia/sleeplessness syndrome

A fascinating case of a middle-aged man complaining of alternating hypersomnia and sleeplessness was described by Reggiani et al. [118]. The hypersomnia episodes, which resembled narcoleptic attacks, were associated with hypotension (down to 80/50 mmHg) while supine, which was made worse by standing. These alternated with episodes of excessive arousal associated with paroxysmal hypertension (up to 215/100 mmHg) and tachycardia which were clinically reminiscent of the clonidine withdrawal syndrome. It was postulated that this patient's problems might be due to abnormal inhibition and stimulation of central alpha$_2$ receptors, which are involved in the regulation of both sympathetic outflow and sleep–wake rhythms. Treatment with clonidine not only eliminated his narcoleptic attacks, but also normalized his blood pressure, and prevented the orthostatic hypotension.

Does blood pressure variability contribute to cardiovascular damage?

It is not known which component of arterial pressure is responsible for vascular damage. Hypertension leads to morbid events by two main processes: first, by causing blood vessels to burst (as in cerebral haemorrhage), and, second, by accelerating the formation of atheromatous plaques. In both cases it is likely that mechanical factors play a major role, although hormonal factors may

contribute independently of blood pressure [119]. As O'Rourke observed [120], physical materials are relatively resistant to continuous levels of stress, and are more susceptible to intermittent stress. If this also applies to the effects of blood pressure on the arterial wall, the mean arterial pressure may be much less important than the rate of change in pressure. Hence, it might be expected, on theoretical grounds, that individuals with increased lability of blood pressure would suffer more vascular damage.

Unfortunately, no definitive answer can be given to this question at present. In experimental animals blood pressure variability can be increased by sectioning the carotid sinus and aortic baroreceptor nerves [121,122]. However, this does not necessarily lead to sustained hypertension, and, so far as is known, does not lead to accelerated vascular damage, although this latter question has received relatively little attention.

In man there is even less information, although there have been case reports of individuals who appear to have increased blood pressure lability, secondary to a greatly impaired baroreflex sensitivity, who also do not have sustained hypertension [40]. A small number of cross-sectional studies have approached this problem, but their findings must be interpreted with great caution because it is difficult to draw causal inferences from them. Kobrin et al. [123] classified elderly hypertensive patients in two groups according to whether or not blood pressure fell during the night. Patients whose pressure did not fall had a higher prevalence of atherosclerotic complications and left ventricular hypertrophy than those whose pressure showed the normal decline. In another study using intra-arterial monitoring Parati et al. [124] found that subjects whose 24-hour variability was higher than the group average were more likely to have target organ damage. In this study, variability was measured over 30 min epochs, so that this would not be influenced by circadian variations in pressure to a great extent. Somewhat similar findings were reported by Pessina et al. [125], using non-invasive ambulatory monitoring. However, it is not clear from these studies which is cause and which is effect, because subjects with more advanced hypertension and more target organ damage are likely to have a diminished baroreflex sensitivity, and hence more labile blood pressure. Our preliminary results suggesting that increased blood pressure variability may be a predictor of cardiovascular morbidity are described in Chapter 13.

Summary and conclusions

Blood pressure variability is not a single entity that can be adequately described by a single number, but has a number of components of different physiological origins and different time courses. In general, the degree of short-term variability increases as the absolute level of pressure increases, but this association is more marked for acute (within-subject) changes in blood pressure than for chronic (or between-subject) changes.

Variability can also be regarded as being comprised of a number of intrinsic rhythms on which other changes, arising from physical and mental activity, are superimposed. The highest frequency rhythm of blood pressure (about 0.25 Hz) is associated with respiration, and is largely mediated by the vagus (parasympathetic) nerves. A somewhat slower rhythm (Mayer waves) occurs at a frequency of 0.1 Hz, and is predominantly due to sympathetically mediated changes in vascular tone; it is more pronounced in the standing than in the sitting position. With the technique of power spectral analysis it is usually possible to detect at least two discrete phasic components of blood pressure and heart rate, corresponding to these two rhythms.

Blood pressure variability is under central nervous system control, and one of its major determinants is baroreflex sensitivity; when this is impaired (e.g. as a result of ageing), blood pressure variability increases.

A number of physical stimuli can produce transient increases in pressure, such as exercise, talking, ingestion of food and drink, and smoking. Changes of mood can also raise pressure, particularly anger and anxiety.

Most measures of spontaneous or induced variability of blood pressure show an increased level in hypertensive patients relative to normotensive subjects. However, when expressed in relative terms (i.e. normalized to the absolute level) the differences are relatively small.

Although variability of pressure does usually vary with the absolute level, the two can change independently of each other. Thus, sensory deprivation in recumbent subjects lowers variability without altering the mean level. Although the haemodynamic mechanisms underlying short-term changes in pressure may differ depending on the type of activity, it appears that blood pressure *per se* is the primary regulated variable, because the blood pressure changes persist after partial blockade of the autonomic nervous system, which may radically alter the underlying haemodynamic mechanism.

While the term 'labile' hypertension has little to commend it, there are certain discrete clinical conditions where blood pressure lability is increased. These include phaeochromocytoma, autonomic neuropathies, baroreceptor denervation, and the hypersomnia/sleeplessness syndrome. A common feature of all these conditions is an interruption of normal sympathetic nervous activity.

Whether or not blood pressure variability contributes to vascular damage independently of the mean level of pressure remains an interesting, but unproven, possibility.

References

1. JACOB HJ, ALPER RJ, BRODY MJ: **Lability of arterial pressure after baroreceptor denervation is not pressure dependent.** *Hypertension* 1989, 14:501–570.

2. MANN S, MILLAR-CRAIG MW, ALTMAN DG, RAFTERY EB, HUNYOR SN: **Blood pressure variability in health, hypertension and autonomic failure.** *Clin Exp Hypertens* [A] 1985, 7:187–194.

3. MANCIA G, FERRARI A, GREGORINI L, *ET AL:* **Blood pressure and heart rate variabilities in normotensive and hypertensive human beings.** *Circ Res* 1983, 53:96–104.

4. PARATI G, POMIDOSSI G, CASADEI R, GROPPELLI A, TRAZZI S, DI RIENZO M, MANCIA G: **Role of heart rate variability in the production of blood pressure variability in man.** *J Hypertens* 1987, 5:557–560.

5. RAWLES JM, WEBSTER J, PETRIE LJ **Linear cardiac output in borderline and sustained hypertension.** *J Hypertens* 1989, 7:63–68.

6. CLEMENT DL, DEPUE N, JORDAENS LJ, PACKET L: **Adrenergic and vagal influences on blood pressure variability.** *Clin Exp Hypertens* [A] 1985, 7:159–166.

7. CLEMENT DL, JORDAENS LJ, HEYNDRICKX GR: **Influence of vagal nervous activity on blood pressure variability.** *J Hypertens* 1984, 2 (suppl 3):391–393.

8. CLEMENT DL, MUSSCHE MM, VANHOUTTE G, PANNIER R: **Is blood pressure variability related to the activity of the sympathetic system?** *Clin Sci* 1979, 57 (suppl):217S–219S.

9. DORNHORST AC, HOWARD P, LEATHART GL: **Respiratory variations in blood pressure.** *Circulation* 1952, 6:553–558.

10. GUYTON AC, SATTERFIELD JH: **Vasomotor waves possibly resulting from CNS ischemic reflex oscillation.** *Am J Physiol* 1952, 170:601–605.

11. MORKIN E, SINGER DH, FISHMAN AP: **Systemic and pulmonary vasomotor waves.** *Am J Physiol* 1965, 209:37–50.

12. HEYMANS C, NEIL E: *Reflexogenic Areas of the Cardiovascular System.* London: Churchill, 1958, pp 180–182.

13. AKSELROD S, GORDON D, UBEL FA, SHANNON DC, BARGER AC, COHEN RJ: **Power spectrum analysis of heart rate fluctuation: a quantitative probe of beat-to-beat cardiovascular control.** *Science* 1981, 213:220–222.

14. POMERANZ B, MACAULAY JB, CAUDILL MA, *ET AL:* **Assessment of autonomic function in humans by heart rate spectral analysis.** *Am J Physiol* 1985, 248:H151–H153.

15. PAGANI M, LOMBARDI F, GUZZETTI S, *ET AL:* **Power spectral density of heart rate variability as an index of sympathovagal interaction in normal and hypertensive subjects.** *J Hypertens* 1984, 2 (suppl 3):383–385.

16. PAGANI M, BROVELLI M, GUZZETTI S, *ET AL:* **Power spectral density of heart rate variability as an index of sympathovagal interaction.** *Eur J Clin Invest* 1984, 14:19.

17. GUZZETTI S, PICCALUGA E, CASATI R, *ET AL:* **Sympathetic predominance in essential hypertension: a study employing spectral analysis of heart rate variability.** *J Hypertens* 1988, 6:711–717.

18. PAGANI M, FURLAN R, DELL'ORTO S, *ET AL:* **Simultaneous analysis of beat by beat systemic arterial pressure and heart rate variabilities in ambulatory patients.** *J Hypertens* 1985, 3 (suppl 3):S83–S85.

19. FURLAN R, CRIVELLARO W, DELL'ORTO S, *ET AL:* **Circadian changes in vascular sympathetic activity in ambulant subjects.** *J Hypertens* 1989, 7 (suppl 6):S30–S31.

20. MANCIA G, CASADEI R. CASTIGLIONI P, DI RIENZO M, PARATI G: **Evaluation of central and reflex cardiovascular control by beat-to-beat analysis of the 24-hour blood pressure signal in man.** *Clin Exp Hypertens* [A] 1988, 10 (suppl 1):193–207.

21. HINES EA, BROWN GE: **A standard test for measuring the variability of blood pressure: its significance as an index of the prehypertensive state.** *Ann Intern Med* 1933, 7:209–217.

22. WATSON RDS, STALLARD TJS, FLINN RM, LITTLER WA: **Factors determining direct arterial pressure and its variability in hypertensive man.** *Hypertension* 1980, 2:333–341.

23. MANCIA G, FERRARI A, GREGORINI L, *ET AL:* **Blood pressure variability in man: its relation to high blood pressure, age, and baroreflex sensitivity.** *Clin Sci* 1980, 59 (suppl):401S–404S.

24. PUDDEY IB, JENNER DA, BEILIN LJ, VANDONGEN R: **Alcohol consumption, age and personality characteristics as important determinants of within-subject variability in blood pressure.** *J Hypertens* 1988, 6 (suppl 4):S617–S619.

25. CONTRADA JR, KRANTZ DS: **Stress, reactivity, and type A behavior: current status and future directions.** *Ann Behav Med* 1988, 10:64–70.

26. DELIUS W, HAGBARTH KE, HONGELL A, WALLIN BG: **Maneuvers affecting sympathetic outflow in human muscle nerves.** *Acta Physiol Scand* 1972, 84:82–94.

27. MANCIA G, FERRARI A, GREGORINI L, ET AL.: Blood pressure variability in man: its relation to high blood pressure, age, and baroreflex sensitivity. *Clin Sci* 1980, 59:401S–410S.

28. MANCIA G, PARATI G, POMIDOSSI G, CASADEI R, DI RIENZO M, ZANCHETTI A: Arterial baroreflexes and blood pressure and heart rate variabilities in humans. *Hypertension* 1985, 8:147–153.

29. FLORAS JS, HASSAN O, VANN JONES J, OSIKOWSKA BA, SEVER PS, SLEIGHT P: Factors influencing blood pressure and heart rate variablity in hypertensive humans. *Hypertension* 1988, 11:273–281.

30. CONWAY J, BOON N, VANN JONES J, SLEIGHT P Mechanisms concerned with blood pressure variability throughout the day. *Clin Exp Hypertens* [A] 1985, 7:153–157.

31. FLORAS JS, HASSAN MO, JONES JV, ET AL.: Baroreceptor reflexes and the control of blood-pressure and plasma noradrenaline in hypertension. In *Arterial Baroreceptors and Hypertension* edited by Sleight P. Oxford: Oxford University Press, 1980, pp 470–475.

32. HILTON SM: Inhibition of the baroreceptor reflex by the brainstem defence centre. In *Arterial Baroreceptors and Hypertension* edited by Sleight P. Oxford: Oxford University Press, 1980, pp 318–323.

33. SLEIGHT P, FOX P, LOPEZ R, BROOKS DE: The effect of mental arithmetic on blood pressure variability and baroreflex sensitivity in man. *Clin Sci Mol Med* 1978, 55 (suppl):381S–382S.

34. CUNNINGHAM DJC, PETERSEN ES, PETO R, SLEIGHT P: Comparison of the effect of different types of exercise on the baroreflex regulation of heart rate. *Acta Physiol Scand* 1972, 86:444–455.

35. COWLEY AW, LIARD JF, GUYTON AC: Role of the baroreceptor reflex in daily control of arterial blood pressure and other variables in dogs. *Circ Res* 1973, 32:564–576.

36. MANCIA G, BERTINIERI G, CAVALLAZZI A, ET AL: Mechanisms of blood pressure variability in man. *Clin Exp Hypertens* [A] 1985, 7:167–178.

37. ALEXANDER N, VELASQUEZ MT, DECUIR M, MARONDE RF: Studies of sympathetic activity in the sinoaortic-denervated hypertensive rats. *Am J Physiol* 1980, 238:H521–H526.

38. ALPER RH, JACOB HJ, BRODY MJ: Regulation of arterial pressure lability in rats with chronic sinoaortic deafferentation. *Am J Physiol* 1987, 253:H466–H474.

39. AKSAMIT TR, FLORAS JS, VICTOR RG, AYLWARD PE: Paroxysmal hypertension due to sinoaortic denervation in humans. *Hypertension* 1987, 9:309–314.

40. KUCHEL O, CUSSON JR, LAROCHELLE P, BUU NT, GENEST J: Case report. Posture- and emotion-induced severe hypertensive paroxysms with baroreceptor dysfunction. *J Hypertens* 1987, 5:277–283.

41. GRIBBIN B, PICKERING TG, SLEIGHT P, PETO R: Effect of age and high blood pressure on baroreflex sensitivity in man. *Circ Res* 1971, 29:424–431.

42. MANCIA G, FERRARI A, LUDBROOK J, ZANCHETTI A: Carotid baroreceptor influences on blood-pressure in normotensive and hypertensive subjects. In *Arterial Baroreceptors and Hypertension* edited by Sleight P. Oxford: Oxford University Press, 1980, pp 484–491.

43. KOTCHEN TA, MORLEY JM, GUTHRIE GP, BERK MR, KNAPP CF, MCFADDEN M: Baroreceptor sensitivity in prehypertensive young adults. *Hypertension* 1989, 13:878–883.

44. LEDOUX JR, DEL BO A, TUCKER LW, HARSHFIELD G, TALMAN WT, REIS DJ: Hierarchic organization of blood pressure responses during the expression of natural behaviors in rat: mediction by sympathetic nerves. *Exp Neurol* 1982, 78:121–133.

45. SOWERS JR: Dopaminergic control of circadian norepinephrine levels in patients with essential hypertension. *J Clin Endocrinol Metab* 1981, 53:1133–1137.

46. REIS DJ, LEDOUX JE: Some central neural mechanisms governing resting and behaviorally coupled control of blood pressure. *Circulation* 1987, 76 (suppl I):2–9.

47. ATHANASSIADIS D, DRAPER GJ, HONOUR AJ, CRANSTON WI: Variability of automatic blood pressure measurements over 24-hour periods. *Clin Sci* 1969, 36:147–156.

48. MANN S, MILLAR-CRAIG MW, MELVILLE DI, BALASUBRAMANIAN V, RAFTERY EB: Physical activity and the circadian rhythm of blood pressure. *Clin Sci* 1979, 57 (suppl):291S–294S.

49. YOUNG MA, ROWLANDS DB, STALLARD TH, WATSON RDS, LITTLER WA: Effect of environment on blood pressure: home versus hospital. *Br Med J* 1983, 286:1235–1236.

50. ROWLANDS DB, STALLARD TJ, WATSON RDS, LITTLER WA: The influence of physical activity on arterial pressure during ambulatory recordings in man. *Clin Sci* 1980, 58:115–117.

51. VAN EGEREN LF: Computer-based monitoring of physical activity. In *Clinical Evaluation and Physiological Monitoring.* edited by Miles L, Broughton R. New York: Raven (in press).

52. GELLMAN M, SPITZER S, IRONSON G, ET AL: Posture, place and mood effects on ambulatory blood pressure. *Psychophysiology* (in press).

53. PALATINI P, MOS L, MUNARI L, ET AL: Beats modulate blood pressure during running. *Am J Hypertens* 1989, 2:872–874.

54. LIND AR, TAYLOR SH, HUMPHREYS PW, KENNELLY BM, DONALD KW: The circulatory effects of sustained voluntary muscle contraction. *Clin Sci* 1964, 27:229–244.

55. PALATINI P, MOS L, MUNARI L, ET AL: Blood pressure changes during heavy-resistance exercise. *J Hypertens* 1989, 7 (suppl 6):S72–S73.

56. LITTLER WA, HONOUR AJ, SLEIGHT P: Direct arterial pressure, heart rate, and electrocardiogram during human coitus. *J Reprod Fertil* 1974, 40:321–331.

57. LITTLER WA, HONOUR AJ, SLEIGHT P: Direct arterial pressure, pulse rate, and electrocardiogram during micturition and defecation in unrestricted man. *Am Heart J* 1974, 88:205–210.

58. FAGAN TC, CONRAD KA, MAR HJ, NELSON L: Effects of meals on hemodynamics: implications for antihypertensive drug studies. *Clin Pharmacol Ther* 1986, 39:255–260.

59. KELBAEK H, MUNCK O, CHRISTENSEN NJ, GODTFREDSEN J: Central haemodynamic changes after a meal. *Br Heart J* 1989, 61:506–509.

60. LIPSITZ LA, NYQUIST RP, WEI JY, ROWE JW: Postprandial reduction in blood pressure in the elderly. *N Engl J Med* 1983, 309:81–83.

61. PEITZMAN SJ, BERGER SR: Postprandial blood pressure decrease in well elderly persons. *Arch Intern Med* 1989, 149:286–288.

62. THOMAS GB, MURPHY EA: Circulatory responses to smoking in healthy young men. *Ann NY Acad Sci* 1960, 90:266–276.

63. ROTH GM, MCDONALD JB, SHEARD C: The effect of smoking cigarettes, and of intravenous administration of nicotine on the electrocardiogram, basal metabolic rate, cutaneous temperature, blood pressure, and pulse rate of normal persons. *JAMA* 1944, 125:751–767.

64. CELLINA GU, HONOUR AJ, LITTLER WA: Direct arterial pressure, heart rate, and electrocardiogram during cigarette smoking in unrestricted patients. *Am Heart J* 1975, 89:18–25.

65. LARBI EB, COOPER RS, STAMLER J: Alcohol and hypertension. *Arch Intern Med* 1983, 143:28–29.

66. ORLANDO J, ARONOW WS, CASSIDY J, PRAKASH R: Effect of ethanol on angina pectoris. *Ann Intern Med* 1976, 84:652–655.

67. GOULD L, ZAHIR M, DEMARTINO A, GOMPRECHT RF: The cardiac effects of a cocktail. *JAMA* 1971, 218:1799–1802.

68. STOTT DJ, BALL SG, INGLIS GC, ET AL: Effects of a single moderate dose of alcohol on blood pressure, heart rate and associated metabolic and endocrine changes. *Clin Sci* 1987, 73:411–416.

69. POTTER JF, WATSON RDS, SKAN W, BEEVERS DG: The pressor and metabolic effects of alcohol in normotensive subjects. *Hypertension* 1986, 8:625–631.

70. POTTER JF, MACDONALD IA, BEEVERS DG: Alcohol raises blood pressure in hypertensive patients. *J Hypertens* 1986, 4:435–441.

71. MALHOTRA H, MEHTA SR, MATHUR D, KHANDELWAL PD: Pressure effects of alcohol in normotensive and hypertensive subjects. *Lancet* 1985, ii:584–586.

72. POTTER JF, BEEVERS DG: Pressor effect of alcohol in hypertension. *Lancet* 1984, i:119–122.

73.   MACMAHON S: Alcohol consumption and hypertension. *Hypertension* 1987, 9:111–121.

74.   SMITS P, THIEN T, VAN'T LAAR A: Circulatory effects of coffee in relation to the pharmacokinetics of caffeine. *Am J Cardiol* 1985, 56:958–963.

75.   ROBERTSON D, FROLICH JC, CARR RK, *ET AL.:* Effects of caffeine on plasma renin activity, catecholamines and blood pressure. *N Engl J Med* 1978, 298:181–186.

76.   IZZO JL, GHOSAL A, KWONG T, FREEMAN RB, JAENIKE JR: Age and prior caffeine use alter the cardiovascular and adrenomedullary responses to oral caffeine. *Am J Cardiol* 1983, 52:769–773.

77.   LANE JD: Caffeine and cardiovascular response to stress. *Psychosom Med* 1983, 45:447–451.

78.   PINCOMB GA, LOVALLO WR, PASSEY RB, WILSON MF: Effect of behavior state on caffeine's ability to alter blood pressure. *Am J Cardiol* 1988, 61:798–802.

79.   VAN DUSSELDORP M, SMITS P, THIEN T, KATAN MB: Effect of decaffeinated versus regular coffee on blood pressure. A 12-week double-blind trial. *Hypertension* 1989, 14:563–569.

80.   PERITI M, SALVAGGIO A, QUAGLIA G, DI MARIZIO L: Coffee consumption and blood pressure: an Italian study. *Clin Sci* 1987, 72:443–447.

81.   FREESTONE S, RAMSAY LE: Effect of coffee and cigarette smoking on the blood pressure of untreated and diuretic-treated hypertensive patients. *Am J Med* 1982, 73:348–353.

82.   JAMES GD, PECKER MS, PICKERING TG, *ET AL.:* The effects of dietary sodium on the average ambulatory and casual blood pressure of borderline hypertensives (in press).

83.   LYNCH JJ, THOMAS SA, LONG JM, MALINOW KL, CHICKADONZ G, KATCHER AH: Human speech and blood pressure. *J Nerv Ment Dis* 1980, 168:526–534.

84.   LONG JM, LYNCH JJ, MACHIRAN NM, THOMAS SA, MALINOW KM: The effect of status on blood pressure during verbal communication. *J Behav Med* 1982, 5:165–172.

85.   MALINOW KL, LYNCH JJ, FOREMAN PJ, FRIEDMANN E, THOMAS SA: Blood pressure increases while signing in a deaf population. *Psychosom Med* 1986, 48:95–101.

86.   FRIEDMAN E, THOMAS SA, KULICK-CIUFFO D, LYNCH JJ, SUGINAHARA M: The effects of normal and rapid speech on blood pressure. *Psychosom Med* 1982, 44:545–553.

87.   THOMAS SA, FRIEDMAN E, LOTTES LS, GRESTY S, MILLER C, LYNCH JJ: Changes in nurses' blood pressure and heart rate while communicating. *Res Nurs Health* 1984, 7:119–126.

88.   LYNCH JJ, LONG JM, THOMAS SA, MALINOW KL, KATCHER AH: The effects of talking on the blood pressure of hypertensive and normotensive individuals. *Psychosom Med* 1981, 43:25–33.

89.   LINDEN W: A microanalysis of autonomic activity during human speech. *Psychosom Med* 1987, 49:562–578.

90.   DEMBROSKI TM, MACDOUGALL JM: Validation of the Vita-Stat automated noninvasive ambulatory blood pressure recording device. In *Cardiovascular Instrumentation* edited by Herd JA, Gotto AM, Kaufmann PG, Weiss SM. NIH Publication, 1984, No 84-1654, pp 55–77.

91.   SCHMIEDER R, RÜDDEL H, LANGEWITZ W, NEUS J, WAGNER O, VON EIFF AW: The influence of monotherapy with oxprenolol and nitrendipine on ambulatory blood pressure in hypertensives. *Clin Exp Hypertens* [A] 1985, 7:445–454.

92.   HARSHFIELD GA, PICKERING TG, KLEINERT HD, BLANK S, LARAGH JH: Situational variation of blood pressure in ambulatory hypertensive patients. *Psychosom Med* 1982, 44:237–245.

93.   PICKERING TG, HARSHFIELD GA, KLEINERT HD, BLANK S, LARAGH JH: Blood pressure during normal daily activities, sleep, and exercise. Comparison of values in normal and hypertensive subjects. *JAMA* 1982, 247:992–996.

94.   JAMES GD, YEE LS, HARSHFIELD GA, BLANK SG, PICKERING TG: The influence of happiness, anger, and anxiety on the blood pressure of borderline hypertensives. *Psychosom Med* 1986, 48:502–508.

95.   JAMES GD, YEE LS, HARSHFIELD GA, PICKERING TG: Sex differences in factors affecting the daily variation of blood pressure. *Soc Sci Med* 1988, 26:1019–1023.

96.   CLARK LA, DENBY L, PREGIBON D, *ET AL:* The effects of activity and time of day on the diurnal variations of blood pressure. *J Chron Dis* 1987, 40:671–681.

97.   JAMES GD, PICKERING TG: Ambulatory blood pressure monitoring: assessing the diurnal variation of blood pressure. *Am J Phys Anthropol* (in press).

98.   FLORAS JS, HASSAN MO, VAN JONES J, OSIKOWSKA BA, SEVER PS, SLEIGHT P: Factors influencing blood pressure and heart rate variability in hypertensive humans. *Hypertension* 1988, 11:273–281.

99.   HARSHFIELD GA, PICKERING TG, JAMES GD, BLANK SG: Blood pressure variability and reactivity in the natural environment. In *Blood Pressure Measurements* edited by Meyer-Sabellek W, Anlauf M, Cotzen R, Steinfeld L. Darmstadt: Steinkopff, 1990, pp 211–216.

100.   SANNERSTEDT R: Hemodynamic response to exercise in patients with arterial hypertension. *Acta Med Scand* 1966, 458 (suppl):1–83.

101.   AMERY C, JULIUS S, WHITLOCK LS, CONWAY J: Influence of hypertension on the hemodynamic response to exercise. *Circulation* 1967, 36:231–237.

102.   MARRACCINI P, PALOMBO C, GIACOMI S, *ET AL:* Reduced cardiovascular efficency and increased reactivity during exercise in borderline and established hypertension. *Am J Hypertens* 1989, 2:913–916.

103.   MONTAIN SJ, JILKA SM, EHSANI AA, HAGBERG JM: Altered hemodynamics during exercise in older essential hypertensive subjects. *Hypertension* 1988, 12:478–484.

104.   PICKERING TG, GERIN W: Reactivity and the role of behavioral factors in hypertension: a critical review. *Ann Behav Med* 1990, 12:3–16.

105.   LYNCH JJ, THOMAS SA, PASKEWITZ DA, MALINOW KL, LONG JM: Interpersonal aspects of blood pressure control. *J Nerv Ment Dis* 1982, 170:143–153.

106.   VAN DER MEIRACKER AH, MAN IN'T VELD AJ, RITSEMA VAN ECK HJ, WENTING GH, SCHALEKAMP MADH: Determinants of short-term blood pressure variability. Effects of bed rest and sensory deprivation in essential hypertension. *Am J Hypertens* 1988, 1:22–26.

107.   SNYDER DW, NATHAN MA, REIS DJ: Chronic lability of arterial pressure produced by selective destruction of the catecholamine innervation of the nucleus tractus solitarii in the rat. *Circ Res* 1978, 43:662–671.

108.   ALPER RH, JACOB HJ, BRODY MJ: Central and peripheral mechanisms of arterial pressure lability following baroreceptor denervation. *Can J Physiol Pharmacol* 1987, 65:1615–1618.

109.   JULIUS S: The blood pressure seeking properties of the central nervous system. *J Hypertens* 1988, 6:177–185.

110.   RAVOGLI A, TRAZZI S, VILLARI A, *ET AL:* Early 24 hour blood pressure elevation in normotensive subjects with parenteral hypertension. *Hypertension* (in press).

111.   ULRYCH M: Changes of general haemodynamics during stressful mental arithmetic and non-stressing quiet conversation and modification of the latter by beta-adrenergic blockade. *Clin Sci* 1969, 36:453–461.

112.   GARAVAGLIA GE, MESSERLI FH, SCHNIDER RE, NUNEZ BD: Antihypertensive therapy and cardiovascular reactivity during isometric stress. *J Hum Hypertens* 1988, 2:247–251.

113.   ANDREN L, HANSSON L: Circulatory effects of noise in essential hypertension. *Acta Med Scand* 1980, 646:69–72.

114.   GUYTON AC: Arterial pressure and hypertension. Philadelphia: W.B. Saunders, 1980, p. 564.

115.   LIARD JF, TARAZI RC, FERRARIO CM, MANGER WM: Hemodynamic and humoral characteristics of hypertension induced by prolonged stellate ganglion stimulation in conscious dogs. *Circ Res* 1975, 36:455–464.

116.   KRIEGER EM: Neurogenic mechanisms in hypertension: Resetting of the baroreceptors. *Hypertension* 1986, 8 (suppl I):7–14.

117.   CORBETT JL, FRANKEL HL, HARRIS PJ: Cardiovascular changes associated with skeletal muscle spasm in tetraplegic man. *J Physiol* 1971, 215:381–431.

118. Reggiani P, Magrini F, Mondadori C, Branzi G, Zanchetti A: Marked blood pressure fluctuations during narcoleptic attacks alternating with abnromal wakefulness: effects of treatment with clonidine. *Curr Heart J* 1989, 10:2–7.
119. Giese J: Renin, angiotensin and hypertensive vascular damage: a review. In *Hypertension Manual* edited by Laragh JH. Yorke. 1973, pp 371–403.
120. O'Rourke MF: Basic concepts for the understanding of large arteries in hypertension. *J Cardiovasc Pharmacol* 1985, 7 (suppl):S14–S21.
121. Cowley AW, Liard JF, Guyton AC: Role of the baroreceptor reflex in daily control of arterial pressure and other variables in the dog. *Circ Res* 1973, 32:564–576.
122. Ferrario CM, McCubbin JW, Page IH: Hemodynamic changes of chronic experimental neurogenic hypertension in unanesthetized dogs. *Circ Res* 1969, 24:911–922.
123. Kobrin I, Oigman W, Kuman A, *et al.*: Diurnal variation of blood pressure in elderly patients with essential hypertension. *J Am Geriatr Soc* 1984, 312:896–899.
124. Parati G, Pomidossi G, Albini F, Malaspina D. Mancia G: Relationship of 24-hour blood pressure mean and variability to severity of target-organ damage in hypertension. *J Hypertens* 1987, 5:93–98.
125. Pessina AC, Palatini P, Sperti G, *et al.*: Evaluation of hypertension and related target organ damage by average day-time blood pressure. *Clin Exp Hypertens* [A] 1985, 7:267–278.

Diurnal, ultradian and seasonal rhythms of blood pressure

The most important and consistent sources of blood pressure variation are the diurnal changes associated with the sleep–wake cycle. This chapter will review what is known about the sources of such variability, how it is altered in disease, and its pathological significance. It will also review cyclical changes of shorter duration (ultradian rhythms) and seasonal changes.

Changes in blood pressure associated with sleep and wakefulness

Sleep is an active process regulated by centres in the brainstem and composed of distinct cycles that recur regularly throughout the course of the night [1]. Two basic varieties are recognized: non-dreaming, or slow-wave sleep [so-called because of low-frequency, high-amplitude waves on the electroencephalogram (EEG)], and dreaming, or rapid eye movement (REM), sleep which occurs when the EEG shows low-voltage, high-frequency activity similar to the pattern of wakefulness. The deepest stages of slow-wave sleep (stages 3 and 4) occur in the first 2 h of sleep; periods of REM sleep occur in 90 min cycles, with episodes lasting longer during the latter part of the night.

Blood pressure changes are closely linked to the level of arousal. During the first hour of sleep there is normally a progressive fall in blood pressure, with the maximal decrease of 15–20% 2 h after sleep onset [2–9], as shown in

Fig. 5.1. This coincides with the deepest stages of slow-wave sleep (stages 3 and 4). During REM sleep the blood pressure is at about the same level as in stage 2 (approximately 10% less than during wakefulness) but is much more variable, with fluctuations of as much as 30 mmHg over a few minutes [2]. Similar surges in pressure mediated by sympathetic vasoconstriction are also seen during K complexes, which are brief periods of arousal during stages 1 and 2 sleep in response to external stimuli [5].

Blood pressure rises immediately on waking. The close association between blood pressure and the level of arousal is further shown by the fact that in a drowsy subject the episodes of alpha rhythm (which signify arousal) are accompanied by surges in arterial pressure [5]. The contrasting effects of sleep and wakefulness on blood pressure were clearly demonstrated in a study by Athanassiadis et al. [8]. They reported that in patients on an accident ward, whose physical activity was limited by plaster casts, blood pressure remained relatively constant during the day, and fell consistently by about 25% during sleep.

Haemodynamic and neurohormonal changes during sleep

The fall in blood pressure during sleep is accompanied by a decreased heart rate. Cardiac output decreases by a modest amount [4], but there may also be vasodi-

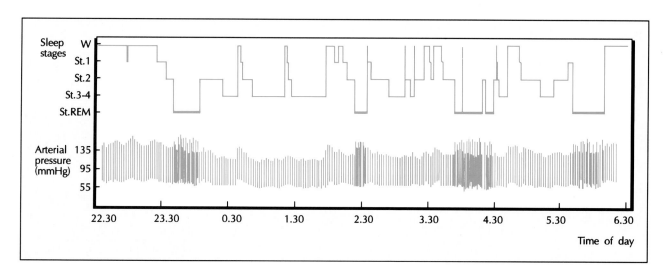

Fig. 5.1. Typical blood pressure changes during sleep in a normal subject. Upper trace shows sleep stages (W, waking; St.l, 2, 3, 4, stages l, 2, 3, 4). Blood pressure is plotted every 60 s, and every 30 s during REM sleep to show increased variability. Reproduced with permission from Coccagna et al., *Electroencephalogr Clin Neurophysiol* 1971, 31:277–281.

latation [9]. Oxygen consumption decreases during the first half of the night, followed by a gradual rise towards morning [10]. Cerebral blood flow has been reported to be increased during sleep [11]. Renal blood flow and glomerular filtration rate fall by as much as 20% [12,13], but there is a much more pronounced decrease in urine flow, which has been attributed to increased tubular reabsorption [12,14]. This nocturnal oliguria is not a direct consequence of sleep, as it can persist independently of the sleep–wake cycle [15], and is not dependent on changes in posture [12]. The composition of the urine also changes: there are large decreases in the excretion of sodium and chloride, but relatively small decreases of potassium and bicarbonate excretion [14].

Plasma potassium also shows a diurnal rhythm, with higher levels in the morning (between 8.00 a.m. and 12 noon) and lower levels at night; the difference between the two levels is about 0.6 mmol/litre [13,16].

Plasma catecholamine levels fall during sleep (Fig. 5.2), which is consistent with a diminished sympathetic activity [17,18]. Urinary catecholamines (both adrenaline and noradrenaline) also show a diurnal rhythm, with the lowest levels at night [19,20]. This rhythm is still apparent in recumbent subjects who remain awake during the night, but it has a smaller amplitude [19]. The diurnal rhythm of noradrenaline (but not of adrenaline) is less pronounced in elderly subjects, who also tend to have higher levels of noradrenaline at all times [21]. This may be related to the fact that nocturnal sleep is more fragmentary in older people.

Plasma renin and aldosterone levels have usually been found to rise steadily at the onset of sleep, and reach their highest levels during the second half of the night [22,23]. It was originally thought that the nocturnal rise in renin levels was not directly related to sleep, since it persisted to some extent in subjects who remained awake during the night [23,24]. In such subjects the blood pressure

does not change, so that the increase of renin release cannot be due to hypotension. It also does not appear to be due to a decreased sodium delivery to the macula densa, as it is not abolished by a saline infusion [23]. However, it can be abolished by beta blockade, and is therefore presumably mediated, at least in part, by the sympathetic nervous system [24]. More recent studies using electroencephalographic monitoring have shown that there is, in fact, a very close linkage between renin levels and the stage of sleep: renin secretion is shut off during episodes of REM sleep [25], which occur mainly during the second half of the night. An important study by Brandenberger *et al.* [26] has shown that when sleep is undisturbed, there is a marked rhythm to renin secretion, such that secretion increases during non-REM sleep, and stops during REM sleep. If the sleep pattern is disturbed, for example by waking, renin secretion is also suppressed (see Fig. 5.3). These findings suggest that there is a single central mechanism regulating both sleep cycles and renin secretion during the night. How it operates is far from clear: the most obvious neural influence on renin secretion is via the sympathetic nervous system, although such nervous activity increases on waking while renin secretion is suppressed.

It might be assumed that the nocturnal rise in aldosterone levels is a consequence of increased renin and angiotensin formation. However, it has been reported that while beta blockade prevents the nocturnal rise in renin levels, that of aldosterone persists [24].

The decrease in blood pressure during sleep is paralleled by increased secretions of growth hormone and prolactin [27,28], whose release is stimulated by endogenous opioids, which also lower blood pressure [29]. Naloxone, a specific opioid inhibitor, has been shown to prevent the fall in systolic pressure that accompanies the onset of sleep, without affecting diastolic pressure or heart rate [30]. This finding suggests that opioids may be involved in the regulation of blood pressure during sleep.

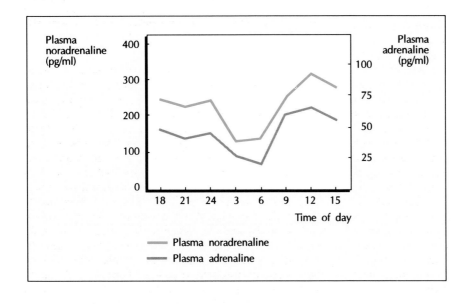

Fig. 5.2. Diurnal variations of plasma noradrenaline and adrenaline. Reproduced with permission from Tofler *et al., N Engl J Med* 1987, 316:1514.

Antidiuretic hormone (ADH) levels rise during the night, which could contribute to the nocturnal oliguria [31]. In one study, plasma atrial natriuretic factor (ANF) was reported to be elevated at night [31], but this does not occur if subjects remain recumbent and awake throughout the 24-hour period [32].

Is there a circadian rhythm of blood pressure?

Recordings made over 24 h in ambulatory subjects, using either invasive [33] or non-invasive recorders [34], have typically shown that blood pressure tends to be highest in the morning, with a gradual decrease over the course of the day, and lowest during the night (Fig. 5.4a). This observation led to the suggestion that there might be an intrinsic circadian rhythm of blood pressure analogous to the circadian pattern of cortisol or body temperature. The case for an intrinsic sinusoidal pattern of blood pressure variation has been argued most forcefully by Halberg *et al.* [35], who found that such curves fitted the blood pressure pattern of subjects kept in a confined environment for a period of several days. It has also been proposed by Raftery and colleagues [33] that there is a gradual increase in blood pressure during the early morning hours (3.00 a.m. to 6.00 a.m.) before the time of waking, and that this increase could contribute to the high incidence of cerebral haemorrhage and myocardial infarction in the early morning. Other workers, however, have presented data which indicate that the apparent sinusoidal pattern of blood pressure is most probably an artefact attributable to the averaging of records from individuals who wake at different times: when the recordings are synchronized to the time of waking, rather than to the time of day, the early morning rise in pressure is no longer seen [36,37]. Instead, blood pressure remains relatively stable during the hour before waking, but rises abruptly at the moment of waking (Fig. 5.5). This pattern is consistent with the changes described earlier [9], in studies where EEG was recorded as well as blood pressure.

Raftery's group found that patients with ventricular pacemakers, and hence fixed heart rates over 24 h, who were studied during normal daily activities, showed a persistent but somewhat diminished diurnal rhythm of blood pressure [38]. They argued that this finding provides further evidence for an intrinsic circadian rhythm. This is a *non sequitur*, however: what they did demonstrate was that blood pressure can vary independently of heart rate, but there is no reason to suppose that the observed changes in blood pressure could not have been produced by changes in activity and arousal. Mancia *et al.* [39] examined the average blood pressure levels over consecutive 30 min periods throughout the 24 h and also found no early-morning increase preceding waking. All the half-hour averages during waking were substantially similar, leading them to conclude that there is no circadian rhythm of blood pressure. The relatively flat profile of blood pressure during the day observed in their study may be attributed to the fact that their patients were hospitalized.

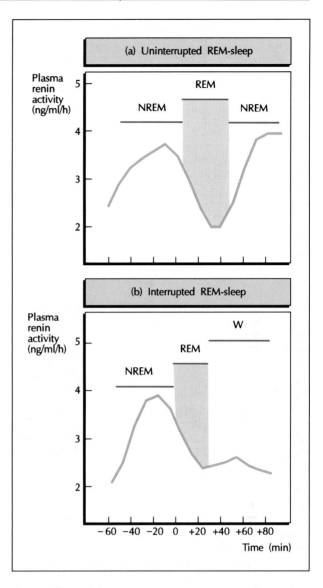

Fig. 5.3. Effects of slow-wave or non-REM (NREM) and REM sleep on plasma renin activity: (a) renin secretion is suppressed during REM sleep; (b) renin also falls on waking (W). Reproduced with permission [26].

The question whether there is an endogenous circadian rhythm of blood pressure, or whether the changes can be accounted for by variations in activity, is an important one. It can best be answered by removing the influence of external stimuli, so that if the rhythm persists, it can be attributed to endogenous factors. This was done in the study by Athanassiadis *et al.* [8], where blood pressure was monitored non-invasively for 24 h in patients in an orthopaedic ward who were immobilized by plaster casts. In this situation the blood pressure showed no evidence of any sinusoidal change, being relatively constant during the day and decreasing during sleep. There were, in effect, two levels of pressure: one corresponding to waking, and the other to sleeping. Similar observations were made in hospitalized patients kept on bed rest by Mann *et al.* [40]. In the latter study, diurnal variations in pressure became more pronounced when subjects were

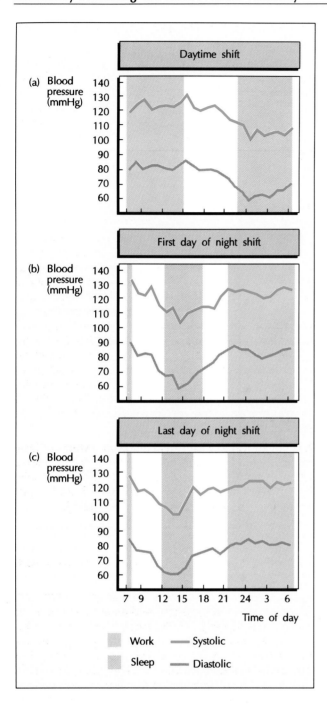

Fig. 5.4. Diurnal rhythms of blood pressure on three different work shifts. Reproduced with permission from Sundberg *et al.* [41].

studied a second time while physically active during the day.

Shift workers

Studies of shift workers have also shown a close linkage between activity and blood pressure. Sundberg *et al.*

[41] monitored 24-hour pressure and heart rate in seven normotensive nurses on three different days. On the first day they worked a normal daytime shift, and showed a typical diurnal pattern, with the highest pressures during work and the lowest pressures at night (see Fig. 5.4). The second recording was made on the first day they worked a night shift, and showed a complete reversal of the diurnal blood pressure pattern, with the lowest blood pressure occurring while they were asleep during the day. The third recording, made a few days later, was similar to the second. In contrast to the immediate reversal of the blood pressure rhythm, the diurnal rhythm of heart rate was not fully reversed by the third recording[1].

Baumgart *et al.* [42] studied industrial workers on both day and night shift, and also found that the diurnal pattern of blood pressure changed immediately the workers switched their shifts. Furthermore, the amplitudes of the diurnal pressure variations were the same on both shifts.

Another study of shift workers was performed by Chau *et al.* [43]. They monitored the 24-hour blood pressures of 15 workers in a chemical factory, who each worked three different shifts: morning (4.00 a.m. to 12 noon); afternoon (12 noon to 8.00 p.m.), and night (8.00 p.m. to 4.00 a.m.). In all cases the highest pressures were seen during the hours of work, but the diurnal patterns of blood pressure were different for the three shifts. The periods of high blood pressure were longer when subjects worked during the morning or night than when they worked during the afternoon, although the average 24-hour pressures were not very different (123/83 mmHg for the morning shifts, 120/79 mmHg for the afternoon, and 124/83 mmHg for the night shift). These differences can presumably be explained by differences in sleep patterns (which were not reported in this study).

The close linkage of the diurnal rhythm of blood pressure to the activity cycle is in marked contrast to some other bodily rhythms, which are more closely linked to an 'internal clock'. Examples of the latter type of rhythm include body temperature, urinary electrolyte excretion, and cortisol secretion. All of these are less easily disrupted by sudden changes in the sleep–wake cycle, although they can eventually be reversed [44–46].

Chronobiological analysis of diurnal blood pressure variations

A large number of biological variables show an intrinsic rhythm with a period of approximately 24 h, hence the term circadian ('around the day') rhythms. Halberg *et al.* [35] have been strong advocates of the use of 'rhythmometry' to analyse human diurnal blood pressure patterns. As shown in Fig. 5.6, the basis of this approach is to analyse the observed patterns as a series of cosine waves, with a basic period of 24 h. A number of terms need to be defined for this analysis. The mesor[2] is the

---

[1]Another example of this dissociation of diurnal rhythms is provided by the urinary excretion of catecholamines and sodium. The former adapts very quickly to a diurnal phase shift, while the latter takes several days [20].

[2]The word mesor is derived from the Midline-Estimating Statistic of Rhythm.

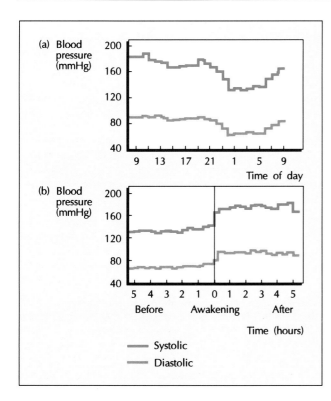

Fig. 5.5. Diurnal rhythm of blood pressure: (a) pooled data for 14 hypertensive subjects, plotted according to clock time; (b) same data plotted according to time of waking. Reproduced with permission from Floras et al. [37].

mean level, which is close (but not necessarily identical) to the average 24-hour blood pressure; the amplitude is the distance from the peak (or trough) to the mesor, which in this case would be the difference between the average 24-hour pressure and the peak pressure [47]; the acrophase defines the timing of the cycle, and is expressed as a phase angle between the reference time (0°) and the peak of the wave. The total cycle time is 360°. The Chronodesm is the confidence interval for the fit of the observed data points to the estimated waveform. On this schema, hypertension can be classified as 'mesor hypertension' when the entire profile is shifted to a higher level, or 'amplitude hypertension'. Ideally, this type of analysis should be performed over periods of more than 24 h, preferably 48 h.

While this approach has a mathematical appeal, it may be criticised on two grounds. First, the available evidence overwhelmingly suggests that blood pressure is not determined by an endogenous rhythm to the extent that, for example, heart rate or plasma cortisol are; and second, it imposes a symmetry that may be more artefactual than real. In this sense, it may be a Procrustean bed[3], where the peak and trough of blood pressure are assumed to be exactly 12 h apart, and also equidistant from the mesor. Neither of these criteria is likely to be met in reality. The fit between the theoretical waveform and the observed data points can be improved by including as many as

four harmonics in the Fourier analysis [48], but the physiological relevance of this is questionable.

The study of shift workers by Chau et al. [43] cited above used an elaborate Fourier analysis procedure to describe the diurnal patterns during the three shifts. A 'high' and 'low' blood pressure span were identified, and a Fourier equation used to fit the data. The simple cosine model (with one harmonic) gave a very poor fit, and four harmonics were, in fact, needed.

Ultradian rhythms

Circadian rhythms normally have a periodicity of approximately 24 h, but ultradian rhythms, with a periodicity of approximately 90 min, may also exist. These ultradian rhythms were first described for REM sleep [49], but may also be apparent during the day. A study using continuous monitoring of heart rate, blood pressure, and cardiac output in conscious dogs showed a 90 min periodicity of all three [50]. It was concluded that the rhythm was due to phasic variations in the level of sympathetic drive to the heart, because this periodicity of both blood pressure and heart rate can be suppressed by clonidine [51]. In dogs the amplitude of this ultradian rhythm of blood pressure may actually exceed the amplitude of the circadian rhythm.

It is not known to what extent ultradian rhythms of heart rate and blood pressure exist in man. It seems reasonable to suppose that they do exist, but may not be readily detectable in studies of free-ranging individuals, because they would be obscured by extraneous stimuli.

Comparison of diurnal patterns in normal and hypertensive subjects

In patients with hypertension the diurnal pattern of blood pressure change is generally similar to the changes occurring in normotensive subjects, except that the entire blood pressure profile is shifted upwards (Fig. 5.7). Thus, the differences between work and home pressures, and between home and sleep pressures, are approximately the same in normotensive and hypertensive subjects (about a 20% decrease during sleep in both cases) when expressed on a percentage basis, although in absolute terms they may be greater in hypertensive subjects [6,52,53]. There is some controversy about whether hypertensive patients with left ventricular hypertrophy (LVH) show the same diurnal variation in blood pressure as those without. According to Raftery [54] the pattern is similar, but a recent study by Verdecchia et al. [55] found that patients whose pressure remained high during the night were more likely to have LVH. What is not clear from this study, however, is whether the develop-

[3]Procrustes was a legendary Greek robber, who forced his victims to lie on an iron bed. If they did not fit the length of the bed, he either stretched them or cut off their legs.

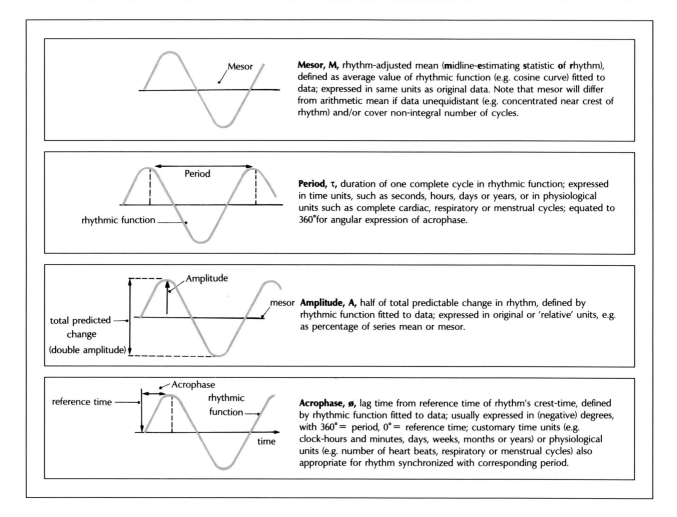

Fig. 5.6. Definitions of rhythm parameters used in the cosine method of analysing the diurnal rhythms of blood pressure and other variables. Reproduced with permission from Halberg *et al.* In *Ambulatory Blood Pressure Monitoring* edited by Weber MA, Drayer JIM, Darmstadt: Steinkopff, 1984, pp 137–156.

ment of LVH affects the diurnal pattern of blood pressure, or whether a persistent elevation in pressure throughout the day and night accelerates the development of LVH.

The diurnal hormonal patterns may also be altered in some patients with hypertension. The nocturnal rise in renin is seen in patients with borderline hypertension, but is absent in those with more severe hypertension [24]. Aldosterone, however, rises in both situations. In hypertensive subjects the decrease in plasma noradrenaline normally seen during sleep still occurs, but is somewhat less pronounced [56], as shown in Fig. 5.8. When hypertensive subjects are studied in the recumbent position for 24 h, with the influence of extraneous stimuli removed, there is a good correlation between plasma noradrenaline and arterial pressure [56]. Diurnal changes in blood pressure have also been reported to correlate with changes in plasma renin activity and in noradrenaline levels [57] in patients with renovascular hypertension. In hypertensive subjects the normal diurnal pattern of sodium excretion, with a pronounced decrease during the night, may be absent or even reversed [58]. This is of potential practical importance because overnight urine collections are sometimes used in lieu of 24-hour collections, and may hence give misleading results.

Sleep-disordered breathing and the sleep apnoea syndrome

A wide spectrum of severity of sleep-disordered breathing has been recognized, with snoring at the benign extreme, and obstructive sleep apnoea at the other. These conditions are relevant to the present discussion not only because they affect the changes in blood pressure occurring during sleep, but also because they are significant risk factors for cardiovascular disease. As a result of the compartmentalization of contemporary medical science, the significance of these risk factors has not been fully appreciated by researchers in the field of cardiovascular disease.

It has often been claimed that snoring is associated with an increased risk of hypertension, CHD and cerebral infarction, independently of blood pressure. Waller and

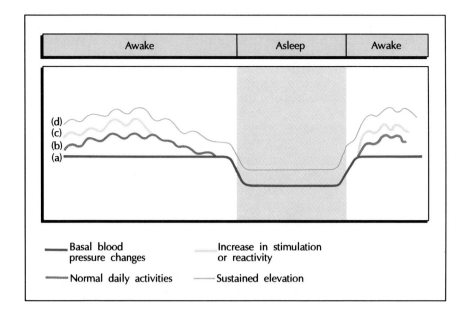

Fig. 5.7. Hypothetical patterns of blood pressure variability: (a) basic pattern of sleep and wakefulness; (b) effects of daily activities superimposed; (c) increased variability could result from increased activity or reactivity; (d) in most hypertensive subjects the pattern is one of sustained elevation of pressure. Reproduced with permission from Pickering, *Circulation* 1987, 76 (monograph 6):I–77.

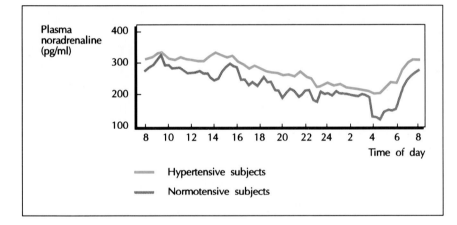

Fig. 5.8. Diurnal rhythms of plasma noradrenaline in normotensive and hypertensive subjects. Reproduced with permission from Tuck *et al., Am J Cardiol* 1985, 55:12.

Bhopal [59] recently reviewed eight studies which examined the association between snoring and vascular disease [60–67]. They reported that snoring is more common in men than in women, and is also associated with increasing age, obesity and smoking. Most of the studies which found an association did not control adequately for these potentially confounding factors, and may also be confounded by the association between sleep apnoea and snoring. Waller and Bhopal concluded that, in the absence of sleep apnoea, there is no conclusive evidence that snoring has any pathophysiological effect on the cardiovascular system.

Hoffenstein *et al.* [68] related daytime blood pressure to nocturnal snoring (evaluated by a microphone on the throat and an oximeter on the ear to measure oxygen saturation) in 372 snorers. They found that blood pressure was related to obesity, the apnoea–hypopnoea index and mean nocturnal oxygen saturation, but not to the amount of snoring itself. They also concluded that the association between snoring and hypertension is indirect.

Sleep apnoea syndrome is a condition that is probably under-diagnosed. The main reason for this is that,

at present, its diagnosis requires an all-night study in a specialized sleep laboratory. However, a number of techniques are being developed which should offer the possibility of diagnosing sleep apnoea by ambulatory monitoring. These include oximetry [69], EEG monitoring [70], and respiratory monitoring [71].

Sleep apnoea mainly effects middle-aged men, and its hallmark is episodic and repetitive apnoeic episodes occurring throughout the night. Characteristic symptoms include daytime sleepiness, snoring, disturbed sleep, morning headaches, and fatigue. There may also be an association with impotence [72].

The sleep apnoea syndrome is conventionally defined by the presence of at least 10 apnoeic episodes per hour (or sometimes 30 per night) lasting 10 s or longer. Such episodes may be of central origin, or due to mechanical obstruction of the airways, or to a combination of the two. Minor degrees of sleep apnoea are not uncommon in normal men, but are quite rare in women before the menopause [73]. However, in post-menopausal women the incidence of sleep-disordered breathing resembles the incidence in men [74]. Approximately 80% of individuals with the sleep apnoea syndrome are obese [75] and approximately 80% are also hypertensive [76–78]. The prevalence of sleep apnoea in hypertensive patients is also quite high, being 30% in one survey [79], and 22% in another [80]. Furthermore, it may be particularly common in patients whose hypertension is refractory to treatment [72]. However, one study of elderly patients found no difference in the prevalence of sleep apnoea between hypertensive and normotensive patients, although it was high in both groups [81]. It has been suggested that the relationship between sleep apnoea and blood pressure at night is a causal one on the basis of the findings that tracheostomy or continuous positive airway pressure (CPAP), which relieve the apnoeic episodes, can also restore the normal nocturnal blood pressure fall, although the effects on daytime hypertension are less consistent [77,82].

The haemodynamic changes which occur during the apnoeic episodes have been well described by Tilkian *et al.* [83], and are outlined in Fig. 5.9. As the apnoea develops there is systemic oxygen desaturation and an abrupt elevation of arterial pressure, without any accompanying tachycardia. In Tilkian's study there were quite marked increases in the level of blood pressure during sleep, the average change being from 139/85 mmHg during wakefulness to 167/105 mmHg during sleep. However, in elderly subjects, apnoeic episodes may be associated with hypotension [81]. Such subjects may show minor breathing disorders while awake. The apparent divergence in the effects of hypoxia on blood pressure during sleep may be explained by the fact that the reflex effect of hypoxia, mediated by the carotid bodies, is vasoconstriction, while the direct effect is vasodilatation. Thus, the net effect of hypoxia may depend on the sensitivity of the chemoreceptor reflexes.

The increases in blood pressure during apnoeic episodes are almost certainly mediated by the sympathetic nervous system. Sympathetic nervous activity (which can be directly recorded from the peroneal nerve) increases markedly during apnoeic episodes [84]. Urine and plasma catecholamines are higher in patients with sleep apnoea compared with normal controls [85]; furthermore, the usual nocturnal fall in catecholamine excretion is absent. After tracheostomy or CPAP treatment the nocturnal catecholamine excretion falls to normal, with the blood pressure [82,86]. Pancreatic polypeptide, which can be assayed in the blood as a marker of vagal activity, increases after the introduction of CPAP [82].

The usual nocturnal decrease in urine and electrolyte excretion is also impaired in patients with sleep apnoea, but normalizes following treatment with CPAP [87,88]. This phenomenon could not be explained by changes

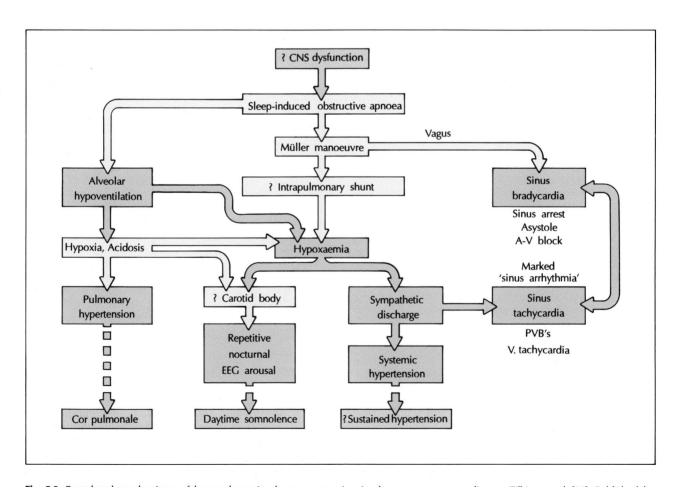

Fig. 5.9. Postulated mechanisms of haemodynamic changes occurring in sleep apnoea, according to Tilkian *et al.* [83]. Published by permission.

in glomerular filtration rate, ADH secretion, or renin and aldosterone levels [88], but may be attributable to high levels of ANF, which are lowered by CPAP [89].

Other conditions in which the normal diurnal pattern of blood pressure is altered: dippers and non-dippers

There are some situations in which the fall in blood pressure during sleep in hypertensive patients may be absent or reversed. Patients showing this phenomenon have been referred to as 'non-dippers', to distinguish them from the normal 'dippers' [90,91]. Such conditions are of interest for several reasons: first, they may be helpful in understanding the regulation of blood pressure during sleep and wakefulness; second, the findings of an absent nocturnal blood pressure fall may be of diagnostic value; and third, it may also have prognostic value. A problem that is sometimes overlooked is that the absence of a nocturnal fall in blood pressure may simply be due to the patient not sleeping, or if non-invasive blood pressure monitoring was used, being aroused by the inflation of the blood pressure cuff. However, in the conditions in which the diurnal rhythm of blood pressure is abnormal there is usually a decrease in heart rate during the night, which should help distinguish the non-dippers from the non-sleepers. These conditions are described below.

Malignant hypertension

Shaw et al. [92] monitored the blood pressure in hospitalized and recumbent patients using a non-portable non-invasive monitor. They divided the patients into two groups according to the fundal changes. The first group was classified as having benign hypertension, although their average daytime pressure was 217/127 mmHg, and most had ECG changes indicating LVH (ECG-LVH). The second group, with malignant hypertension, all had grade 3–4 retinopathy, and somewhat higher pressures (238/135 mmHg). Blood pressure fell during sleep in the benign group by 15/9 mmHg, but showed no change in the malignant group. Since there was considerable overlap in the blood pressures of patients in the two groups, these differences cannot be attributed simply to the height of the blood pressure. The heart is also unlikely to be the culprit, since most of the patients in both groups had ECG-LVH, and none were in overt heart failure. There was also overlap in renal function (measured as blood urea). The authors therefore suggested that the difference might have occurred because the peripheral resistance was 'fixed' in the patients with malignant hypertension. This seems unlikely, however, because the range of blood pressures seen over the whole 24 h was approximately the same in the two groups.

Secondary hypertension

According to Hany et al. [93] the circadian blood pressure variability is blunted in patients with secondary hypertension. They based this statement on a study which included patients with renal parenchymal disease, renovascular hypertension, primary aldosteronism, phaeochromocytoma, Cushing's disease, and polycystic kidneys. Since there were so few patients in the different categories, it was not possible to say whether they all showed similar diurnal rhythms of blood pressure, and as we shall see below, the probability is that they did not. Thus, to state that secondary hypertension is characterized by an abnormal diurnal rhythm of blood pressure is almost certainly a gross over-simplification. Gosse et al. [94] suggested that the circadian variation in blood pressure in hypertensive patients is determined more by the severity of hypertension than by its cause. While this would be consistent with the absence of a nocturnal fall in blood pressure in patients with malignant hypertension, it does not explain Hany's results, and has not been found in other studies [95].

Renovascular hypertension

In contradiction to the conclusions of Hany et al. [93] described above, two studies which included patients with renovascular hypertension did not report any consistent differences in the diurnal rhythm of blood pressure when the subjects were compared with essential hypertensive patients [94,95].

Chronic renal disease

Baumgart et al. [96] studied patients with chronic renal disease, and compared them with patients with similar blood pressures and taking comparable medications, but normal renal function. They were divided into three groups (chronic renal parenchymal disease, on chronic haemodialysis, and following renal transplantation). In all three groups there was marked attenuation of the nocturnal blood pressure fall in comparison with their control groups. The decrease in heart rate was still present, although somewhat attenuated.

The common factor in these patients was the presence of azotaemia, although the mechanism of the abnormal blood pressure profile was unexplained. There may be an element of autonomic neuropathy, and we have shown that baroreflex sensitivity is impaired in such patients [97]. In the transplant patients prednisone therapy was another contributing factor.

Phaeochromocytoma

Patients in whom phaeochromocytoma is suspected are obvious candidates for ambulatory monitoring. The classic paroxysmal elevations in blood pressure have been detected in about 25% of 24-hour studies in patients in whom the diagnosis is proved [98], and so it may be necessary to study a patient on more than one occasion to detect them. Littler and Honour [99] were the first to report that the nocturnal fall in blood pressure may be absent (in two of the three patients they studied). In a subsequent study of eight patients Imai et al. [98] found that this was the exception rather than the rule: in their patients the nocturnal fall was smaller than in patients with either treated or untreated essential hypertension, but still present. Their findings are of great theoretical interest because in such patients urinary catecholamine levels are usually greatly elevated throughout the day and night [100]. One interpretation of this finding is that the nocturnal fall in blood pressure may depend more on catecholamines released from sympathetic nerve terminals than on circulating levels.

There have been occasional reports of cyclical variations in blood pressure in patients with phaeochromocytoma [101,102]. Ganguly *et al.* [102] described one such case who was admitted to hospital in a state of marked dehydration with cyclical variations in pressure ranging from 240/140 mmHg to 100/80 mmHg every 5–10 min. The increases in pressure were accompanied by a reflex bradycardia. Rehydration of the patient with intravenous saline abolished the oscillations of blood pressure. While such oscillations bear some resemblance to Mayer waves, they have a much slower period (see Chapter 4).

Pre-eclamptic toxaemia
During normal pregnancy there is a normal fall in blood pressure during sleep [103], but in patients with preeclamptic toxaemia this fall may be absent or reversed with an increase in pressure during sleep [104–109].

In pre-eclampsia the normal hormonal patterns may be altered: although both renin and angiotensin II levels are generally lower than in normal pregnancies, angiotensin II levels show a smaller decrease during the night. Plasma noradrenaline shows a normal pattern, but plasma adrenaline may rise. Thus, it has been suggested that the nocturnal rise in blood pressure in these patients might be caused by either the relative elevation in adrenaline or angiotensin II levels [109].

Miyamoto *et al.* [110] have reported that pre-eclamptic women have higher blood pressures at night (10.00 p.m.) than during the day (10.00 a.m.), in contrast with women having a normal pregnancy, who had lower pressures at night. Heart rate also remained higher at night in the pre-eclamptic patients. Miyamoto *et al.* also found an abnormal pattern of thermal conductivity of the skin in the pre-eclamptic patients. This was measured as the time taken for a thermistor on the skin to equilibrate with the body's core temperature, and is thought to be a measure of blood flow. In the pre-eclamptic patients conductivity was higher at night than during the day, which, since the blood pressure was also higher, was interpreted to indicate a fluid shift from extravascular to intravascular compartments.

Cushing's syndrome
Munakata *et al.* [111] studied 15 patients with Cushing's syndrome (11 of pituitary origin and four of adrenal origin) and found that the normal nocturnal fall in blood pressure was absent, although the usual decrease in heart

rate persisted. Blood pressure gradually rose between 12 midnight and early morning, reaching a peak at about the time of waking. That this phenomenon was attributable to glucocorticoids was supported by the finding that patients with chronic glomerulonephritis or systemic lupus erythematosus also had no nocturnal fall in blood pressure when treated with prednisone, but a normal fall when untreated [112], as shown in Fig. 5.10. The diurnal rhythm of heart rate was unaffected by glucocorticoids in these patients and the diurnal rhythm of blood pressure was normal in patients with primary aldosteronism. It was suggested that the disturbance of glucocorticoid metabolism might influence the blood pressure via effects on the sympathetic nervous system, for example by modulating the synthesis of noradrenaline [113] or by enhancing the vascular responsiveness to catecholamines [114].

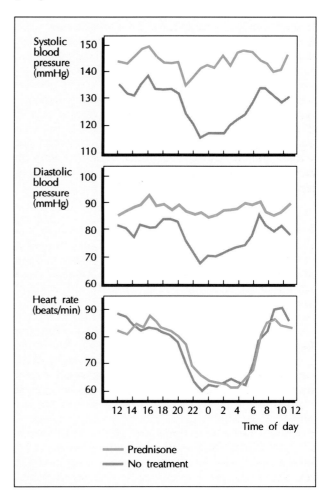

Fig. 5.10. Effects of prednisone administration on the diurnal rhythm of blood pressure in patients with chronic renal disease. Reproduced with permission [112].

Orthostatic hypotension
Patients suffering from idiopathic orthostatic hypotension have been found to exhibit a paradoxical elevation of pressure during the first part of the night, and the

lowest pressures of the day during the morning, when they are typically most symptomatic [115]. These pressure changes are associated with less consistent changes in heart rate, which may decrease during the night, or show little change. The nocturnal rise in pressure cannot be explained purely on the basis of recumbency, because it is also seen in patients who are recumbent for the full 24 h. This increase in pressure is associated with a nocturnal polyuria, which has been attributed to a pressure natriuresis.

Orthostatic hypotension is also a feature of the Shy-Drager syndrome, which differs from idiopathic orthostatic hypotension in that there are also sphincter disturbances and Parkinsonian features. Some of these patients may also have sleep apnoea, but even in those who do not, the blood pressure increases during the night [116].

Diabetes mellitus with autonomic neuropathy
Autonomic neuropathy is not an uncommon complication of insulin-dependent (type I) diabetes, and has been attributed to interruption of both vagal and sympathetic control of the circulation. The former is manifested by a relatively fixed heart rate, and the latter by orthostatic hypotension. In common with patients with idiopathic orthostatic hypotension, blood pressure remains high during the night [117]. The diurnal pattern of water and sodium excretion is also abnormal, with a relative increase during the night in comparison with normal subjects and diabetics without neuropathy [118].

Congestive heart failure
Caruana et al. [119] studied patients with congestive heart failure, all of whom had experienced a previous myocardial infarction. Neither blood pressure nor heart rate showed much change during the night, particularly in those patients who had the lowest ejection fractions.

Cardiac transplantation
Cardiac denervation is another situation where pressure increases at night. This has been observed in patients with cardiac transplants [117,120,121]. The nocturnal bradycardia is still present. The mechanism is unexplained, but could, in part, be due to increased venous filling of the heart associated with recumbency.

Seasonal variations in blood pressure

Blood pressure tends to be about 5 mmHg higher in winter than in summer in temperate climates. The effect appears to be a direct consequence of changes in environmental temperature, and is more marked in older than in younger subjects [122,123]. It has also been observed in children, however [124].

In an epidemiological study conducted in England [125] it was concluded that the seasonal effects could largely be accounted for by the ambient temperature at the time of blood pressure measurement. However, another study suggests that this may not be the whole story. Hata et al. [126] investigated three groups of subjects: normotensives and patients with either borderline or established hypertension. The study was conducted in Japan where the temperature ranged from 5°C in winter to 29°C in summer. The subjects were studied after resting for two hours in a room whose temperature was virtually the same during winter and summer. The normotensives had the same blood pressure in both seasons, although their 24-hour urinary excretion of sodium and noradrenaline was higher in winter. The two groups of hypertensive patients showed similar seasonal changes of sodium and noradrenaline, but in both cases the pressures were higher (by 8–10 mmHg) in the winter than in the summer. Thus, a possible explanation for this phenomenon is that sodium intake is higher (or sodium loss, via sweating, lower) in winter, and sympathetic activity is also higher.

In a study of the long-term reproducibility and seasonal effect on ambulatory blood pressure, Giaconi et al. [127] studied 22 patients with untreated borderline hypertension on two occasions 6 months apart: once in the summer, and once in the winter (the order was varied in different subjects). Their results are summarized in Fig. 5.11. With the exception of the clinic systolic pressures, all the readings were significantly higher in the winter than in the summer.

	Summer	Winter	Difference
Outdoor temperature	24.9°C	12.0°C	$P < 0.001$
Clinic			
systolic BP	No change	No change	NS
diastolic BP	84 ± 9 mmHg	89 ± 9 mmHg	$P < 0.01$
Ambulatory			
systolic BP	121 ± 11 mmHg	125 ± 9 mmHg	$P < 0.025$
diastolic BP	81 ± 7 mmHg	86 ± 6 mmHg	$P < 0.0005$
BP, blood pressure.			

Fig. 5.11. Seasonal changes of ambulatory and clinic blood pressure. Data from [127].

We have also examined the seasonal variations in blood pressure variability measured during ambulatory monitoring [128]. Overall, the variability was slightly, but not significantly, greater in summer (perhaps because the subjects were more active), but the effects of specific activities and moods on blood pressure were significantly greater in winter.

Summary and conclusions

As with many other physiological variables, there is a pronounced diurnal variation in blood pressure, with the peak levels usually occurring during the morning and the lowest levels during sleep. These changes appear to be very closely linked to the level of arousal and sympathetic nervous activity rather than to an underlying circadian rhythm. Thus, in shift workers the diurnal blood pressure rhythm parallels the timing of sleep and wakefulness.

In hypertensive patients, the diurnal rhythm is usually preserved, but re-set at a higher level of pressure, without much change in amplitude. An ever-growing number of conditions have been described in which this pattern is lost, however, with an absent or diminished nocturnal fall in pressure. There is a spectrum of breathing abnormalities which interfere with the normal pattern of sleep, most prominent of which is the sleep apnoea syndrome. This may originate from central causes or from mechanical instability of the airways leading to periodically obstructed breathing, hypoxia, and hypertension. It appears to be associated with daytime hypertension, for reasons which are unclear.

The mechanisms by which other pathological conditions cause a persistently elevated pressure at night are not understood, but they appear to operate without any gross interference with the pattern of sleep, and in many cases without impairing the fall in heart rate. In some cases, such as Cushing's syndrome and the administration of corticosteroids, an endocrine mechanism may be postulated, while in others autonomic neuropathy may be responsible.

Finally, seasonal variations in blood pressure have been reported, with higher levels in the winter than in the summer, at least in temperate climates. These variations may be due to increased sympathetic activity and a more positive sodium balance in the winter.

References

1. KLEITMAN N: *Sleep and Wakefulness.* Chicago: University of Chicago Press, 1963.
2. SNYDER F, HOBSON JA, MORRISON DF, *ET AL.:* Changes in respirations, heart rate, and systolic blood pressure in human sleep. *J Appl Physiol* 1964, 19:417–422.
3. COCCAGNA G, MANTOVANI M, BRIGNANI F, *ET AL.:* Arterial pressure changes during spontaneous sleep in man. *Electroencephalogr Clin Neurophysiol* 1971, 31:277–281.

4. KHATRI IM, FRIES ED: Hemodynamic changes during sleep. *J Appl Physiol* 1967, 22:867–873.
5. RICHARDSON DW, HONOUR AJ, GOODMAN AC: Changes in arterial pressure during sleep in man. *Hypertension* 1968, 16:62–78.
6. LITTLER WA, HONOUR AJ, CARTER RD, SLEIGHT P: Sleep and blood pressure. *Br Med J* 1975, 3:346–348.
7. PICKERING TG: Sleep, circadian rhythms and cardiovascular disease. *Cardiovasc Rev Reports* 1980, 1:37–47.
8. ATHANASSIADIS D, DRAPER GJ, HONOUR AJ, CRANSTON WI: Variability of automatic blood pressure measurements over 24-hour periods. *Clin Sci* 1969, 36:147–156.
9. BRISTOW JD, HONOUR AJ, PICKERING TG, SLEIGHT P: Cardiovascular and respiratory changes during sleep in normal and hypertensive subjects. *Cardiovasc Med* 1969, 3:476–486.
10. RYAN T, MLYNCZAK S, ERICKSON T, MAN SFP, MAN GCW: Oxygen consumption during sleep: influence of sleep stage and time of night. *Sleep* 1989, 12:201–210.
11. TOWNSEND RE, PRINZ PN, ABRIST WD: Human cerebral blood flow during sleep and waking. *J Appl Physiol* 1973, 35:620–625.
12. STANBURY SW, THOMPSON AE: Diurnal variations in electrolyte excretion. *Clin Sci* 1951, 10:267–293.
13. WESSON LG: Electrolyte excretion in relation to diurnal cycles of renal function. *Medicine* 1964, 43:547–592.
14. SIROTA JH, BALDWIN DW, VILLAREAL H: Diurnal variations of renal function in man. *J Clin Invest* 1950, 29:187–192.
15. MILLS JN: Diurnal rhythm in urine flow. *J Physiol* 1950, 113:528–536.
16. MOORE-EDE MC, BRENNAN MF, BALL MR: Circadian variation of intercompartmental potassium fluxes in man. *J Appl Physiol* 1975, 38:163–170.
17. DOLLERY CT, HAMILTON CA, MALING TJB: Changes in sleep pattern, blood pressure, heart rate, and plasma noradrenaline after night-time administration of slow release clonidine. *Clin Sci* 1979, 57:509–514.
18. WATSON RDS, REID JL, HAMILTON CA, LITTLER WA: Plasma noradrenaline, physical activity and systolic blood pressure in hypertension. *Clin Sci Mol Med* 1978, 54:26P.
19. TOWNSHEND MM, SMITH AJ: Factors influencing the urinary excretion of free catecholamines in man. *Clin Sci* 1973, 44:253–265.
20. BING RF, HARLOW J, SMITH AJ, TOWNSHEND MM: The urinary excretion of catecholamines and their derivatives in primary hypertension in man. *Clin Sci Mol Med* 1977, 52:319–323.
21. PRINZ PN, HALTER J, BENEDETTI C, RASKIND M: Circadian variation of plasma catecholamines in young and old men: relation to rapid eye movement and slow wave sleep. *J Clin Endocrinol Metabol* 1979, 49:300–304.
22. BREVER H, KAULHAUSEN H, MÜHLBAUER W: Circadian rhythm of the renin-angiotensin-aldosterone system. In *Chronobiological Aspects of Endocrinology.* Symposia Medica Hoechst. 9. Stuttgart: Schattauer Verlag, 1974, pp 101–109.
23. MODLINGER RS, SCHARIF-ZADEH K, ERTEL NH, *ET AL.:* The circadian rhythm of renin. *J Clin Endocrinol Metab* 1976, 43:1276–1282.
24. STUMPE KO, KOLLOCH R, VETTER H, *ET AL.:* Acute and long-term studies of the mechanisms of action of beta-blocking drugs in lowering blood pressure. *Am J Med* 1976, 60:853–865.
25. MULLEN PE, JAMES VHT, LIGHTMAN SL, LINSELL C, PEART WS: A relationship between plasma renin activity and the rapid eye movement phase of sleep in man. *J Clin Endocrinol Metab* 1980, 50:466–469.
26. BRANDENBERGER G, FOLLENIUS M, SIMON C, EHRHART J, LIBERT JP: Nocturnal oscillations in plasma renin activity and REM-NREM sleep cycles in humans: a common regulatory mechanism? *Sleep* 1989, 11:242–250.
27. TAKAHASHI Y, KIPNIS DM, DAUGHADAY WH: Growth hormone secretion during sleep. *J Clin Invest* 1968, 47:2079–2090.
28. SASSIN JF, FRANTZ AG, KAPEN S, WEITZMAN ED: The nocturnal rise of human prolactin is dependent on sleep. *J Clin Endocrinol Metab* 1975, 37:436–440.

29. LAMBIE M, SCHMITT H, VINCENT M, REMOND G: Central cardiovascular effects of morphinomimetic peptides in dogs. *Eur J Pharmacol* 1977, 46:67.

30. RUBIN P, BLASCHKE TF, GUILLEMINAULT C: Effect of naloxone, a specific opioid inhibitor on blood pressure fall during sleep. *Circulation* 1981, 63:117–121.

31. DONCKIER J, ANDERSON JV, YEO T, BLOOM SR: Diurnal rhythm in the plasma concentration of atrial natriuretic peptide. *N Engl J Med* 1986, 315:710–711.

32. RICHARDS AM, TONOLO G, FRASER R, ET AL.: Diurnal changes in plasma atrial natriuretic peptide concentrations. *Clin Sci* 1987, 73:489–495.

33. MILLAR-CRAIG MW, BISHOP CN, RAFTERY EB: Circadian variation of blood-pressure. *Lancet* 1978, i:795–797.

34. CLARK LA, DENBY L, PREGIBON D, ET AL.: The effects of activity and time of day on the diurnal variations of blood pressure. *J Chron Dis* 1987, 40:671–681.

35. HALBERG F, HALBERG E, HALBERG J, HALBERG F: Chronobiologic assessment of human blood pressure variation in health and disease. In *Ambulatory Blood Pressure Monitoring* edited by Weber MA, Drayer JIM. Darmstadt: Steinkopff, 1984, pp 137–156.

36. LITTLER WA, WATSON RDS: Circadian variation in blood pressure. *Lancet* 1978, i:995–996.

37. FLORAS JS, JONES JV, JOHNSTON JA, BROOKS DE, HASSAN MO, SLEIGHT P: Arousal and the circadian rhythm of blood pressure. *Clin Sci Mol Med* 1978, 55 (suppl) :395S–397S.

38. DAVIES AB, GOULD BA, CASHMAN PMM, RAFTERY EB: Circadian rhythm of blood pressure in patients dependent on ventricular demand pacemakers. *Br Heart J* 1984, 52:93–98.

39. MANCIA G, FERRARI A, GREGORINI L, ET AL.: Blood pressure and heart rate variability in normotensive and hypertensive human beings. *Circ Res* 1983, 53:96–104.

40. MANN S, MILLAR-CRAIG MW, MELVILLE DI, BALASUBRAMANIAN V, RAFTERY EB: Physical activity and the circadian rhythm of blood pressure. *Clin Sci* 1979, 57 (suppl) :291S–294S.

41. SUNDBERG S, KOHVAKKA A, GORDIN A: Rapid reversal of circadian blood pressure rhythm in shift workers. *J Hypertens* 1988, 6:393–396.

42. BAUMGART P, WALGER P, FUCHS G, DORST KG, VETTER H, RAHM KH: Twenty-four hour blood pressure is not dependent on endogenous circadian rhythm. *J Hypertens* 1989, 7:331–334.

43. CHAU HP, MALLION JP, DE GAUDEMARIS R, ET AL.: Twenty-four hour ambulatory blood pressure in shift workers. *Circulation* 1989, 80:341–347.

44. LEWIS PR, LOBBAN MC: Dissociation of diurnal rhythms in human subjects on abnormal time routines. *J Exp Physiol* 1957, 42:371–386.

45. KLEITMAN N, KLEITMAN E: Effect of non-24-hour routine living on oral temperature and heart rate. *J Appl Physiol* 1953, 6:283–291.

46. MILLS JN, STANBURY SW: Persistent 24-hr renal excretory rhythm on a 12-hr cycle of activity. *J Physiol* 1952, 117:22–37.

47. PORTALUPPI F, MONTANARI L, CAPANNA M, FERLINI M: Chronobiologic vs. sphygmomanometric assessment of hypertension in a hospital setting. *Clin Cardiol* 1989, 12:380–383.

48. BOUSQUET F, CHAU NP, PONCELET P, WAREMBOURG A, CARRE A: Essai de classification typologique du profil de pression sur 24 heures chez le sujet agé par analyze de Fourier. *Arch Mal Coeur* 1988, 81 (suppl H7A):255–259.

49. ASERINSKY E, KLEITMAN N: Regularly occurring periods of eye motility, and concomitant phenomena, during sleep. *Science* 1953, 118:273–274.

50. SHIMADA SG, MARSH DJ: Oscillations in mean arterial pressure in conscious dogs. *Circ Res* 1979, 44:692–700.

51. LIVNAT A, ZEHR JE, BROTEN TP: Ultradian oscillations in blood pressure and heart rate in free-running dogs. *Am J Physiol* 1984, 246:R817–R824.

52. PICKERING TG, HARSHFIELD GA, KLEINERT HD, BLANK S, LARAGH JH: Blood pressure during normal daily activities, sleep, and exercise. Comparison of values in normal and hypertensive subjects. *JAMA* 1982, 247:992–996.

53. MESSERLI FH, GLADE LB, VENTURA HO, ET AL.: Diurnal variations of cardiac rhythm, arterial pressure, and urinary catecholamines in borderline and established essential hypertension. *Am Heart J* 1982, 104:109–113.

54. RAFTERY EB: Understanding hypertension. The contribution of direct ambulatory blood pressure monitoring. In *Ambulatory Blood Pressure Monitoring* edited by Weber MA, Drayer JIM. Darmstadt: Steinkopff, 1984, pp 105–116.

55. VERDECCHIA P, SCHILLACA G, GUERRERI M, ET AL.: Circadian blood pressure changes and left ventricular hypertrophy in essential hypertension. *Circulation* 1990, 81:528–536.

56. SOWERS JR: Dopaminergic control of circadian norepinephrine levels in patients with essential hypertension. *J Clin Endocrinol Metab* 1981, 53:1133–1137.

57. MASLOWSKI AH, NICHOLLS MG, ESPINER EA, IKRAM H, BONES PJ: Mechanisms in human renovascular hypertension. *Hypertension* 1983, 5:597–602.

58. DYER AR, STAMLER R, GRIMM R, ET AL.: Do hypertensive patients have a different diurnal pattern of electrolyte excretion? *Hypertension* 1987, 10:417–424.

59. WALLER PL, BHOPAL RS: Is snoring a cause of cardiovascular disease? An epidemiological review. *Lancet* 1989, i:143–146.

60. LUGARESI E, CIRIGNOTTA F, COCCAGNA G, PIANA C: Some epidemiological data on snoring and cardiocirculatory disturbance. *Sleep* 1980, 3:221–224.

61. MONDINI S, ZUCCONI M, CIRIGNOTTA F, ET AL.: Snoring as a risk factor for cardiac and circulatory problems: an epidemiolgocal study. In *Sleep/Wake Disorders: Natural History, Epidemiology, and Long-term Evolution* edited by Guilleminault C, Lugaresi E. New York: Raven Press, 1983, pp 99–105.

62. KOSHENVUO M, KAPRIO J, TEHKIVI T, PARTINEN M, HEIKKILA K, SARMA S: Snoring as a risk factor for ischaemic heart disease and stroke in man. *Br Med J* 1987, 294:160–169.

63. GISLASON T, ABERG H, TAUBE A: Snoring and systemic hypertension — an epidemiological study. *Acta Med Scand* 1987, 221:415–421.

64. ERKINJUNTTI T, SULKAVA R, PALOMAKI H, TILVIS R: Snoring and dementia. *Age Ageing* 1987, 16:305–310.

65. PARTINEN M, PALOMAKI H: Snoring and cerebral infarction. *Lancet* 1985, ii:1325–1326.

66. KOSKENVUO M, KAPRIO J, PARTINEN M, LANGINVAINIO H, SARNA S, HEIKKILA K: Snoring as a risk factor for hypertension and angina pectoris. *Lancet* 1985, ii:893–896.

67. NORTON DG, DUNN EV: Snoring as a risk factor for disease: an epidemiological survey. *Br Med J* 1985, 291:630–632.

68. HOFFENSTEIN V, RUBINSTEIN I, MATEIKA S, SLUTSKY AS: Determinants of blood pressure in snorers. *Lancet* 1988, ii:992–994.

69. STRADLING J, APPS M, CALVERLY P, CHADWICK G, MCNICHOLAS W: Adequacy of oximetry-alone studies for the diagnosis of sleep and breathing disorders. *J Amb Mon* 1989, 2:197–201.

70. IVES JR: Ambulatory EEG monitoring: current state of the art of event type recorders and their future applications. *J Amb Mon* 1989, 1:183–189.

71. ANCOLI-ISRAEL S: The use of a modified Respitrace-Medilog portable system in the evaluation of sleep apnea. *J Amb Mon* 1988, 1:267–278.

72. HIRSHKOWITZ M, KARACAN I, GURAKAR A, WILLIAMS RL: Hypertension, erectile dysfunction, and occult sleep apnea. *Sleep* 1989, 12:223–232.

73. BLOCK AJ, BOYSEN PG, WYNNE JW, HUNT LA: Sleep apnea, hypopnea and oxygen desaturation in normal subjects. *N Engl J Med* 1979, 300:513–517.

74. BLOCK AJ, WYNNE JW, BOYSEN PG: Sleep-disordered breathing and nocturnal oxygen desaturation in postmenopausal women. *Am J Med* 1980, 69:75–79.

75. GUILLEMINAULT C, DEMENT WC: Sleep apnea syndrome and related sleep disorders. In *Sleep Disorders: Diagnosis and Treatment* edited by Williams RL, Karacan I. New York: Wiley, 1978, pp 9–28.

76. BURACK B, POLLACK C, BORAWIECKI B: The hypersommia-sleep apnea syndrome (HSA): a reversible major cardiovascular hazard. *Circulation* 1977, 56 (suppl III):177.

77. GUILLEMINAULT C, SIMMONS FB, MOTTA J: Obstructive sleep apnea syndrome and tracheostomy: long-term follow-up experience. *Arch Intern Med* 1981, 141:985–988.

78. GUILLEMINAULT C, TILKIAN A, DEMENT W: The sleep apnea syndromes. *Annu Rev Med* 1976, 27:465–484.

79. KALES A, BIXLER EO, CADIEUX RJ, ET AL.: Sleep apnea in a hypertensive population. *Lancet* 1984, ii:1005–1008.

80. LAVIE P, BEN-YOSEF R, RUBIN A-H: Prevalence of sleep apnea syndrome among patients with essential hypertension. *Am Heart J* 1984, 108:373–376.

81. MCGINTY D, BEAHM E, STERN N, LITTNER M, SOWERS J, REIGE W: Nocturnal hypotension in older men with sleep-related breathing disorders. *Chest* 1988, 94:305–311.

82. JENNON P, WILDSCHIODTZ G, CHRISTENSEN NJ, SCHWARTZ T: Blood pressure, catecholamines, and pancreatic polypeptide in obstructive sleep apnea with and without nasal continuous positive airway pressure (CPAP) treatment. *Am J Hypertens* 1989, 2:847–852.

83. TILKIAN AG, GUILLEMINAULT C, SCHROEDER JS, LEHRMAN KL, SIMMONS FB, DEMENT WC: Hemodynamics in sleep-induced apnea studies during wakefulness and sleep. *Ann Intern Med* 1976, 85:714–719.

84. HEDNER J, EJNELL H, SELLGREN J, HEDNER J, WALLIN G: Is high and fluctuating muscle sympathetic nerve activity in the sleep apnoea syndrome of pathogenetic importance for the development of hypertension? *J Hypertens* 1988, 6 (suppl 4):529–531.

85. CLARK RW, BOUDOULAS H, SCHAAL SF, SCHMIDT HS: Adrenergic hyperreactivity and cardiac abnormality in primary disorders of sleep. *Neurology* 1980, 30:113–119.

86. FLETCHER EC, MILLAR J, SCHAAF JW, FLETCHER JG: Urinary catecholamines before and after tracheostomy in obstructive sleep apnea in hypertension. *Sleep* 1987, 10:35–44.

87. KRIEGER J, IMBS J-L, SCHMIDT M, KURTZ D: Renal function in patients with obstructive sleep apnea — effects of nasal continuous positive airway pressure. *Arch Intern Med* 1988, 148:1337–1340.

88. WARLEY ARH, STRADLING JR: Abnormal diurnal variation in salt and water excretion in patients with obstructive sleep apnea. *Clin Sci* 1988, 74:183–185.

89. KRIEGER J, LAKS L, WILCOX I, ET AL.: Atrial natriuretic peptide release during sleep in patients with obstructive sleep apnea before and during treatment with nasal continuous positive airway pressure. *Clin Sci* 1989, 77:407–411.

90. O'BRIEN E, SHERIDAN J, O'MALLEY K: Dippers and non-dippers (letter). *Lancet* 1988, ii:397.

91. PICKERING TG: The clinical significance of diurnal blood pressure variations: dippers and nondippers. *Circulation* 1990, 81:700–702.

92. SHAW DB, KNAPP MS, DAVIES DH: Variations in blood pressure in hypertensives during sleep. *Lancet* 1963, i:797–798.

93. HANY S, BAUMGART P, FRIELINGSDORF J, VETTER H, VETTER W: Circadian blood pressure variability in secondary and essential hypertension. *J Hypertens* 1987, 5 (suppl 5):487–489.

94. GOSSE P, JULLIEN E, REYNAUD P, DALLOCCHIO M: Variations circadiennes de la tension artérielle. Importance de la sévérité et non de la cause de l'hypertension artérielle. *Arch Mal Coeur* 1988, 81 (suppl HTA):247–250.

95. REEVES RA, JOHNSON AM, SHAPIRO AP, TRAUB YM, JACOB R: Ambulatory blood pressure monitoring: methods to assess severity of hypertension, variability and sleep changes. In *Ambulatory Blood Pressure Monitoring* edited by Weber MA, Drayer JIM. Darmstadt: Steinkopff, 1984, pp 27–34.

96. BAUMGART P, WALGER P, GEMEN S, VON EIFF M, RAIDT H, RAHN KH: Blood pressure elevation during the night in chronic renal failure, hemodialysis and after renal transplantation. *Nephron* (in press).

97. PICKERING TG, GRIBBIN B, OLIVER DO: Baroreflex sensitivity in patients on long-term haemodialysis. *Clin Sci* 1972, 43:645–657.

98. IMAI Y, ABE K, MIURA Y, ET AL.: Hypertensive episodes and circadian fluctuations of blood pressure in patients with phaeochromocytoma: studies by long-term blood pressure monitoring based on a volume-oscillometric method. *J Hypertens* 1988, 6:9–15.

99. LITTLER WA, HONOUR AJ: Direct arterial pressure, heart rate, and electrocardiogram in unrestricted patients before and after removal of a phaeochromocytoma. *Quart J Med* 1979, 43:441–449.

100. GANGULY A, HENRY DP, YUNE HY, ET AL.: Diagnosis and localization of urinary norepinephrine excretion during sleep, plasma norepinephrine concentration and computerized axial tomography (CT scan). *Am J Med* 1979, 67:21–26.

101. MATSUGUCHI H, TSUNEOYSHI M, TAKESHITA A, NAKAMURA M, KATO T, ARAWKA A: Noradrenaline secreting glomus jugulare tumor with cyclic changes of blood pressure. *Arch Intern Med* 1975, 135:1110–1113.

102. GANGULY A, GRIM CE, WEINBERGER MH, HENRY DP: Rapid cyclic fluctuations of blood pressure associated with an adrenal pheochromocytoma. *Hypertension* 1984, 6:281–284.

103. SELIGMAN SA: Diurnal blood pressure variation in pregnancy. *Obstet Gynecol* 1971, 79:417–422.

104. WERKO L, BRODY S: The blood-pressure in toxaemia of pregnancy. Spontaneous diurnal variability. *J Obst Gynaecol Br Comm* 1953, 60:180–185.

105. REDMAN CWG, BEILIN LJ, BONNAR J: Reversed diurnal blood pressure rhythm in hypertensive pregnancies. *Clin Sci Mol Med* 1976, 51:687S–689S.

106. MURNAGHAN GA: Hypertension in pregnancy. *Postgrad Med J* 1976, 52 (suppl 7):123–126.

107. MURNAGHAN GA, MITCHELL RH, RUFF S: Circadian variation of blood pressure in pregnancy. In *Pregnancy Hypertension* edited by Bonnar HJ, MacGillivray J, Symonds M. Proceedings of the First Congress of the International Society for the Study of Hypertension in Pregnancy. MTP Press, 1978, pp 107–112.

108. RUFF SC, MITCHELL RH, MURNAGHAN GA: Long term variations of blood pressure in normotensive pregnancy and pre-eclampsia. In *Pregnancy Hypertension* edited by Sammour M, Symonds M, Zuspan F, El-Tomi N. Proceedings of the Second Congress of the International Society for the Study of Hypertension in Pregnancy. Ain Shams University Press, 1981, pp 129–143.

109. BEILIN LJ, DEACON J, MICHAEL CA, ET AL.: Diurnal rhythms of blood pressure, plasma renin activity, angiotensin II and catecholamines in normotensive and hypertensive pregnancies. *Clin Exp Hypertens* [B] 1983, 2:271–293.

110. MIYAMOTO S, SHIMOKAWA H, SAKAI K, MATSUMOTO N, NAKANO H: A possible explanation for nocturnal hypertension in preeclamptics. *Clin Exp Hypertens* [B] 1989, 8:495–506.

111. MUNAKATA M, IMAI Y, ABE K, ET AL.: Involvement of the hypothalamo-pituitary-adrenal axis in the control of circadian blood pressure rhythm. *J Hypertens* 1988, 6 (suppl 4):44-46.

112. IMAI Y, ABE K, SASAKI S, ET AL.: Exogenous glucocorticoid eliminates or reverses circadian blood pressure variations. *J Hypertens* 1989, 7:113–120.

113. HAMET P: Endocrine hypertension: Cushing's syndrome, acromegaly, hyperparathyroidism, thyrotoxicosis, and hypothyroidism. In *Hypertension* edited by Genest J, Kuchel O, Hamet P, Cantin M. New York: McGraw-Hill, 1983, pp 964–976.

114. KALSNER S: Mechanism of hydrocortisone potentiation of responses to epinephrine and norepinephrine in rabbit aorta. *Circ Res* 1969, 24:383–395.

115. MANN S, ALTMAN DG, RAFTERY EB, BANNISTER R: Circadian variation of blood pressure in autonomic failure. *Circulation* 1983, 68:477–483.

116. MARTINELLI P, COCCAGNA G, RIZZUTO N, LUGARESI E: Changes in systemic arterial pressure during sleep in Shy-Drager syndrome. *Sleep* 1981, 4:139–146.

117. REEVES RA, SHAPIRO AP, THOMPSON ME, JOHNSEN AM: Loss of nocturnal decline in blood pressure after cardiac transplantation. *Circulation* 1986, 73:401–408.

118. BELL GM, REID W, EWING DJ, ET AL: Abnormal diurnal urinary sodium and water excretion in diabetic autonomic neuropathy. *Clin Sci* 1987, 73:259–265.

119. CARUANA M, LAHIRI A, CASHMAN PMM, ALTMAN DG, RAFTERY EB: Effects of chronic congestive heart failure secondary to coronary artery disease on the circadian rhythm of blood pressure and heart rate. *Am J Cardiol,* 1988, 62:755–759.

120. WENTING GJ, MEIRACKER AH, SIMONS ML, ET AL: Circadian variation of heart rate but not of blood pressure after heart transplantation. *Transplant Proc* 1987, 19:2554–2555.

121. SEHESTED J, MEYER-SABELLEK W, HETZER R: Reversed circadian variation of blood pressure in heart transplant patients? In *Blood Pressure Measurements* edited by Meyer-Sabellek W, Antauf M, Gotzen R, Steinfeld L. Darmstadt: Steinkopff, 1990, pp 211–216.

122. BRENNAN PJ, GREENBERG G, MIALL WE, THOMPSON SG: Seasonal variations in arterial blood pressure. *Br Med J* 1982, 285:919–923.

123. KHAW K-T, BARRETT-CONNOR E, SUAREZ L: Seasonal and secular variation in blood pressure in man. *J Cardiac Rehabil* 1984, 4:440–444.

124. JENNER DA, ENGLISH DR, VANDONGEN R, BEILIN LJ, ARMSTRONG BK, DUNBAR D: Environmental temperature and blood pressure in 9-year old Australian children. *J Hypertens* 1987, 5:683–686.

125. HELLER RF, ROSE G, TUNSTALL PEDOE HD, CHRISTIE GS: Blood pressure measurement in the United Kingdom Heart Disease Prevention Project. *J Epidemiol Commun Health* 1978, 32:235–238.

126. HATA T, OGIHARA T, MARUYAMA A, ET AL: The seasonal variation of blood pressure in patients with essential hypertension. *Clin Exp Hypertens* [A] 1982, 4:341–354.

127. GIACONI S, PALOMBO C, GENOVESI-EBERT A, MARABOTTI C, VOLTERVANI D, GHIONE S: Long-term reproducibility and evaluation of seasonal influences on blood pressure monitoring. *J Hypertens* 1988, 6 (suppl 4):64–66.

128. JAMES GD, YEE LS, PICKERING TG: Seasonal differences in daily blood pressure variation. *Soc Sci Med* (in press).

6 Diurnal variations in cardiovascular morbidity

The importance of diurnal variations in cardiovascular variables such as blood pressure is underlined by the finding of a pronounced diurnal variation in morbid events, for both coronary and cerebrovascular disease. There is generally a relative lack of morbid events occurring during the night, and a relative excess during the day. In this chapter the circadian distribution of cardiovascular events will be reviewed, together with some possible underlying mechanisms.

Myocardial infarction

In 1963 Pell and d'Alonzo examined the diurnal distribution of myocardial infarcts in 1331 employed men [1]. Only 12% of attacks occurred during sleep, while 23% occurred at work. The fatality rate was highest during the night (38%), and lowest (22%) between 9.00 a.m. and 12 noon. It was suggested that this was because of the greater availability of prompt medical care during the day. Tunstall Pedoe et al. [2] found that as many infarcts occurred between 8.00 a.m. and 8.00 p.m. as between 8.00 p.m. and 8.00 a.m., but that there was a relative deficit of attacks in the early morning hours, and a peak at the time of getting up and going to work. Similar findings were reported by Johansson [3], and also by Muller et al. for 703 patients [4] in the Multicenter Investigation of Limitation of Infarct Size (MILIS) trial, in whom the onset of the infarction was estimated from the plasma creatine kinase curves. This method of estimating the time at which the infarction began avoids the possible bias of failure to report the onset of pain during sleep. The incidence of infarctions was 1.26 times higher between the hours of 6.00 a.m. and 12 noon than at other times, and was lowest between 6.00 p.m. and 6.00 a.m. (Fig. 6.1). Muller et al. [4] reported a similar trend in 703 cases of non-fatal myocardial infarction. A number of studies have indicated that there may be a secondary peak in the evening at around 7.00 p.m. [1–3].

Hjalmarson et al. [5] analysed the largest series of all — 4796 patients — and were able to identify subgroups of patients in whom the peak incidence of infarctions was modified or absent. For the whole group there was a peak at around 9.00 a.m., and a secondary peak at around 8.00 p.m. They divided the 24-hour period into four quarters (12 midnight – 6.00 a.m., 6.00 a.m. – 12 noon; 12 noon – 6.00 p.m., and 6.00 p.m. – 12 midnight). Subgroup analyses revealed some interesting, although modest, differences. Women had a higher incidence of infarctions than men during the 6.00 p.m. – 12 midnight period (26.7 versus 24.6%), perhaps reflecting their greater level of activity at night. Smokers also had a more pronounced evening peak than non-smokers. The most pronounced evening peak was seen in patients with a history of congestive heart failure, perhaps reflecting their abnormal blood pressure rhythm (see Chapter 5). The evening peak was also prominent in diabetics, possibly for the same reason.

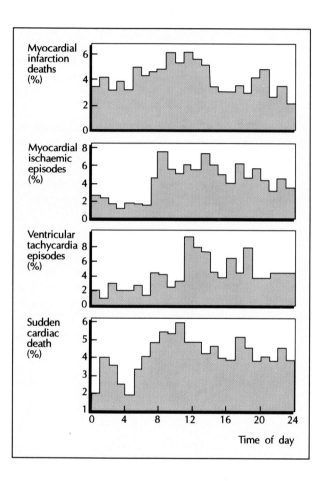

Fig. 6.1. The diurnal variation in cardiac morbid events plotted as consecutive hourly percentages throughout the day and night. In absence of a diurnal rhythm approximately 4% per hour would be expected. Data for myocardial infarction are from Muller et al. [4], for mycoardial ischaemic episodes (ST/ECG changes) from Mulcahy et al. [29], for ventricular tachycardia from Lucente et al. [50], and for sudden cardiac death from Muller et al. [21].

Non-Q-wave myocardial infarction

In marked contrast to the studies reviewed above, the Diltiazem Reinfarction study reported no significant diurnal variation in the onset of non-Q-wave myocardial infarction in a series of 540 patients, in all of whom the diagnosis was verified by cardiac enzyme changes [6], as shown in Fig. 6.2. Subgroup analysis showed a tendency for women and diabetics to have their infarcts in the afternoon. This difference with Q-wave (transmural) myocardial infarction is of interest because the pathophysiology is also different: after a Q-wave infarct there is usually a complete occlusion of the infarct-related artery, whereas this is much less common after a non-Q-wave infarct [7].

Factors contributing to the diurnal rhythm

A number of factors could contribute to the diurnal rhythm of myocardial infarction. The morning hours represent a time of peak physical and mental activity, when many people are at work. Data from the MILIS study [4] indicate that drinking coffee or smoking cigarettes are unlikely to be major factors, because the diurnal rhythm was still observed in those who did neither of these. The level of physical activity at the time of onset does not appear to be able to account for the diurnal rhythm [8].

The diurnal pattern of infarctions corresponds to the pattern of several other cardiovascular variables such as blood pressure, heart rate, and plasma catecholamines [9]. However, diurnal variations in some components of the clotting system are perhaps of greater relevance to the thrombotic process. Platelet aggregability to either adenosine diphosphate (ADP) or adrenaline shows a peak during the morning hours [10,11]. This increased aggregability occurs as a consequence of the increased physical activity on getting up in the morning, because in subjects who stay in bed until 12 noon, it is delayed until the time that they get up [10,11]. Other activities such as public speaking [12], smoking [13], and exercise [14], which are also associated with an increased

sympathetic activity, also increase platelet aggregability. Of the various stimuli which could increase platelet aggregability, the most important one producing the morning rise appears to be assumption of the upright posture [11].

The fibrinolytic activity of plasma has also been found to show a diurnal rhythm, with the lowest activity occurring in the early morning hours [15]. Two major components of the fibrinolytic system, tissue-type plasminogen activator (t-PA) and its fast-acting inhibitor (PAI), show opposite rhythms [16]. The activity of t-PA is greatest during the day (265% of the 24-hour average level), and barely detectable at night (1% of the average). In comparison the activity of PAI is greatest during the night (201% of the 24-hour average), and lower during the day (55% of the average level). This antifibrinolytic activity in the early morning hours might also contribute to the higher incidence of thrombotic cardiovascular events. Similar changes have been reported in patients with CHD [17]. The diurnal variations of some other blood clotting indices have also been investigated. In patients with stable angina, fibrinopeptide A (a product of fibrinogen cleavage by thrombin), beta-thromboglobulin and platelet factor IV (both indices of platelet activation), do not show a significant circadian rhythm [18].

Effects of beta blockade

The morning peak of myocardial infarctions is not seen, or is dampened, in populations of patients studied while receiving beta-blocking agents, suggesting a major pathogenic role for the sympathetic nervous system [19,20]. In the study by Hjalmarson *et al.* [5] the morning

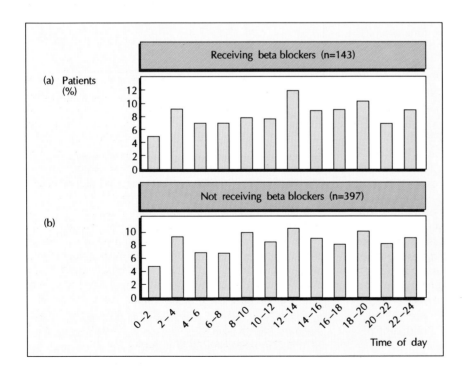

Fig. 6.2. Absence of a diurnal rhythm in the onset of non-Q-wave myocardial infarction in patients (a) receiving beta blockers or (b) not receiving beta blockers. Reproduced with permission [6].

peak was diminished by beta blockers, and the evening peak was enhanced.

Sudden cardiac death

Myers and Dewar [8] analysed the circumstances of death in 100 men who died suddenly and unexpectedly from CHD. Significantly fewer deaths occurred during the night between 2.00 a.m. and 6.00 a.m. than at other times, and the peak incidence was between 6.00 p.m. and 10.00 p.m. In a much larger series of 2203 cases Muller et al. [21] found a statistically significant diurnal rhythm, with a peak between 10.00 a.m. and 11.00 a.m. and a trough between 1.00 a.m. and 6.00 a.m. (Fig. 6.1).

The circadian variation in the incidence of sudden cardiac death was also observed in the Framingham Study by Willich et al. [22]. In 429 individuals the peak incidence was between 7.00 a.m. and 9.00 a.m., the lowest incidence occurring during the night. These authors also attempted to determine whether the diurnal variation in sudden death was merely a reflection of the known periodicity of myocardial infarction. On this basis, and assuming that one-third of sudden cardiac deaths are due to myocardial infarction [23], they estimated that primary sudden cardiac death (i.e. not due to infarction) also had a circadian periodicity, with a peak incidence between 6.00 a.m. and 12 noon.

In the study of Muller et al. [21] there was no detectable diurnal rhythm for deaths occurring in hospital. This finding would be consistent with a role for physical activity or sympathetic arousal, since these patients were presumably in bed during the day. Further support for the importance of sympathetic arousal has been provided by a recent analysis of the Beta-Blocker Heart Attack Trial (BHAT), in which the morning increase in sudden cardiac death was observed in the placebo-treated group, but not in the group treated with propranolol [24].

There are two main theories concerning the aetiology of sudden cardiac death. First, it has been suggested that it may be caused by sudden fissuring of an atheromatous plaque causing coronary artery occlusion [25], and, second, that it may be a primary arrhythmic event [26]. It seems likely that both occur, and both types could be related to increased levels of autonomic and physical activity. The reported prevalence of these two types varies quite widely from one publication to another, and a recent analysis by Davies et al. [27] suggested that this may depend on the population studied. In their autopsy series of 168 patients who died suddenly, 73% had a recent coronary thrombosis. A thrombosis was more likely to be the cause of death in patients with single-vessel disease or a history of chest pain preceding their demise; a primary arrhythmic event (inferred from the absence of an acute lesion) was more likely in patients with three-vessel disease or an old infarct.

Angina

In patients with symptomatic stable angina and coronary artery disease the incidence of episodes is greatest during the day, and falls off in the late afternoon and evening [28,29]. Few attacks occur during the night. This distribution corresponds to a true circadian periodicity, and parallels the diurnal changes in heart rate [28].

The diurnal rhythm of angina may be partly attributable to the greater level of physical activity during the day, but other factors may also contribute. Yasue et al. [30] found that attacks of symptomatic angina and ST segment depression occurring during exercise testing can be induced at a lower threshold in the morning than in the afternoon [30]; others, however, have not found any such difference [31]. Joy et al. [32] exercised patients with stable angina at three times of the day (8.00 a.m., 12 noon and 4.00 p.m.) and found greater heart rates and ST changes for the same level of exercise in the afternoon than in the morning. Similar changes were seen in patients on propranolol [32].

Variant angina

In some patients angina may occur as a result of coronary vasospasm (Prinzmetal angina) in the absence of fixed coronary artery disease. Some authors have reported a diurnal rhythm of episodes in such patients [33–35], whereas others have not [36]. As shown in Fig. 6.3, this rhythm may be very different from classic angina, because there is an increased incidence which precedes waking. Yasue et al. [37] have proposed that coronary artery tone may be increased in the morning hours, on the grounds that major coronary arteries show greater dilatation in response to nitroglycerine in the morning than in the afternoon.

Nocturnal angina

Although angina is more common during the day, in some patients it may occur during the night. However, there is disagreement about whether such episodes are more likely to occur during REM sleep than at other times [38–41]. Quyyumi et al. [42] have described two haemodynamic patterns. In patients with variant angina, who do not have significant coronary artery stenosis, and in whom the pain is provoked by coronary artery spasm rather than by an atheromatous stenosis, there was no evidence of arousal or increased heart rate preceding the ischaemic episodes. It is therefore most probable that such episodes were due to decreased myocardial oxygen supply occurring as a result of spasm. In patients with severe obstructive coronary artery disease the ST segment changes are usually preceded by bodily movement, arousal, and increases in heart rate. Although Quyyumi et al. did not measure blood pressure, it is possible that this also increased, and that the ischaemia was primarily due to increased myocardial oxygen demand.

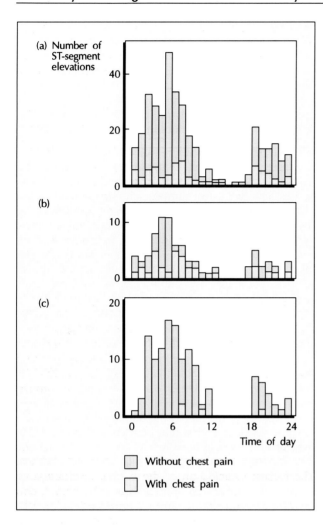

Fig. 6.3. The diurnal rhythm of episodes of silent and symptomatic ischaemia in patients with variant angina. (a) Distribution of all episodes; (b) patients with one to five episodes per day; (c) patients with 31 or more episodes. Reproduced with permission [34].

The opposite view, that reduced coronary flow is the dominant mechanism, has been proposed by Figueras *et al.* [43], on the grounds that the ischaemic threshold during atrial pacing was much higher than during spontaneous nocturnal angina (during the former, heart rate could be increased by 90% before pain occurred, whereas during the latter it occurred with an increase of only 10%). Furthermore, their patients with nocturnal angina also had strongly positive ergonovine tests.

In patients with nocturnal angina there is a pronounced diurnal rhythm of fibrinopeptide A (FPA), which parallels the incidence of anginal episodes (both peaking between 12 midnight and 6.00 a.m.). That this is a consequence, rather than a cause, of the angina was shown by the fact that heparin blocks the changes of FPA without affecting the anginal attacks [18].

Silent myocardial ischaemia

There is growing interest in the phenomenon of silent myocardial ischaemia [characterized by ischaemic ST segment changes on the ECG without symptoms], which occurs much more commonly than symptomatic episodes. As with symptomatic angina, episodes of silent ischaemia occur most commonly between 6.00 a.m. and 12 noon [44,45], as shown in Fig. 6.1. When this distribution is corrected for the time of awakening there is an abrupt increase in episodes on waking [44], as shown in Fig. 6.4. This finding is very similar to the synchronization of the increase in blood pressure with the time of waking shown in Fig. 5.5.

The mechanisms of silent ischaemia are probably somewhat different from those of classic angina, even though the two commonly occur in the same patient. A number of studies have shown that silent ischaemic episodes are not necessarily preceded by any increase in

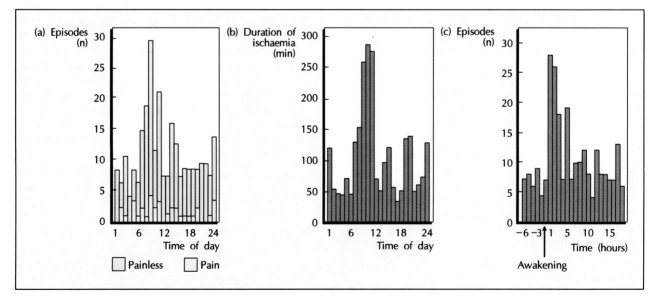

Fig. 6.4. (a) The diurnal rhythm of episodes of silent and symptomatic ischaemia in patients with coronary artery disease; (b) total duration of ischaemic episodes by time of day, and (c) the number of episodes adjusted to the time of waking. Reproduced with permission [44].

heart rate, and also occur at a lower heart rate than exertional angina [28,29,45]. The diurnal distribution of silent ischaemic episodes cannot be wholly explained by changes in physical activity, although this may certainly be a factor [44].

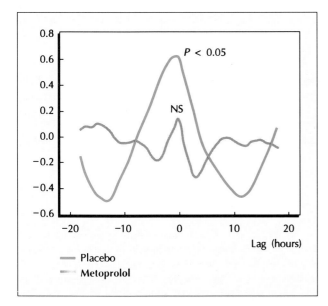

Fig. 6.5. Cross-correlation relationships between heart rate and silent ischaemia (ST/ECG changes) in patients before and after treatment with metoprolol. The y axis shows the degree of correlation between the two variables as a function of lag (i.e. separation in time between the two, measured in hours). The peak at a lag of zero indicates that changes in the two tend to occur simultaneously. Reproduced with permission [48].

Effects of anti-anginal treatment

Evidence that the morning peak of ischaemic episodes is due to increased sympathetic nervous activity is provided by the observation that the diurnal rhythm of such episodes is greatly attenuated by a beta-adrenergic blocker such as atenolol, but not by a calcium antagonist such as nifedipine [46]. The morning peak of silent ischaemia can also be suppressed by metoprolol, which also lowers heart rate and blood pressure, but has no effect on the increase in platelet aggregability [47,48], suggesting that the beneficial effect of metoprolol is due to a reduction in oxygen demand.

Lambert *et al.* [48] used Fourier analysis and cross-correlation techniques to investigate the relationships between heart rate and ischaemic episodes in patients monitored for 72 h, both before and after metoprolol treatment. In the untreated state a marked cross-correlation was observed between the two variables, indicating a tight coupling between them (Fig. 6.5).

Metoprolol both diminished the heart rate variations and the number of ischaemic episodes, and also eliminated the cross-correlation between them (Fig. 6.5). These results suggest that the majority of silent ischaemic episodes can be related to changes in heart rate (or to whatever is producing these changes), and that the residual ischaemia persisting after beta blockade is related to other pathophysiological mechanisms.

The importance of heart rate as a determinant of myocardial ischaemia was demonstrated in a somewhat different way in a study by Quyyumi *et al.* [49] which compared the effects of atenolol and pindolol. The former lowered heart rate to a similar extent during the day and the night, while the latter (by virtue of its intrinsic sympathomimetic activity) lowered heart rate during the day, and produced a slight increase at night. Atenolol produced a similar reduction of ischaemic episodes during the day and night, while pindolol only reduced the daytime episodes.

Arrhythmia

Sudden cardiac death may result from a malignant ventricular arrhythmia, and it is of interest that ventricular tachycardia shows a similar circadian distribution with a peak incidence between 8.00 a.m. and 2.00 p.m. [50,51], as shown in Fig. 6.1.

Stroke

The earliest examination of the diurnal distribution of stroke was carried out by Marshall [52], who found thrombotic strokes to be most common during the night (12 midnight to 6.00 a.m.), but observed no significant diurnal pattern for cerebral haemorrhage. In a second study, Agnoli *et al.* [53] obtained quite different results, finding a peak incidence of non-embolic stroke between 6.00 a.m. and 2.00 p.m. In neither of these studies was computed tomography available to determine whether the strokes were thrombotic or haemorrhagic. More recently, Tzementzis *et al.* [54] examined the question in 557 patients, including 194 with subarachnoid haemorrhage, 118 with intra-cerebral haemorrhage, and 245 with thrombo-embolic stroke. The diagnosis was confirmed in all cases by computed tomography scanning. All three types of stroke had a peak incidence between 10.00 a.m. and 12 noon. With subarachnoid haemorrhage there appears to be a second peak between 6.00 p.m. and 8.00 p.m. (see Fig. 6.6).

Haemorrhagic strokes (both subarachnoid and intra-cerebral) were rare during the night, but this trend was less marked for thrombotic strokes. Subarachnoid haemorrhage was significantly more likely to occur during activities which are likely to cause an acute elevation in blood pressure, such as defaecation, sexual intercourse, and sporting activities. Thrombotic strokes were significantly more likely to occur during quiet activities, such as sitting, reading, or sleeping.

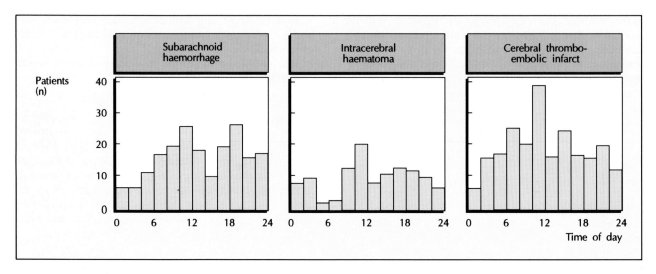

Fig. 6.6. The diurnal variation of cerebrovascular morbid events plotted as consecutive 2-hourly numbers of events throughout the day and night. Reproduced with permission [54].

Increased physical and mental activity as triggers of thrombotic events

While it has not yet been demonstrated conclusively that the diurnal rhythm of thrombotic events is due to the rest–activity cycle rather than to endogenous circadian rhythms, there is strong circumstantial evidence that this is the case. Muller *et al.* [55] have reviewed the mechanisms by which physical and mental activity might act as triggers for the development of acute thrombotic events. While their discussion was directed primarily at coronary thrombosis, it could apply equally well to cerebral thrombosis.

Their arguments can be summarized as follows. It is now established that most myocardial infarctions occur as a consequence of an acute coronary thrombosis developing on an atheromatous plaque [56], which in many cases may have caused a relatively mild stenosis (i.e. less than 60% of the luminal diameter of the artery) before the thrombosis occurred [57]. The acute event that leads to the thrombosis is generally thought to be rupture of the plaque surface, which exposes a thrombogenic focus of collagen to the blood [25]. It is proposed that this will only happen to a plaque that is already 'vulnerable', perhaps as a result of a minor disruption of the endothelium. While such plaque ruptures could occur at random, the diurnal variation of thrombotic events would favour the view that surges in physical or mental activity could trigger them. Some of the potential physiological mechanisms are summarized in Fig. 6.7. The most important mediators are likely to be increases in arterial pressure, coronary artery tone or blood coagulability. The response of normal coronary arteries to many of these stimuli may be to dilate. However, segments diseased with atheromatous plaques show a paradoxical vasoconstriction, due to the loss of endothelium-derived relaxing factor [58]. Thus, it is no longer appropriate to talk of a 'fixed' coronary artery stenosis, because it is becoming increasingly clear that such lesions can behave in a very dynamic way.

Muller *et al.* further suggested that there may be an inverse relationship between the degree of plaque vulnerability and the intensity of the trigger stimulus needed to produce plaque rupture, and that combinations of stimuli might interact, as we saw in Chapter 4 for smoking and caffeine, for example.

The consequences of an acute thrombosis may depend on the severity of the underlying stenosis. It has been suggested recently that sudden cardiac death is more likely to occur if the stenosis was mild enough not to

Possible triggers	Blood pressure	Heart rate	Coronary vascular resistance	Plasma catecholamines	Platelet aggregability	Fibrinolytic activity
Upright posture	−	↑	?	↑	↑	↑
Exercise	↑	↑	↑	↑	↑	↑
Cold exposure	↑	↑	↑	↑	↑	↑
Smoking	↑	↑	↑	↑	↑	↑
Mental stress	↑	↑	↑	↑	↑	↑

Fig. 6.7. Physiological changes produced by possible triggers of coronary thrombosis. Adapted by permission from [55].

induce ischaemia and the formation of collateral circulation [59]. When the stenosis is more severe, ischaemia may initially be silent. Most patients with silent ischaemia develop symptoms of angina before they die or have a myocardial infarction [60]. Acute thrombosis in a more severely stenosed artery may cause unstable angina rather than sudden death, because of the protective effect of the collateral circulation.

The role of blood pressure changes

The relationship of the circadian pattern of cardiovascular morbid events to changes in blood pressure has so far received little attention. None of the non-invasive ambulatory blood pressure monitors currently available in the USA can monitor the ECG and ST segment changes concurrently with blood pressure. The intra-arterial technique is ideally suited to studying patients with myocardial ischaemia, because ischaemic episodes may be fleeting, and the intermittent readings taken by the non-invasive devices may miss the changes. However, this technique has almost exclusively been used by hypertension specialists, who do not appear to be very interested in studying patients with cardiac disease, while the cardiologists who have carried out most of the work described in this chapter seem unenthusiastic about measuring blood pressure.

Systolic pressure is one of the major determinants of myocardial oxygen demand, and its diurnal variations generally parallel the changes in heart rate, the other major determinant. Thus, it is likely that the diurnal rhythm of blood pressure is an important determinant of ischaemic events, as well as of haemorrhagic events, which may be even more closely related to it.

Diastolic pressure is important for maintaining coronary artery flow and myocardial oxygen supply. It is possible that in some patients with nocturnal angina the level of diastolic pressure during sleep may fall below the critical level needed for coronary perfusion, for it has been observed that patients treated with beta blockers may have diastolic pressures as low as 30 or 40 mmHg during the night [61].

It is important to appreciate that there may be a dissociation between the diurnal rhythms of heart rate and blood pressure. In Chapter 5 a number of pathological conditions have been described in which heart rate decreases during the night, but blood pressure remains high. One might speculate that in such patients the 'protective' effect of sleep is diminished.

Summary and conclusions

All the morbid events of sudden onset which can be attributed to the hypertensive process show an unequal distribution throughout the day and night, with the majority of episodes occurring between the hours of 6.00 a.m. and 12 noon, and relatively few during the night. These include thrombotic events (myocardial and cerebral thrombosis), ischaemic events (angina and silent is-

chaemia), haemorrhagic events (subarachnoid and cerebral haemorrhage), arrhythmias (ventricular tachycardia), and sudden cardiac death.

Although the mechanisms precipitating the individual events are of course different, a common link appears to be activation of the sympathetic nervous system accompanying the increased physical and mental activity which occurs on getting up in the morning. Thus, there is a strong link between changes in heart rate and episodes of myocardial ischaemia, and treatment with beta blockers has been shown to abolish the circadian rhythms of myocardial ischaemia and infarction. In the heart, this sympathetic activation leads to increased myocardial oxygen demand, and may result in ischaemia distal to an atheromatous stenosis. Coronary artery vasomotor tone is also affected, however, leading to changes in oxygen supply. Both factors may change at the same time, or separately, and changes in oxygen supply may determine why some patients get angina during the night. There are also diurnal changes in blood clotting factors, such as platelet aggregability and fibrinolytic activity, which may contribute to the triggering of thrombotic events.

References

1. PELL S, D'ALONZO CA: Immediate mortality and five-year survival of employed men with a first myocardial infarction. *N Engl J Med* 1964, 270:915–922.
2. TUNSTALL PEDOE H, CLAYTON D, MORRIS JN, BRIGDEN W, MCDONALD L: Coronary heart attacks in east London. *Lancet* 1975, ii:833–838.
3. JOHANSSON BW: Myocardial infarction in Malmo 1960–1968. *Acta Med Scand* 1972, 191:505–515.
4. MULLER JE, STONE PH, TURI ZG, ET AL: Circadian variation in the onset of acute myocardial infarction. *N Engl J Med* 1985, 313:1315–1322.
5. HJALMARSON A, GILPIN EA, NICOD P, ET AL: Differing circadian patterns of symptom onset in subgroups of patients with acute myocardial infarction. *Circulation* 1989, 80:267–275.
6. KLEIMAN NS, SCHECHTMAN KB, YOUNG PM, ET AL: Lack of diurnal variation in the onset of non-Q wave infarction. *Circulation* 1990, 81:548–555.
7. DE WOOD MA, STIFTER WF, SIMPSON CS, ET AL: Coronary arteriographic findings soon after non-Q wave myocardial infarction. *N Engl J Med* 1986, 315:417–423.
8. MYERS A, DEWAR HA: Circumstances attending sudden deaths from coronary artery disease with coroner's necropsies. *Br Heart J* 1975, 37:1133–1143.
9. TURTON MB, DEEGAN T: Circadian variations of plasma catecholamines, cortisol and immunoreactive insulin concentrations in supine subjects. *Clin Chim Acta* 1974, 55:389–397.
10. TOFLER GH, BREZINSKI D, SCHAFER AI, ET AL: Concurrent morning increase in platelet aggregability and the risk of myocardial infarction and sudden cardiac death. *N Engl J Med* 1987, 316:1514–1518.
11. BREZINSKI DA, TOFLER GH, MULLER JE, ET AL: Morning increase in platelet aggregability associated with assumption of the upright posture. *Circulation* 1988, 78:35–40.
12. LEVINE SP, TOWELL BL, SUAREZ AM, KNIERIEM LK, HARRIS MM, GEORGE JN: Platelet activation and secretion associated with emotional stress. *Circulation* 1985, 71:1129–1134.
13. PITTILO RM, CLARKE JMF, HARRIS D, ET AL: Cigarette smoking and platelet adhesion. *Br J Haematol* 1984, 58:627–632.
14. HARRISON MJG, EMMONS PR, MITCHELL JRA: The variability of human platelet aggregation. *J Atheroscler Res* 1967, 7:197–205.
15. ROSING DR, BRAKMAN P, REDWOOD DR, ET AL: Blood fibrinolytic activity in man: diurnal variation and the response to varying intensities of exercise. *Circ Res* 1970, 27:171–184.
16. ANDREOTTI F, DAVIES GJ, HACKETT DR, ET AL: Major circa-

dian fluctutions in fibrinolytic factors and possible relevance to time of onset of myocardial infarction, sudden cardiac death and stroke. *Am J Cardiol* 1988, 62:635–637.

17. ANGLETON P, CHANDLER WL, SCHMER G : Diurnal variation of tissue-type plasminogen activator and its rapid inhibitor (PAI-1). *Circulation* 1989, 79:101–106.

18. OGAWA H, YASUE H, OSHIMA S, OKUMURA K, MATSUYAMA K, OBATA K : Circadian variation of plasma fibrinopepetide A level in patients with variant angina. *Circulation* 1989, 80:1617–1626.

19. PETERS RW, MULLER JE, GOLDSTEIN S, BYINGTON R, FRIEDMAN LM AND BHAT STUDY GROUP : Propranolol and the circadian variation in the frequency of sudden cardiac death: the BHAT experience. *Circulation* 1988, 76 (suppl IV):364.

20. WILLICH SN, LINDERER T, WEGCHEIDER K, SCHRODER R AND THE ISAM STUDY GROUP : Increased risk of myocardial infarction in the morning (abstract). *J Am Coll Cardiol* 1988, 11:28A.

21. MULLER JE, LUNDER PL, WILLICH SN, ET AL: Circadian variation in the frequency of sudden cardiac death. *Circulation* 1987, 1:131–138.

22. WILLICH SN, LEVY D, ROCCO MB, TOFLER GH, STONE PH, MULLER JE : Circadian variation in the incidence of sudden cardiac death in the Framingham Heart Study population. *Ann J Cardiol* 1987, 60:801–806.

23. HINKLE LE, THALER HT : Clinical classification of cardiac deaths. *Circulation* 1982, 65:457-464.

24. PETERS RW, MULLER JE, GOLDSTEIN S, BYINGTON R, FRIEDMAN LR : Propranolol and the morning increase in the frequency of sudden cardiac death (BHAT Study). *Am J Cardiol* 1989, 63:1518–1520.

25. DAVIES M, THOMAS AC : Plaque fissuring — the cause of acute myocardial infarction, sudden ischaemic death, and crescendo angina. *Br Heart J* 1985, 53:363–373.

26. LOCUM B : Sudden cardiac death: the major challenge confronting contemporary cardiology. *Am J Cardiol* 1979, 43:313–328.

27. DAVIES MJ, BLAND JM, HANGARTNER JRW, ANGELINI A, THOMAS AC : Factors influencing the presence or absence of acute coronary artery thrombi in sudden ischaemic death. *Eur Heart J* 1989, 10:203–208.

28. NADEMANEE K, INTARACHOT V, JOSEPHSON MA, SINGH BN : Circadian variation in occurrence of transient overt and silent myocardial ischaemia in chronic stable angina and comparison with Prinzmetal angina in men. *Am J Cardiol* 1987, 60:494–498.

29. MULCAHY D, KEEGAN J, CREAN P, ET AL: Silent myocardial ischaemia in chronic stable angina: a study of its frequency and characteristics in 150 patients. *Br Heart J* 1988, 60:417–423.

30. YASUE H, OMOTE S, TAKIZAWA A, ET AL: Pathogenesis and treatment of angina pectoris at rest as seen from its response to various drugs. *Jpn Circ J* 1978, 42:1–10.

31. KHUMI NS, RAFTERY EB : Lack of diurnal variation in maximum symptom-limited exercise test response in chronic stable angina. *Am J Cardiol* 1988, 61:38–42.

32. JOY M, POLLARD CM, NUNAN TO : Diurnal variation in exericse responses to angina. *Br Heart J* 1982, 48:156–160.

33. YASUE H, OMOTE S, TAKIZAWA A, NAGAO M, MIWA K, TANAKA S : Circadian variation of exercise capacity in patients with Prinzmetal variant angina: role of exercise-induced coronary arterial spasm. *Circulation* 1979, 59:938–947.

34. WATERS DD, MILLER D, BOUCHARD A, BOSCH X : Circadian variation in variant angina. *Am J Cardiol* 1984, 54:61–64.

35. ARAKI H, KOIWAYA Y, NAKAGAKI O, NAKAMURA M : Diurnal distribution of ST-segment elevation and related arrhythmias in patients with variant angina: a study by ambulatory ECG monitoring. *Circulation* 1983, 67:995–1000.

36. SPECCHIA G, DISERVI S, FALCONE C, ET AL: Significance of exercise-induced ST-segment elevation in patients without myocardial infarction. *Circulation* 1981, 49:46–53.

37. YASUE H, TOUYAMA M, KATO H, TANAKA S, AKIYAMA F : Prinzmetal's variant form of angina as a manifestation of alpha-adrenergic receptor-mediated coronary artery spasm: documentation by coronary arteriography. *Am Heart J* 1976 91:148–155.

38. MURAO S, HARUMI K, KATAYAMA S, MASHIMA S, SHIMONURA K, MURAYAMA M : All-night polygraphic studies of nocturnal angina pectoris. *Jpn Heart J* 1972, 13:295–306.

39. NOWLIN JB, TROYER WG, COLLINS WS, ET AL: The association of nocturnal angina with dreaming. *Ann Intern Med* 1965, 63:1040–1046.

40. CHIERCHIA S, GUAZZELLI M, MAGINI C, MASERI A : Absence of correlation of nocturnal angina with sleep stages. *Circulation* 1978, 58 (suppl II):194.

41. FARACON I, WILLIAMS RL, TAYLOR WJ : Sleep characteristics of patients with angina pectoris. *Psychosomatics* 1969, 10:280–284.

42. QUYYUMI AA, EFTHIMIOV J, QUYYUMI A, MOCKUS LJ, SPIRO SG, FOX KM : Nocturnal angina: precipitating factors in patients with coronary artery disease and those with variant angina. *Br Heart J* 1986, 56:346–352.

43. FIGUERAS J, CORTADELLAS J, BALDA J, CINCA J : Nocturnal angina in patients with fixed coronary stenosis. Increased coronary vasoconstrictive sensitivity with independence of pacing ischaemic threshold. *Eur Heart J* 1989, 10:903–909.

44. ROCCO MB, BARRY J, CAMPBELL S, ET AL: Circadian variation of transient myocardial ischaemia in patients with coronary artery disease. *Circulation* 1987, 75:395–400.

45. CAMPBELL S, BARRY J, REBECCA GS, ET AL: Active transient myocardial ischaemia during daily life in asymptomatic patients with positive exercise tests and coronary artery disease. *Am J Cardiol* 1986, 57:1010–1016.

46. MULCAHY D, KEEGAN J, CUNNINGHAM D, ET AL: Circadian variation of total ischaemic burden and its alteration with antianginal agents. *Lancet* 1988, ii:755–759.

47. WILLICH SN, POHJOLA-SINTONEN S, BHATIA SJS, ET AL: Suppression of silent ischaemia by metoprolol without alteration of morning increase of platelet aggregability in patients with stable coronary artery disease. *Circulation* 1989, 79:557–565.

48. LAMBERT CR, COY K, IMPERI G, PEPINE CJ : Influence of beta-adrenergic blockade by time series analysis on circadian variation of heart rate and ambulatory myocardial ischaemia. *Am J Cardiol* 1989, 64:835–839.

49. QUYYUMI A, WRIGHT C, MOCKUS L, FOX KM : Effect of partial agonist activity in β blockers in severe angina pectoris: a double blind comparison of pindolol and atenolol. *Br Med J* 1984, 289:951–953.

50. LUCENTE M, REBUZZI AG, LANZA GA, ET AL.: Circadian variation of ventricular tachycardia in acute myocardial infarction. *Am J Cardiol* 1988, 62:670–674.

51. TWIDALE N, TAYLOR S, HEDDIE WF, AYRES BF, TONKIN AM : Morning increase in the time of onset of sustained ventricular tachycardia. *Am J Cardiol* 1989, 64:1204–1206.

52. MARSHALL J : Diurnal variation in occurrence of strokes. *Stroke* 1977, 8:230–231.

53. AGNOLI A, MANFREDI M, MOPSSUTO L, PRINCINELLI A : Rapport entre les rhythmes-hemeroncytaux de la tension artérielle et la pathogénie de l'insuffisance cérébrale vasculaire. *Rev Neurol* 1975, 131:597–606.

54. TSEMENTZIS SA, GILL JS, HITCHCOCK ER, GILL SK, BEEVERS DG : Diurnal variation of and activity during the onset of stroke. *Neurosurgery* 1985, 17:901–904.

55. MULLER JE, TOFLER GH, STONE PH : Circadian variation and triggers of onset of acute cardiovascular disease. *Circulation* 1989, 79:733–743.

56. DE WOOD MA, SPRES J, NORSKE R, ET AL: Prevalence of total coronary occlusion during the early hours of transmural myocardial infarction. *N Engl J Med* 1980, 303:897–902.

57. BROWN BG, GALLERY CA, BADGER RS, ET AL: Incomplete lysis of thrombus in the moderate underlying atherosclerotic lesion during intra-coronary infusion of streptokinase for acute myocardial infarction: quantitative angiographic observations. *Circulation* 1986, 73:653–661.

58. LUDMER PL, SELWYN AP, SHOOK TL, ET AL: Paradoxical vasoconstriction induced by acetylcholine in atherosclerotic coronary arteries. *N Engl J Med* 1986, 315:1046–1051.

59. EPSTEIN SE, QUYYUMI AA, BONOW RO : Sudden cardiac death without warning. Possible mechanisms and implications for screening asymptomatic populations. *N Engl J Med* 1989, 321:320–323.

60. ERIKSSEN J : Prognostic importance of silent ischaemia during long-term follow-up of patients with coronary artery disease. *Herz* 1987, 12:359-358.

61. FLORAS JS : Antihypertensive treatment, myocardial infarction, and nocturnal myocardial ischaemia. *Lancet* 1988, ii:994–996.

7 Clinic measurement of blood pressure and white coat hypertension

Measurement of blood pressure in the clinic or physician's office has been the cornerstone on which our understanding of the risks associated with hypertension and the benefits from its treatment is based. For practical reasons, such measurements are made relatively infrequently in any individual patient, so that if clinical decisions are to be made on the basis of them, it must be assumed that they are representative of that individual's true level of pressure. In this chapter we shall examine the validity of this assumption.

There are two aspects of this problem. First, there is the random variability of blood pressure, which will introduce variation in successive measurements; second, and probably more importantly, there may be a systematic distortion of clinic readings due to the peculiar psychological circumstances of the physician's office. This phenomenon results in a spurious elevation in clinic blood pressure, and has been termed white coat hypertension, and also office or cuff hypertension.

Nearly 50 years ago Ayman and Goldshine [1] observed that in 34 cases of hypertension blood pressures recorded by the patients at home were invariably lower than pressures recorded by the physicians at their offices — in some cases by as much as 70/36 mmHg. They further emphasized that these differences were not transient, because they persisted over an average period of observation of 104 weeks of clinic measurements, and 23 weeks of home measurement. Their observations have two major implications.

First, since the differences between the home and clinic pressures cannot be explained on the basis of differences in physical activity, they indicate that psychological factors may be responsible. Second, they raise the possibility that patients who show this response may be misclassified as being hypertensive on the basis of their clinic pressures. Since the clinical practice of diagnosing and treating hypertensive patients has almost exclusively been based on clinic measurements of pressure, it is of both theoretical and practical importance to gain a better understanding of this phenomenon.

The variability of clinic pressures

The variations in blood pressure when measured in the clinic can be surprisingly large. Following their study of the phenomenon (described below) Armitage and Rose [2] wrote:

'The clinician should recognize that the patient whose diastolic pressure has fallen 25 mm from the last oc-

casion has not necessarily changed in health at all; or, if he is receiving hypotensive therapy, that there has not necessarily been any response to treatment.'

It is appropriate to consider the variability as being of three kinds: variations between subjects; variations between successive readings made on the same occasion; and variations between occasions. All three types of variability are likely to be influenced by a number of factors, such as the circumstances of measurement (e.g. clinic or laboratory), the interval between measurements, and the individuals being studied (e.g. randomly selected individuals in a population survey or newly diagnosed hypertensive patients in a clinic). Our review of the subject will focus on four studies. The first was conducted by Armitage and Rose in 10 normotensive subjects in the laboratory where they worked; two readings were taken on 20 occasions over a 6-week period by a single trained observer [2]. The second is an analysis by Armitage et al. [3] of a population study of seven men who had one or two readings taken annually over a 4-year period. The third is the Framingham Heart Study, in which three readings were taken every 2 years on 10 occasions [4], and the fourth is a study by Watson et al. of 32 newly diagnosed hypertensive patients who had two readings taken on 12 occasions [5].

Variation between subjects

Both systolic and diastolic pressure are distributed normally in the population but with a skew or tail at the upper end of the range. Armitage et al. [3] pointed out that some of the variance can be explained by the fact that such population studies are usually based on readings made on a single occasion. In their survey the standard deviation was 20.2 mmHg for systolic pressure and 12.0 mmHg for diastolic pressure when a single set of readings was used. However, if the average of 4 years' readings (one or two per year) was taken the standard deviations were reduced to 17.4 and 10.7 mmHg, respectively. This difference can be attributed to the increased reliability of multiple readings.

Variation between occasions; regression to the mean

In their laboratory study of normotensive individuals Armitage and Rose [2] found highly significant differences in blood pressure measured on different occasions. There was no consistent pattern of change in systolic pressure, which had a standard deviation of 4.7 mmHg, whereas diastolic pressure fell by 12 mmHg between the first and 20th occasion, with a standard de-

Author	Subjects	Interval	Occasions	Reliability	SDD (mmHg)	Reference
Llabre *et al.*	74 (NT)	1–2 days	5	G* 0.73/0.61	5/4	8
	24 (HT)			G* 0.63/0.59	8/5	
Armitage and Rose	10 (NT)	2–3 days	20	–	6/6	2
Watson *et al.*	32 (HT)	1 week	12	–	10/7	5
Marolf *et al.*	31 (HT)	1 week	3	–	11/8	9
James *et al.*	27 (NT & HT)	2 weeks	2	0.94/0.87	10/7	10
Des Combes *et al.*	101 (HT)	3 months	2	0.82/0.79	–	11
Armitage *et al.*	50 (NT)	1 year	4	–	9/7	3
Kannel *et al.*	782 men (NT & HT)	2 years	10	0.67/0.60	12/8	4
	1001 women (NT & HT)	2 years	10	0.79/0.69	13/8	4

NT, normotensive; HT, hypertensive; Interval, interval between visits (occasions); Occasions, number of occasions of measurement; Reliability, correlation coefficient for systolic and diastolic pressure; G*, generalizability coefficient; SDD, standard deviation of the difference between occasions for systolic and diastolic pressure.

Fig. 7.1. Reliability of clinic blood pressure measurements repeated over occasions of varying intervals.

viation of 5.5 mmHg. Not surprisingly, in their population survey they found a greater variance, with a standard deviation of 9.1 mmHg for systolic pressure and 7.1 mmHg for diastolic pressure [3]. The corresponding values for the laboratory study (using only a single reading on each occasion) were 6.3 and 6.2 mmHg, respectively. The Framingham Study [4] found that the blood pressure on one occasion was highly correlated with the pressure on another: for men the correlation between the pressures at entry to the study with the pressures at examination 2 (2 years later) was 0.67 for systolic pressure and 0.60 for diastolic pressure, and with the pressure at examination 10 (18 years later) was 0.47 for systolic pressure and 0.38 for diastolic pressure. Similar correlations were reported for women.

Figure 7.1 summarizes the results of some studies which have addressed the question of the reliability (reproducibility) of clinic pressures, with intervals between occasions ranging from 1 day to 2 years. Two measures of reliability have generally been used: the test–retest correlation (reliability) coefficients, and the SDD. As shown in Fig. 7.1 there is a tendency for the SDD to be somewhat greater in hypertensive individuals than in normotensive individuals, and to increase with longer intervals between successive occasions. These numbers are important for the comparison with the reliability of ambulatory pressures, reviewed in Chapter 9.

In the rather special circumstances of the newly diagnosed, but untreated, hypertensive patient attending a clinic, Watson *et al.* [5] found a significant decrease in both systolic and diastolic pressure over the first three visits (of 5.8 and 4.0 mmHg, respectively), but no consistent change between visits 4 and 12 (Fig. 7.2).

Such 'within-subject' variation may be due to the statistical artefact labelled regression to the mean. If subjects with high blood pressure are selected for a study or treat-

ment on the basis of the initial screening, they will tend to have lower readings on the second occasion. The magnitude of this decrease can be estimated from the known variability of blood pressure, and has been dealt with mathematically by Gardner and Heady [6]. Another factor contributing to the decrease in pressure shown in Fig. 7.2 is the habituation of the orienting and defence responses, which are described in more detail below.

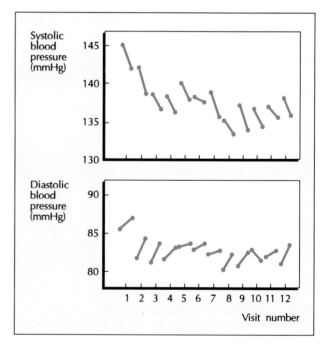

Fig. 7.2. Paired readings of systolic and diastolic pressure taken during 12 consecutive clinic visits. Reproduced with permission [5].

Conversely, subjects initially identified as having low blood pressure will tend to show an increase in pressure over time. The extent of this regression has been estimated [7] using data obtained in the Framingham study over a 4-year period before antihypertensive treatment was widely available, as shown in Fig. 7.3. While regression to the mean can account for a major part of this, at least two other factors are involved. First is the tendency of blood pressure to increase with age, which is just under 1 mmHg per year, and second is the habituation of the orienting response, which will be difficult to disentangle from regression to the mean.

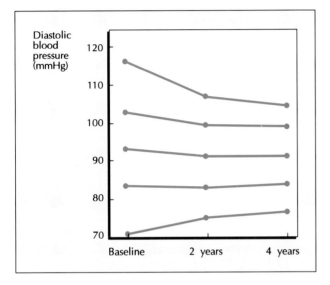

Fig. 7.3. Changes in blood pressure over a 4-year period plotted according to the initial level of blood pressure. Data are from Framingham Study, and published with permission [7].

Two studies incorporating serial measurements of clinic, ambulatory and home pressures [9,10] have shown that this decrease in clinic pressure does not reflect any change in the true pressure. In our own study [10], we observed that clinic pressures decreased in hypertensive patients, but not in normotensive subjects. The ambulatory and home pressures were lower than the clinic pressures, and showed no consistent change over a two-week period. In the second study [9], hypertensive patients were monitored over a period of a week, during which time clinic pressures decreased, but again without any change in home or ambulatory pressures.

Variation between readings

A significant decrease between the first and second readings of systolic pressure was found in the laboratory and survey studies of Armitage *et al.* [2,3], and the hypertension clinic study of Watson *et al.* [5] (by 3, 3.6, and 2 mmHg, respectively). However, either no consistent change or a small increase in diastolic pressure was seen. Armitage and Rose emphasized that the range of differences between the two readings was quite high (about 25 mmHg for both systolic and diastolic pressure). In their survey study the standard deviation of the differ-

ences was 9.5 mmHg for systolic pressure and 7.8 mmHg for diastolic pressure [3]. One of the analyses performed in the Framingham study was to see whether the lability of blood pressure on any one occasion was a repeatable characteristic of individual subjects. It was not: no significant correlations existed between the standard deviations measured on different occasions [4]. However, it was found that the variability of systolic pressure increased with age. In men the standard deviation was 6.7 mmHg at ages 35–39 years and 8.7 mmHg at ages 60–64 years; similar findings were reported for women.

The variation in blood pressure between occasions is consistently greater than the variation between successive readings made on a single occasion [2,3]. Armitage and Rose [2] estimated from their laboratory study how much the variance of measurements could be reduced either by increasing the number of readings per occasion or by increasing the number of occasions. As shown in Fig. 7.4, both procedures help to reduce the variance, but increasing the number of occasions is more effective. Thus, four readings taken on one occasion would give a variance of 91.5/74.0, while one reading taken on four occasions would give a variance of only 74.7/53.3. Similar conclusions were reached by Llabre *et al.* [8], who took three readings with a Dinamap recorder on 5 days. They found greater variance of blood pressure on different days than between readings taken on the same day. Their data indicated that two readings of systolic pressure taken on two different days may be sufficient to generalize across days, whereas two readings taken on three days would be needed for a reliable estimate of diastolic pressure. This type of analysis may be of particular relevance to the comparison of home and ambulatory measurements, because home readings may be equivalent to a few readings made on each of a large number of occasions, while ambulatory recordings would be more akin to a larger number of readings made on one occasion.

Casual and basal blood pressure

In a series of papers published in the 1940s, Smirk introduced the concept of casual and basal blood pressures [12–15]. His idea was that the casual or clinic blood pressure had two independent components: the basal and the supplemental pressures. The basal pressure was measured with the subject seated in a quiet warm room, with multiple readings being taken by a single observer over half an hour. The first set of readings constituted the casual pressure, and the last set the basal pressure. The difference between the two was the supplemental pressure.

In normotensive subjects the basal pressure was typically lower than the casual pressure by about 15/16.5 mmHg (systolic/diastolic pressure), while in patients with essential hypertension a greater difference was observed, of about 36/18.5 mmHg [13]. In neither group was there any significant correlation between the basal and the supplemental pressures [15]. It was proposed that the basal pressure represented the structural or fixed elements of an individual's hypertension, while the supplemental

Number of readings per occasion	Number of occasions	Variance of blood pressure (mmHg)	
		Systolic	Diastolic
1	1	104.9	82.1
2	1	96.0	76.7
4	1	91.5	74.0
∞	1	87.1	71.3
1	2	84.8	62.9
1	4	74.7	53.3
1	∞	64.8	43.7

Fig. 7.4. Effect of the precision of estimate of the blood pressure by increasing the number of readings per occasion and/or the number of occasions. Reproduced with permission [2].

pressure was the elevation attributable to the effects of physical and mental activity.

The relative values of casual and basal blood pressures in the prediction of morbidity in hypertensive patients are reviewed in Chapter 13.

The unreliability of clinic pressures: white coat hypertension

The discrepancy between casual and basal pressure, or between clinic and home blood pressure, presents the clinician with an important question: which measure of pressure is closest to the 'true' level of pressure? For practical purposes, the true pressure may be regarded as the average level over a prolonged period of time, which is generally thought to be the most important determinant of target organ damage. This question can best be answered by recording blood pressure over 24 h, using ambulatory monitoring. In one of the first studies using this technique, published in 1964, Kain *et al.* [16] found that clinic pressures were usually higher than the average daytime pressures, and concluded:

> 'Single casual pressures are apt to reflect temporary rises in pressure resulting from stimuli from the central nervous system due to the presence of the physician, the medical environment, or other personal factors, and therefore may not reliably indicate the net daily 'load', because pressures may be lower at other times'.

Thus, this and many subsequent studies using ambulatory blood pressure recordings confirm the suspicion generated from studies examining the differences between clinic blood pressures and pressures taken by patients at home. That is to say, some aspect of the physician taking the blood pressure in the clinic represents an event of sufficient psychological magnitude to result in physiological alterations which cause spuriously high

blood pressure readings in some individuals. In order to examine these issues, we compared clinic and ambulatory blood pressures in three groups of subjects: normotensive individuals, and patients with either borderline or established hypertension [17,18]. In the normal subjects we found no difference between the average clinic and 24-hour levels, but in both groups of hypertensive patients the clinic pressures were higher. As shown in Fig. 7.5, which is based on data from 66 patients with established hypertension, 578 with borderline hypertension and 58 normotensive subjects, the disparity between the average clinic pressures of the three groups was much greater than between the corresponding ambulatory pressures [18].

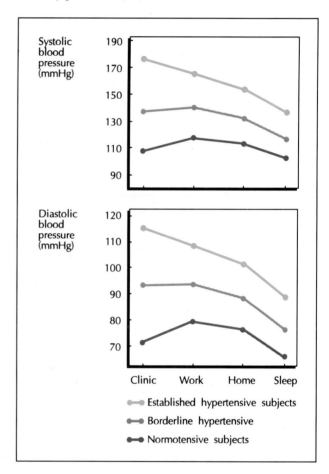

Fig. 7.5. Comparison of clinic and ambulatory (work, home and sleep) pressures in three groups of subjects. Reproduced with permission [18].

We divided the 24-hour period into the three major components of work, home and sleep, and found that pressures tended to be highest at work, intermediate at home and lowest during sleep (Fig. 7.5). The blood pressure at work was generally similar to the pressure in the clinic, but we also found [19] that the correlation between the two was not very close (r = 0.53 for systolic pressure, and r = 0.51 for diastolic pressure). The correlation between clinic and ambulatory pressures was closer for the normotensive subjects than for the hypertensive subjects.

The traditional argument used in defence of clinic pressures is that they represent the patient's response to the stresses of everyday life; we were unable to verify this in our study [20]. Patients with white coat hypertension did not show any greater variability of blood pressure during ambulatory monitoring, nor did their response to stress, as measured by the difference between home and work blood pressures, appear to be any different from patients with sustained hypertension. An extreme example of this phenomenon is shown in Fig. 7.6. This patient, a 64-year-old woman, had persistently elevated clinic pressures for several years, often reaching 180/120 mmHg. Her home pressures, in contrast, had been as low as 120/80 mmHg. Her technique of self-monitoring was shown to be accurate when she took her own pressures in the clinic with her own machine, where she also recorded very high readings. Her ambulatory blood pressures were closer to the home than to the clinic pressures, and echocardiography revealed no evidence of target organ damage.

White coat hypertension appears to be distinct from 'cuff-inflation hypertension', which is described in Chapter 2.

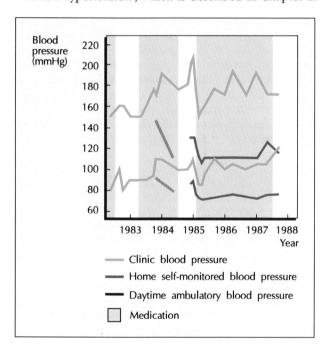

Fig. 7.6. White coat hypertension in a 64-year-old woman.

Definition of white coat hypertension
The broad definition of white coat hypertension is a persistently elevated clinic blood pressure and a normal pressure at other times. Its precise definition is inevitably arbitrary, like any other category of hypertension. It should be emphasized that it cannot be defined on the basis of a single clinic visit: many individuals have a relatively high blood pressure when first seen which, as we have discussed above, decreases with repeated visits. In

our own practice, we have only applied the term to patients diagnosed as being hypertensive before being referred to our Centre whose clinic pressure remained elevated on the second and third visits.

White coat hypertension cannot be diagnosed simply on the basis of clinic and home pressures, because the pressure might be high at work, for example. We have used a cut-off point of 90 mmHg diastolic pressure for the clinic pressures [20], on the grounds that this is the most widely accepted criterion. To establish that the blood pressure is normal outside the clinic requires the use of ambulatory monitoring, and the definition of a cut-off point for the upper limit of the normal range. We chose the 90th percentile of the daytime blood pressure as the upper limit, based on recordings made in 37 normal volunteers: this was 134/90 mmHg. To be classified as white coat hypertensive individuals, our patients had to have both systolic and diastolic ambulatory pressures below these levels.

Prevalence of white coat hypertension
We also attempted to determine the prevalence of white coat hypertension [20]. By the criteria described above, 21% of patients with borderline hypertension (clinic diastolic pressures between 90 and 104 mmHg) had both systolic and diastolic pressures which were below this level during the ambulatory recording. These patients were thus defined as having white coat hypertension. In patients with more advanced hypertension (clinic diastolic pressure above 105 mmHg), we found a much lower prevalence of white coat hypertension (of 5%). The actual levels of pressure recorded in the three groups of subjects are shown in Fig. 7.7.

Similar findings have been reported by other workers. Krakoff *et al.* [21] monitored 60 patients with mild hypertension, all of whom had been advised to take antihypertensive medication on the basis of their clinic pressures. Their average clinic pressure was 155/100 mmHg, while the average ambulatory pressure was 131/82 mmHg; 38% had ambulatory pressures below 130/85 mmHg. Using somewhat different criteria (clinic systolic or diastolic pressure at least 10 mmHg higher than daytime ambulatory pressures), Lerman *et al.* [22] found the prevalence to be 39% in their clinic population of 98 patients.

White coat hypertension may be even more common in elderly patients with isolated systolic hypertension. Ruddy *et al.* [23] compared the clinic and ambulatory pressures of 81 patients with systolic hypertension (defined as a systolic pressure above 160 mmHg and a diastolic pressure below 90 mmHg) with age-matched normotensive controls, all aged 60 years or more. Of the systolic hypertensive patients, 42% had ambulatory pressures within the normotensive range. Lerman *et al.* [22] found that their white coat hypertensive individuals were on average 9 years older than patients with sustained hypertension.

	Normal volunteers	Borderline hypertensive individuals	Essential hypertensive individuals
Clinic			
Physician	117/77 ± 14/9	150/96 ± 15/4	168/111 ± 6/6
Technician	111/73 ± 13/10	140/95 ± 14/8	154/105 ± 20/10
Ambulatory			
Awake	116/78 ± 11/7	139/93 ± 14/8	147/101 ± 13/9
Work	119/80 ± 13/7	143/97 ± 13/8	152/102 ± 15/10
Home	115/76 ± 11/7	136/91 ± 14/8	144/99 ± 14/10
Sleep	102/64 ± 10/6	121/96 ± 14/0	120/81 ± 15/10

Fig. 7.7. Comparison of blood pressures recorded in the clinic by a physician and a technician and by ambulatory recording. Reproduced with permission from Pickering *et al., JAMA* 1988, **259**:225–228.

The influence of interpersonal interactions on blood pressure

The interactions between doctor and patient have been the subject of a number of studies published in the last 30 years, and are of crucial importance in the examination of the home–clinic differences. In 1943 Alam and Smirk [12] noted that during the measurement of the basal blood pressure (measured by a physician taking multiple readings over half an hour), if a second physician entered and started to take the readings the blood pressure immediately increased to approach the casual level. Furthermore, it was immaterial which physician played the role of the second observer. Similar observations were made in normotensive subjects, but with less striking pressure differences. One of the first comparative studies was conducted by Stevenson *et al.* [24], who reported that hypertensive and normotensive subjects showed a similar increase in pressure during an emotionally neutral task (a two-step exercise test), but during a stressful interview the increase was much greater in hypertensive subjects. Thaler *et al.* [25] presented a series of 'doctor–patient' stories to different groups of patients, including some with hypertension and some with peptic ulcer. The hypertensive subjects made significantly more negative statements about the stories than the ulcer patients, and thought that 'doctors were potential or actual agents of danger'. McKegney and Williams [26] and Williams *et al.* [27] measured the blood pressure response to a personal interview, a word association test, and thematic apperception tests. They concluded that the blood pressure response was greatest for the interview, and that the extent of the response was a function of the degree of interpersonal interaction rather than the novelty of the situation. Shapiro *et al.* [28] described a study which was designed to evaluate the effect of a new antihypertensive agent. They found that the blood pressures recorded by the physician were consistently lower during the initial phase of the study, when for a variety of reasons the physician's enthusiasm was much higher than during the latter phases. These differences were attributed to changes in the doctor–patient relationship. A later study by Sapira *et al.* [29] used a film in which

scenes of a doctor interacting with a patient in either a friendly ('good doctor') or hostile ('bad doctor') fashion were shown to hypertensive patients and normal controls. The hypertensive patients denied seeing any differences between the two scenes, which were quite obvious to the normotensive individuals. Blood pressure changes were relatively minor, but when the subjects were interviewed afterwards about their attitudes, the hypertensive patients showed much greater increases in pressure than the normotensive individuals. The original interpretation of these findings was that hypertensive patients show a perceptual defect, but a simpler explanation may be that they were familiar with the physician in the film, and did not want to admit that there was a difference between the two scenes. Further evidence that the perception of the physician as an authority figure could affect the patient's blood pressure comes from a study by Reiser *et al.* [30], for which the subjects were army recruits, and the experimenter either a captain or a private. Although the experimental protocol was otherwise identical, consistently greater increases in pressure occurred in the presence of the captain than in the private. Lynch has demonstrated that the increase in blood pressure that occurs during talking is greater if the person being addressed is perceived as having a higher status [31].

The influence of a physician's presence on the patient's blood pressure has been demonstrated most elegantly by the study of Mancia's group [32,33], using continuous intra-arterial recording of pressure in hospitalized patients. When the physician approached the patient and put a blood pressure cuff on the arm there was an immediate rise in pressure which lasted throughout the procedure of taking a reading, with a gradual return to baseline over a period of several minutes. Repeat visits by the same physician were not associated with any habituation of this response. In a similar study, the average change in pressure evoked by the physician was 23/18 mmHg, which was approximately twice as high as when the pressure was taken by a nurse [33], as shown in Fig. 7.8. In a study of intra-arterial pressure using radiotelemetry in hospitalized patients, Irving *et al.* [34] commented that when patients were being examined by medical staff, their systolic pressures might increase by 30–50 mmHg and their diastolic pressures by 20–30 mmHg [34].

In our own study [20], clinic pressures were recorded not only by a physician (usually male) but also by a technician (usually female). As shown in Fig. 7.7, the technician's readings were not only lower than the physician's, but also closer to the daytime average recorded during ambulatory monitoring. These observations are consistent with the earlier findings of Mancia's group that physicians provoke a greater 'white coat effect' than nurses.

The results of these studies suggest that the nature of the interaction between the patient and the physician, who is often interpreted as an authority figure and the potential harbinger of bad news, is sufficient to raise the blood pressure by a significant amount. Occasionally these elevations in blood pressure do not habituate.

Factors contributing to the white coat effect

In our own study [20], we found that white coat hypertension was more likely to occur if the patient was female, young and non-obese, all of which are factors associated with a relatively benign prognosis. Sokolow's group [35] also found white coat hypertension to be more common in women, but reported a weak positive correlation with

age. Mancia's group, however, found no association with either the age or the sex of the patient. Lerman et al. [22] found no association with sex, but did with age. Laughlin et al. [36], in their comparison of clinic and home pressures, found that patients showing the greatest differences tended to be younger, but that there were no sex differences. In elderly patients, Ruddy et al. [23] found the prevalence to be equally high in men and women. Family history does not appear to be a factor, according to one study [22].

Although these results seem to be somewhat conflicting, the two largest studies [20,35] both showed an increased prevalence of white coat hypertension in women. It is probable that these findings are determined by a number of subtle psychosocial factors. It is possible, for example, to interpret the association of the white coat effect with sex on the basis of traditional male and female roles. Most patients during medical examination adopt a somewhat submissive psychological stance, and allow the physician to assume an authoritative position. Given traditional sexual stereotypes in our society, it is not unreasonable to conclude that women might view these interactions with their doctor in a slightly different, and perhaps a more anxiety-provoking way than would a man with a male physician. Further support for the possible role of status or authority in determining clinic blood pressure elevations comes from our previous discussion of the effects of psychosocial status on blood pressure.

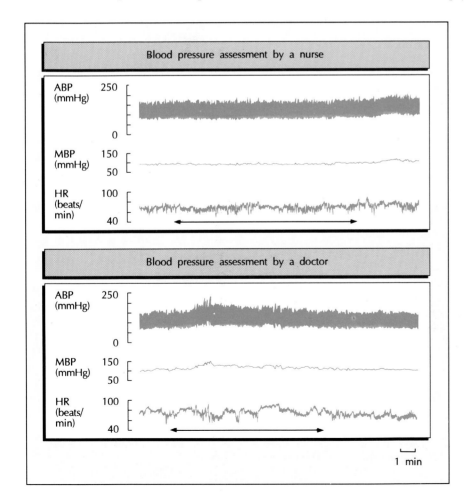

Fig. 7.8. Continuous intra-arterial readings of blood pressure (ABP) taken from one arm while a nurse or a doctor took an auscultatory measurement of blood pressure from the other arm. MBP, mean blood pressure; HR, heart rate. Reproduced with permission from Mancia et al. Hypertension 1987, 9:209–215.

For example, it has been reported that the race of the examiner may also influence the level of blood pressure recorded [37]. Irrespective of the psychological influences which may be responsible for the observed effect, it is clear that sex, and possibly other characteristics, play a role in determining the actual elevations in blood pressure observed during the blood pressure measurement procedure. Comstock [38] has suggested, on the basis of a large epidemiological survey of blood pressure, that the blood pressure of a subject tends to be higher when the examiner is of the opposite sex. Similar findings have been reported in a study of college students by McCubbin *et al.* [39].

There are as yet no available data concerning the white coat effect on male patients exposed to female physicians. Nonetheless, the persistent observation that the sex of the patient and physician is a determinant of clinic blood pressure measurements indicates that the psychosocial nature of the patient–doctor interaction is a significant component of the clinical evaluation which should not be ignored.

Personality

The personality of the patient is another potential factor which may contribute to the white coat effect. It might be expected that patients who show the white coat effect would be generally more anxious, but this is not necessarily the case. In the study of Laughlin *et al.* [36], there was no correlation between the clinic and home differences and the score on the Taylor Manifest Anxiety Scale. In another recent study by Schneider *et al.* [40], patients with borderline hypertension in the clinic were divided into two groups, according to whether their home pressures were raised or normal. The latter group, with normal home and raised clinic pressures, would be equivalent to our patients with white coat hypertension. The two groups did not differ in scores on psychometric tests measuring state and trait anxiety. Gerardi *et al.* [41] administered psychometric tests to three groups of hypertensive patients: white coat hypertensive individuals, patients with similar clinic and home pressures, and those with higher home pressures. The white coat hypertensive patients did not score any higher on either state or trait anxiety than the other two groups. Lerman *et al.* [22] found that white coat hypertensive patients reported less anger than sustained hypertensive patients but did not differ on measures of anxiety, health worry or health stress. We have seen white coat hypertension in a senior officer of the Israeli Air Force, whose blood pressure was lower while being monitored flying an F-16 fighter than when taken in the clinic.

Physiological factors: blood pressure lability and reactivity

An important consideration is whether the white coat effect is merely a manifestation of an increased lability of blood pressure; several studies have addressed this issue. Two studies using non-invasive ambulatory monitoring

found no greater variability of blood pressure over 24 h in white coat hypertensive subjects compared with patients with sustained hypertension or normotensive controls [20,23]. However, it should be admitted that non-invasive ambulatory monitoring gives only a crude estimate of true blood pressure variability. Two studies have used intra-arterial monitoring. In the first, Floras *et al.* [42] classified 59 hypertensive patients according to whether their ambulatory pressure (measured by continuous intra-arterial recording) was similar to, or much lower than, their clinic pressure. Blood pressure variability during the ambulatory monitoring was identical in the two groups, as was the response to a commonly used reactivity task — mental arithmetic.

In the second study, of hospitalized patients, Parati *et al.* [43] measured the blood pressure response to a physician entering the patient's room and taking a conventional auscultatory measurement of blood pressure. Although this provoked very significant pressor responses in many patients, the extent of these responses showed no correlation with either blood pressure reactivity (to four different stressors, including mental arithmetic and the cold pressor test) or variability over 24 h, as shown in Fig. 7.9.

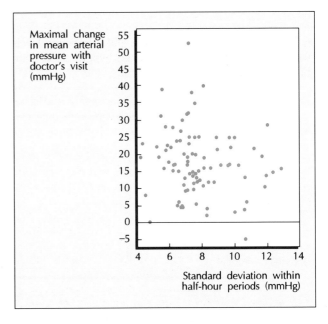

Fig. 7.9. Lack of relationship between pressor response to doctor's visit and short-term variability of blood pressure during intra-arterial ambulatory monitoring in hospitalized patients, expressed as the standard deviation of mean arterial pressure within half-hour periods. Reproduced with permission (Parati *et al.*, *J Hypertens* 1988, 6:481–488).

A third study [41], using non-invasive blood pressure measurement, claimed that white coat hypertensive subjects may show an increased blood pressure reactivity to mental arithmetic. These patients were classified on the basis of their home (not ambulatory) pressures. While they did show a greater reactivity than patients who showed no difference between their home and clinic pressures, it was not greater than in patients who had higher home and clinic pressures. Their reactivity to two other tests (cold pressor and a stressful imagery task) was no greater than in either of the other two groups. Thus, none of these three studies offers any support to the idea that the white coat effect is a manifestation of a generalized cardiovascular hyper-reactivity.

The sensitivity of the baroreceptor reflexes is one factor which regulates the blood pressure response to an acute pressor stimulus (such as a physician), such that a greater response would be elicited in patients with less sensitive reflexes. However, in the study of Floras et al. [42] the opposite was found; the subjects with white coat hypertension had a higher baroreflex sensitivity than those with sustained hypertension. Since a reduced reflex sensitivity is a consequence of sustained hypertension, this finding would also be consistent with a generally normal cardiovascular system in the white coat hypertensive patients.

There is also some indirect evidence that sympathetic nervous activity is normal. Floras et al. [42] found no difference in heart rate or in plasma noradrenaline levels measured both at rest and during exercise. In a study of young hypertensive patients evaluated by home and clinic pressures, Saito et al. [44] found that the patients with white coat hypertension (normal home pressures) had normal 24-h urine noradrenaline and adrenaline levels, whereas the patients with sustained hypertension (high home pressures) had elevated levels. Ruddy et al. [23] also found no differences in heart rate (either in the clinic or during ambulatory monitoring) in white coat hypertensive subjects. Furthermore, plasma renin activity was the same as in patients with sustained hypertension.

These findings suggest that the white coat effect is highly specific to the clinic situation, rather than reflecting some generalized constitutional or physiological disturbance. However, a discordant note has been sounded by Julius et al. [45] in a population study from Tecumseh in Michigan. On the basis of self-monitored home readings and readings made at a single clinic visit (but no ambulatory readings), they defined one population of 'white coat hypertensives', who had an elevated clinic pressure and normal home pressures, and another population of 'sustained hypertensives' who had high home pressures. Both hypertensive groups had higher heart rates, higher systemic vascular resistance, and higher triglyceride and insulin levels than the normotensive subjects. However, the population that they labelled as having white coat hypertension (who comprised 55% of the total 'hypertensive' population) probably bears little resemblance to the patients identified in clinical studies.

Psychophysiologists have distinguished between stimulus specificity and response specificity, and the general consensus is that hypertensive individuals tend to exhibit the latter. The white coat effect, however, appears to be an instance of a high degree of stimulus specificity.

The orienting and defence responses

It is appropriate at this stage to consider what the mechanism of the white coat effect might be. Two types of autonomic arousal in response to external stimuli have been described in animal experiments, which appear to have their counterparts in human studies. The first is the orienting reflex or alerting response, which is characterized by an elevation in blood pressure, but not necessarily in heart rate, in response to a novel stimulus, and which habituates with repeated exposure [46]. The second is the defence reaction, first described by Hess in 1949 [47], which is characterized by an increase in both blood pressure and heart rate in response to a threatening stimulus, and which does not habituate. Since the white coat effect, by definition, also does not habituate, it might more closely resemble the defence response, although it is not clear to what extent these two patterns of response are really distinct from each other. We have reviewed above the evidence that the patient's perception of the physician as a potentially threatening figure has an important effect on the patient's blood pressure, and that this may be more important than the novelty of the situation.

The haemodynamic pattern of the defence reaction has been studied in man and, as in animals, it is characterized by an increase in blood pressure, heart rate and cardiac output [48,49]. There may, however, be a biphasic response pattern: animal studies have shown that when a cat is preparing to fight another cat [50], or when dogs are subjected to avoidance conditioning, the initial response preceding the conditioning period is a rise in blood pressure mediated by vasoconstriction and a decreased heart rate and cardiac output [51].

The haemodynamic pattern underlying the white coat effect has not been characterized. Although there may be a pronounced tachycardia in some younger patients, in the majority of our patients with white coat hypertension the higher blood pressures obtained by a physician than with a nurse are not usually accompanied by higher heart rates.

A hypothesis: white coat hypertension as a conditioned response

An alternative explanation is that while the white coat effect originates as part of the defence reflex, it becomes perpetuated through classic conditioning. The subject who initially exhibits a large pressor response is told by the physician that his or her blood pressure is a matter of concern, and needs to be re-checked. At that point, the specifics of the blood pressure measurement situation, including the interaction with the physician, the physician's characteristics, the clinic setting and the feeling of the blood pressure cuff around the arm, become symbolically associated with danger, and thus become conditioned stimuli for a subsequent conditioned response. The possibility that the clinic setting, the procedure, and the particular physician might be associated with bad news concerning medical well-being becomes incorporated into the patient's psychological outlook. On subsequent visits, the stimuli associated with this 'danger' elicit autonomic arousal, leading to blood pressure elevations. The habituation which might be anticipated on the second visit, and the relaxed feelings associated with familiar surroundings, do not emerge. Indeed, with each visit the fear, arousal and attendant blood pressure elevation are reinforced. Often adding to the cycle is the patient's feeling that blood pressure measurement is a test to be either passed or failed. Failure in this case means an inability to relax and allow the doctor to get low readings. This failure compounds the situation to the point where the clinical evaluation assumes significant anxiety-inducing properties, with important physiological sequelae.

The two contrasting patterns — habituation leading to a diminution of the defence or orienting response, and conditioning leading to a perpetuation of it as the white coat effect — are illustrated schematically in Fig. 7.10.

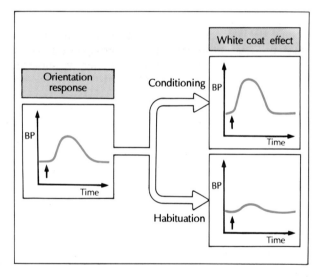

Fig. 7.10. Hypothetical development of the white coat effect. When blood pressure (BP) is first taken there is a pressor response due to the orienting or defence response. In the majority of patients this habituates with repeated exposure, but in some it may become perpetuated as a conditioned response.

This is not at all a novel conceptualization of symptomatology. It is a common observation that patients who have had unpleasant experiences in a physician's office subsequently respond to the office setting, the instruments and the assistants with an aversive emotional response. For example, cancer patients in need of repeated intravenous injections of chemotherapeutic agents often respond with nausea, anxiety and fear in anticipation of the actual procedure themselves.

This point was well illustrated by a letter published in the *New England Journal of Medicine* [52]:

'Oncologist-induced vomiting: the Igvid syndrome:

'To the Editor: I am an oncologist in clinical practice in Milwaukee, and I saw a patient at a local shopping mall three years after she had received adjuvant chemotherapy for breast cancer. She promptly threw up after seeing me, and I can assure you I am not that bad to look at. I presume that this happened because of a conditioned reflex associated with her past chemotherapy.

'Since I would not like to be remembered as someone who causes vomiting, I would like to name this syndrome the Igvid syndrome ('Divgi' backwards) because I think I would rather be considered the antithesis of someone who induces vomiting (i.e., pleasant).

'Ajit B. Divgi, M.D.'

The acquisition of these anticipatory symptoms is adequately explained by classic conditioning principles. The considerable evidence to support the idea that cardiovascular responses can be classically conditioned has been reviewed by Cohen and Randall [53]. They concluded that the rules which govern cardiovascular conditioning are the same as those described for classic conditioning. What is being suggested here, with respect to white coat hypertension, is that it is a highly stimulus-specific response which is acquired, and perhaps can also be treated, according to these same classic conditioning principles.

A recently reported study [54] lends support to this proposed mechanism. Twenty-nine young men who were found to have elevated blood pressures on a routine examination were randomly divided into two groups. The first group was sent a letter telling them that their pressure was too high, and the second group was sent a neutral letter. On the second examination the blood pressure in the first group was 16/10 mmHg higher than in the second group throughout a 45 min testing period. In another study Rudd *et al.* [55] identified 765 subjects with previously unidentified hypertension and randomized them to two groups, one of which received 'traditional' information about hypertension as the 'silent killer' while the other was given more reassuring information. At follow-up the prevalence of high readings was somewhat greater in the traditional group than in the reassurance group.

In an experimental study of healthy individuals Linden *et al.* [56] obtained quite different results. Normotensive patients attending a family practice clinic had their blood pressure measured and were then randomized to receive no information about their blood pressure, to be told it was normal, or to be told that it was 'on the high side'. The blood pressure was then re-checked, but there was no difference between the three groups. Furthermore, it made no difference whether the feedback was provided by a doctor or a nurse. Similar results were obtained in university students studied in a laboratory setting.

There are several possible reasons for the negative findings of the studies of Linden *et al.* First, it may be that people are not so easily fooled, and that telling a healthy individual that his or her pressure is on the high side may be an insufficiently strong stimulus. The consequences might be different in patients who are referred specifically for evaluation of their blood pressure. Second, it is possible that the effects of feedback are delayed, and might only be apparent at the time of the next visit. Third, it may be only a subset of individuals who are susceptible.

An anecdotal example may further illustrate this phenomenon. A previously normotensive young woman underwent a routine physical examination for an employment check-up. She felt extremely anxious during the examination, and was told that her blood pressure was significantly elevated, and required further work-up and treatment. Ever since that occasion she has been aware of palpitations and flushing coming on whenever she has her blood pressure checked by a physician, whereas a visit to a dentist provokes no such response.

Clinical implications and prognosis of white coat hypertension

The potential implications of this phenomenon are huge. If we are correct in our estimate of a 20% prevalence rate of white coat hypertension in patients with mild hypertension, it raises the possibility that 10 million people in the United States are misclassified as being hypertensive. An urgent need is to understand the prognosis for such patients: are they at increased risk of cardiovascular morbidity or not? Our knowledge of the natural history of mild hypertension indicates that although such patients are at significantly increased risk compared to their normotensive peers, in absolute terms this risk is still small. If left untreated, the majority of such people will live a normal life-span without any ill effects from their blood pressure. Another major consideration is that the results of the trials of treatment for mild hypertension have been very disappointing. These have been briefly reviewed in Chapter 1, with the paradoxical conclusion that treatment of mild hypertension benefits the population, but not the individual patient. One solution to this dilemma is to attempt to stratify patients within this population according to their level of risk. Our working hypothesis is that patients with white coat hypertension represent a low-risk group for whom antihypertensive medication may not be necessary.

At present, the evidence supporting this view is not conclusive, but is at least consistent with it. The only published prospective study of morbidity related to ambulatory pressures was conducted by Perloff et al. [57,58]. Although they did not attempt to define a subgroup with white coat hypertension, they found that patients whose ambulatory pressure was low relative to their clinic pressure were at lower risk than those with higher ambulatory pressures. Ambulatory pressures added to the prognostic value of clinic pressure in patients who were under the age of 50 years, had an initial diastolic pressure below 105 mmHg, and had experienced no prior morbid event. These are all characteristics which we would associate with white coat hypertension. In older patients with more advanced hypertension the ambulatory pressures were not of additional value over the clinic pressures.

We have been following a group of patients with borderline hypertension initially evaluated with clinic and ambulatory measurements of blood pressure. An initial analysis of 739 patients followed prospectively for an average duration of 5 years has been carried out. We observed a prevalence of cardiovascular morbid events of 2.1% in patients with white coat hypertension, and 4.4% in those with sustained hypertension (Pickering et al., in preparation).

These prospective observations of a relatively low level of cardiovascular risk in white coat hypertension are supported by cross-sectional studies of target organ damage. In one of the first studies using ambulatory monitoring, Sokolow et al. [35] had observed that patients with no evidence of target organ damage had a greater difference between clinic and home pressure than patients with target organ damage. In the study of Floras et al. [42], there was evidence of target organ damage in 64% of the patients with sustained hypertension, but in only 19% of those with white coat hypertension. Since impaired baroreflex sensitivity is a consequence rather than a cause of hypertension, this would also explain why the white coat patients had a higher baroreflex sensitivity. Further evidence for an absence of target organ damage in patients with white coat hypertension comes from a study by White et al. [59] of three groups of subjects: normotensive subjects, white coat hypertensive subjects, and sustained hypertensive patients. None of the hypertensive patients had ever been treated. Cardiac structure and function were evaluated by echocardiography, radionuclide cineangiography and exercise testing. All three tests showed differences between the normotensive subjects and the patients with sustained hypertension, but the patients with white coat hypertension resembled the normotensive subjects (Fig. 7.11).

Implications for treatment

Clinic blood pressure measurements have traditionally been used not only for diagnosing hypertension but also for evaluating the response to treatment. One of the concerns in this respect has been the placebo effect, which can be defined in the present context as a decrease in pressure that occurs as a result of the expectation of the patient rather than from any physiological effect of the treatment. If it is accepted that there is an increase in pressure in the clinic setting as a result of the white coat effect, a decrease in clinic pressure following the initiation of treatment could occur either because the white coat effect is dampened or because the overall level of pressure is reduced [60]. The former case might be regarded as a placebo effect. The two could only be distinguished, however, if clinic pressures were supplemented by other measures such as home reading or ambulatory recording. Corcoran et al. [61] found that pharmacological treatment had no effect on the clinic–home differ-

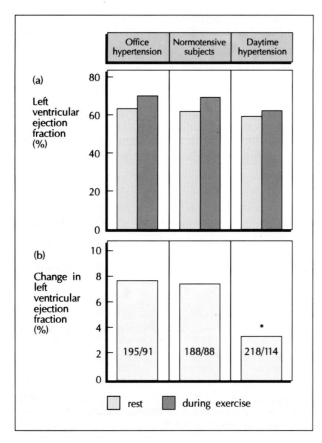

Fig. 7.11. (a) Left ventricular ejection fraction at rest and during exercise in patients with white coat hypertension (Office hypertension), in patients with sustained hypertension (Daytime hypertension), and in normotensive subjects. (b) Change of left ventricular ejection fraction with exercise in the same three groups. Peak blood pressure during exercise is also shown. *P < 0.05 versus other groups. Reproduced with permission [59].

ences: for patients on no treatment, home pressures were 22/14 mmHg lower than clinic pressures; for those being treated with reserpine or hydralazine home pressures were lower by 16/10 and 21/14 mmHg, respectively. Most of the studies which have compared the effect of pharmacological treatment on clinic and ambulatory pressure have shown that the reduction in ambulatory pressure is at least as great as the effect on clinic pressure [62,63]. Coats *et al.* [64] concluded that the white coat effect was attenuated by a beta blocker (atenolol) but not by a calcium antagonist (nifedipine), while Elijovich and Laffer [65] found that it was unaffected by either class of agent. This implies that the white coat effect persists in patients who are receiving treatment. The most likely physiological mediator of the phenomenon is the sympathetic nervous system, so that it might be expected that it would be suppressed by sympatholytic agents. The fact that this is not the case is another testimony to its potency. This subject is discussed further in Chapter 10.

Behavioural treatments of hypertension, using techniques such as biofeedback and relaxation training, have been the subject of numerous studies, most of which have claimed a therapeutic effect [66,67]. These procedures all require the subject to focus for brief periods of time on reducing the level of autonomic arousal. If blood pressure reductions are observed in the clinic, there is a strong possibility that such reductions are achieved as a result of this learned behaviour pattern, and that the patient has learned to suppress the white coat effect without necessarily affecting blood pressure at other times. For this reason, it is essential that a technique such as ambulatory monitoring be used to evaluate the therapeutic effectiveness of such treatments. So far, despite the large number of studies using clinic measurements of blood pressure, hardly any have used ambulatory monitoring. One study that did was conducted by Jacob *et al.* [68], who compared the response to pharmacological treatment with either a beta blocker or a diuretic and to non-pharmacological treatment with relaxation training. Relaxation training produced a modest reduction in clinic blood pressures, but was without any significant effect on ambulatory pressures. The beta blocker, however, lowered blood pressure equally in the two situations.

It is worth mentioning at this juncture the specific implications for behavioural treatment which result from this conceptualization of white coat hypertension. It is proposed that the white coat effect begins as a defence reaction and is acquired and maintained by classic conditioning. It is not the result of generalized anxiety, nor of generalized hyper-reactivity of the sympathetic nervous system; it is highly stimulus-specific. Therefore, it may be more efficiently extinguished using a circumscribed systematic desensitization procedure rather than the more traditional relaxation or stress management procedures usually employed to treat high blood pressure non-pharmacologically.

Summary and conclusions

Clinical measurements of blood pressure have always been the standard method for the evaluation of the hypertensive patients, and are likely to continue to be so for the foreseeable future. They are, however, subject to a number of sources of error, which limit the degree to which they represent the true blood pressure. The spontaneous variability of blood pressure is such that there is considerable variation in readings taken in the same subject both within the same occasion, and between different occasions. In patients initially diagnosed as hypertensive there is a tendency for clinic pressure to fall with repeated visits, because of both regression to the mean and habituation to the measurement procedure.

In hypertensive patients a clinic visit evokes a variable pressor response, which further reduces the reliability of the clinic readings. In some patients this may result in white coat hypertension, which is defined as a persistently elevated clinic pressure but normal pressure at other times. This occurs in about 20% of patients with mild hypertension and may result in significant misclassification of hypertension. Such patients do not appear to be generally more anxious than others, nor to show a general increase in blood pressure variability. It is hypothesized that the white coat effect is relatively specific to the clinic situation, and arises by a conditioning mechanism which perpetuates the defence or orienting responses. The effect is evoked more potently by a physician than by a nurse.

It is also hypothesized that white coat hypertension is a benign condition. Such patients typically show less evidence of target organ damage than patients with similar clinic pressures but sustained hypertension. Furthermore, the limited prospective data suggests that the risk of cardiovascular morbidity is relatively low.

References

1. AYMAN D, GOLDSHINE AD: **Blood pressure determinations by patients with essential hypertension: the difference between clinic and home readings before treatment.** *Am J Med Sci* 1940, 200:465–474.
2. ARMITAGE P, ROSE GA: **The variability of measurements of casual blood pressure. I. A laboratory study.** *Clin Sci* 1966, 30:325–335.
3. ARMITAGE D, FOX W, ROSE GA, TINKER CM: **The variability of measurements of casual blood pressure. II. Survey experience.** *Clin Sci* 1966, 30:337–334.
4. KANNEL WB, SORLIE P, GORDON T: **Labile hypertension: a faulty concept?** *Circulation* 1980, 61:1183–1187.
5. WATSON RDS, LUMB R, YOUNG MA, STALLARD TJ, DAVIES P, LITTLER WA: **Variation in cuff blood pressure in untreated outpatients with mild hypertension: implications for initiating antihypertensive treatment.** *J Hypertens* 1987, 5:207–211.
6. GARDNER MJ, HEADY JA: **Some effects of within-person variability in epidemiological studies.** *J Chron Dis* 1973, 26:781–795.
7. MACMAHON S, PETO R, CUTLER J *ET AL*: **Blood pressure, stroke, and coronary heart disease. Part I. Prolonged differences in blood pressure: prospective observational studies corrected for the regression dilution bias.** *Lancet* 1990, 335:765–774.
8. LLABRE MM, IRONSON GH, SPITZER SB, GELLMAN MD, WEIDLER DJ, SCHNEIDERMAN N: **Blood pressure stability of normotensive and mild hypertensives in different settings.** *Health Psychol* 1988 7 (suppl):127–137.
9. MAROLF AP, HANY S, BATTIG B, VETTER W: **Comparison of casual, ambulatory and self-determined blood pressure measurement.** *Nephron* 1987, 47 (suppl 1):142–145.
10. JAMES GD, PICKERING TG, YEE LS, HARSHFIELD GA, RIVA S, LARAGH JH: **The reproducibility of average ambulatory, home, and clinic pressures.** *Hypertension* 1988, 11:545–549.
11. DES COMBES BJ, PORCHET M, WAEBER B, BRUNNER HR: **Ambulatory blood pressure recordings. Reproducibility and unpredictability.** *Hypertension* 1984, 6:110–114.
12. ALAM GM, SMIRK FH: **Casual and basal blood pressures. I. In British and Egyptian men.** *Br Heart J* 1943, 5:152–155.
13. ALAM GM, SMIRK FH: **Casual and basal blood pressures. II. In essential hypertension.** *Br Heart J* 1943, 5:156–160.
14. GATMAN M, AMIN M, SMIRK FH: **Casual and basal blood pressures. III. In renal hypertension.** *Br Heart J* 1943, 5:161–162.
15. SMIRK FH: **Casual and basal blood pressures. IV. Their relationship to the supplemental pressure with a note on statistical implications.** *Br Heart J* 1944, 6:174–182.
16. KAIN HK, HINMAN AT, SOKOLOW M: **Arterial blood pressure measurements with a portable recorder in hypertensive patients. I. Variability and correlation with 'casual' pressures.** *Circulation* 1964, 30:882–892.
17. PICKERING TG, HARSHFIELD GA, KLEINERT HD, BLANK S, LARAGH JH: **Blood pressures during normal daily activities, sleep, and exercise. Comparison of values in normal and hypertensive subjects.** *JAMA* 1982, 247:992–996.
18. HARSHFIELD GA, PICKERING TG, JAMES GD, BLANK SG: **Blood pressure variability and reactivity in the natural environ-**

ment. In *Blood Pressure Measurement. New techniques in Autonomic and 24-hour Indirect Monitoring* edited by Meyer-Sabellek W, Anlauf M, Cotzen R, Steinfeld L. Darmstadt: Steinkopff, 1990, pp 241–252.
19. HARSHFIELD GA, PICKERING TG, KLEINERT HD, BLANK S, LARAGH JH: **Situational variations of blood pressure in ambulatory hypertensive patients.** *Psychosom Med* 1982, 44:237–244.
20. PICKERING TG, JAMES GD, BODDIE C, HARSHFIELD GA, BLANK S, LARAGH JH: **How common is white coat hypertension?** *JAMA* 1988, 259:225–228.
21. KRAKOFF LR, EISON H, PHILLIPS RH, LEIMAN SH, LEV S: **Effect of ambulatory pressure monitoring on the diagnosis and cost of treatment for mild hypertension.** *Am Heart J* 1988, 116:1152–1154.
22. LERMAN CE, BRODY DS, HUI T, LAZARO C, SMITH DG, BLUM MJ: **The white-coat hypertension response: prevalence and predictors.** *J Gen Intern Med* 1989, 4:225–231.
23. RUDDY MC, BIALY GB, MALKA ES, LACY CR, KOSTIS JB: **The relationship of plasma renin activity to clinic and ambulatory blood pressure in elderly people with isolated systolic hypertension.** *J Hypertens* 1988, 6 (suppl 4), S412–S415.
24. STEVENSON IP, DUNCAN CH, FLYNN JT, WOLF S: **Hypertension as a reaction pattern to stress. Correlation of circulatory hemodynamics with changes in the attitude and emotional state.** *Am J Med Sci* 1952, 224:286–299.
25. THALER M, WEINER H, REISER MR: **Exploration of the doctor–patient relationship through projective techniques. Their use in psychosomatic illness.** *Psychosom Med* 1957, 19:228–239.
26. MCKEGNEY FP, WILLIAMS RB: **Psychological aspects of hypertension. II. The differential influence of interview variables on blood pressure.** *Am J Psychiatry* 1967, 123:1539–1545.
27. WILLIAMS RB, KIMBALL CP, WILLIARD HN; **The influence of interpersonal interaction on diastolic blood pressure.** *Psychosom Med* 1972, 34:194–198.
28. SHAPIRO AP, MYERS T, REISER MF, FERRIS EB: **Comparison of blood pressure response to Veriloid and to the doctor.** *Psychosom Med* 1964, 16:478–487.
29. SAPIRA JD, SCHEIB ET, MORIARTY R, SHAPIRO AP: **Differences in perception between hypertensive and normotensive populations.** *Psychosom Med* 1971, 33:239–250.
30. REISER MF, REEVES RB, ARMINGTON J: **Effect of variations in laboratory procedure and experimenter upon the ballistocardiogram, blood pressure, and heart rate in healthy young men.** *Psychosom Med* 1958, 17:185–199.
31. LONG J, LYNCH JJ, MACHIRAN NM *ET AL*: **The effect of status on blood pressure during verbal communications.** *J Behav Med* 1982, 5:165–172.
32. MANCIA G, BERTINIERI G, GRASSI G *ET AL*: **Effects of blood pressure measurement by the doctor on patient's blood pressure and heart rate.** *Lancet* 1983, ii:695–697.
33. MANCIA G, PARATI G, POMIDOSSI G, GRASSI G, CASADEI R, ZANCHETTI A: **Alerting reaction and rise in blood pressure during measurement by physician and nurse.** *Hypertension* 1987, 9:209–215.
34. IRVING JB, BRASH HM, KERR F, KIRBY BJ: **The value of ambulatory monitoring in borderline and established hypertension.** *Postgrad Med J* 1976, 52 (suppl 7):137–139.
35. SOKOLOW M, PERLOFF D, COWAN R: **Contribution of ambulatory blood pressure to the assessment of patients with mild to moderate elevations of office blood pressure.** *Cardiovasc Rev Reports* 1980, 1:295–303.
36. LAUGHLIN KD, SHERRARD DH, FISHER L: **Comparison of clinic and home blood pressure levels in essential hypertension and variables associated with clinic — home differences.** *J Chron Dis* 1979, 33:197–206.
37. MURPHY JK, ALPERT BS, MOES DM, SOMES GW: **Race and cardiovascular reactivity. A neglected relationship.** *Hypertension* 1986, 8:1075–1083.
38. COMSTOCK GW: **An epidemiologic study of blood pressure levels in a biracial community in the Southern United States.** *Am J Hygiene* 1957, 65:271–315.

39. MCCUBBIN JA, WILSON JF, BRUEHL S, BRADY M, CLARK K, KORT E: Gender effects on blood pressures obtained during an on campus screening. *Psychosom Med* (in press).

40. SCHNEIDER RH, EGAN BM, JOHNSON EH *ET AL*: Anger and anxiety in borderline hypertension. *Psychosom Med* 1986, 48:242–248.

41. GERARDI RJ, BLANCHARD EB, ANDRASIK F: Psychological dimensions of 'office hypertension'. *Behav Res Ther* 1985, 23:609–612.

42. FLORAS JS, JONES JV, HASSAN MO, OSIKOWSKA B, SEVER PS, SLEIGHT P: Cuff and ambulatory blood pressure in subjects with essential hypertension. *Lancet* 1981, ii:107–109.

43. PARATI G, POMIDOSSI G, CASADEI R, *ET AL*: Limitations of laboratory stress tesing in the assessment of subjects' cardiovascualr reactivity to stress. *J Hypertens* 1986, 4 (suppl 6):S51–S53.

44. SAITO I, TAKESHITA E, HAYASHI S *ET AL*: Comparison of clinic and home blood pressure levels and the role of the sympathetic nervous system in clinic-home differences. *Am J Hypertens* 1990, 3:219–224.

45. JULIUS S, MEJIA A, JONES K *ET AL*: 'White coat' versus 'sustained' borderline hypertension in Tecumseh, Michigan. *Hypertension* (in press).

46. SOKOLOW YN: *Perception and the Conditional Reflex.* New York: Pergamon, 1963.

47. HESS WB: *Das Zwischenhern.* Basel: Schwade Verlag, 1949.

48. BROD J, FENCL VS, HEJL Z, JIRKA J: Circulatory changes underlying blood pressure elevation during acute emotional stress (mental arithmetic) in normotensive and hypertensive subjects. *Clin Sci* 1959, 18:269–279.

49. STEAD EA, WARREN JV, MERRILL AJ, BRANNON ES: The cardiac output in male subjects as measured by the technique of right atrial catheterization. Normal values with observations on the effect of anxiety and tilting. *J Clin Invest* 1945, 24:290–298.

50. ADAMS DB, BUCCELLI G, MANCIA G, ZANCHETTI A: Relation of cardiovascular changes in fighting to emotion and exercise. *J Physiol* 1971, 212:321–335.

51. ANDERSON DE, TOSHEFF JG: Cardiac output and total peripheral resistance changes during preavoidance in the dog. *J Appl Physiol* 1973, 34:650–654.

52. DIVGI AB: Oncologist-induced vomiting. The Igvid Syndrome. *N Engl J Med* 1989, 320:189 (letter).

53. COHEN DH, RANDALL DC: Classical conditioning of cardiovascular responses. *Annu Rev Physiol* 1983, 46:187–197.

54. ROSTRUP M, KHELDSEN SE, AMUNDSEN R, EIDE I: Does awareness of hypertension per se influence blood pressure, heart rate, plasma catecholamines, and response to cold pressor test? *J Hypertens* 1988, 6 (suppl 4):S743–S744.

55. RUDD P, PRICE MG, GRAHAM LE *ET AL*: Consequences of work-site hypertension screening. Differential changes in psychosocial function. *Am J Med* 1986, 80:853–860.

56. LINDEN W, HERBERT CP, JENKINS A, RAFFLE V: Should we tell them when their blood pressure is up? *Can Med Assoc J* 1989, 141:409–415.

57. PERLOFF D, SOKOLOW M, COWAN R: The prognostic value of ambulatory blood pressure. *JAMA* 1983, 249:2793–2798.

58. PERLOFF D, SOKOLOW M, COWAN RM, JUSTER RP: Prognostic value of ambulatory blood pressure measurements: further analyses. *J Hypertens* 1989, 7 (suppl 3):S3–S10.

59. WHITE WB, SCHULMAN P, MCCABE EJ, DEY HM: Average daily blood pressure, not office blood pressure, determines cardiac function in patients with hypertension. *JAMA* 1989, 261:873–872.

60. PICKERING TG, HARSHFIELD GA, DEVEREUX RB, LARAGH JH: What is the role of ambulatory blood pressure monitoring in the management of hypertensive patients? *Hypertension* 1985, 7:171–177.

61. CORCORAN AC, DUSTAN HP, PAGE IH: The evaluation of antihypertensive procedures, with particular reference to their effects on blood pressure. *Ann Intern Med* 1955, 43:1161–1177.

62. GOULD BA, MANN S, DAVIES AB, ALLMAN GD, RAFTERY EB: Does placebo lower blood pressure? *Lancet* 1981, ii:1377–1381.

63. WAEBER B, NUSSBERGER J, BRUNNER HR: Shortcomings of office blood pressure in assessing antihypertensive therapy. *Clin Exp Hypertens [A]* 1985, 7:291–298.

64. COATS AJS, CONWAY J, SOMERS VK, ISEA JE, SLEIGHT P: Ambulatory pressure monitoring in the assessment of antihypertensive therapy. *Cardiovasc Drugs Ther* 1989, 3:303–311.

65. ELIJOVICH F, LAFFER CL: Magnitude, reproducibility, and components of the pressor response to the clinic. *Hypertension* 1990, 15 (suppl I):I161–I164.

66. POLEFRONE J, MANUCK SB, LARKIN KT, FRANCIS ME: Behavioral aspects of arterial hypertension and its treatment. In *Medical Factors and Psychological Disorders* edited by Morrison RL, Bellack AS. Plenum, 1987, pp 203–229.

67. LEHMAN JW, BENSON H: The non-pharmacological treatment of hypertension. In *Hypertension* edited by Genest J, Kuchel O, Hamet P, Cantin M. New York: McGraw Hill, 1983, pp 1238–1245.

68. JACOB RG, SHAPIRO AP, REEVES AP, JOHNSEN AM, MCDONALD RH, COBURN PC: Relaxation therapy for hypertension. Comparison of effects with concomitant placebo diuretic, and β-blocker. *Arch Intern Med* 1986, 146:2335–2350.

8   Self-monitoring of blood pressure

The potential for hypertensive patients to have their blood pressures measured at home, either by using self-monitoring or by having a family member make the measurements, was first demonstrated in 1940 by Ayman and Goldshine [1]. Home monitoring has the theoretical advantage of being able to overcome the two main limitations of clinic readings: the small number of readings that can be taken, and the white coat effect. It also provides a simple and cost-effective means for obtaining a large number of readings which are at least representative of the natural environment in which patients spend a major part of their day.

Although the technique has been readily available for many years, it has taken a surprisingly long time to find its way into general clinical practice. This is in part due to the fact that no clear guidelines have been established for the interpretation of home readings. Nevertheless, the scene is rapidly changing, spurred on by the aggressive marketing of electronic self-monitoring devices and the increasing awareness of the fallibility of clinic readings.

Comparison of home and clinic pressures

The original observation of Ayman and Goldshine that home pressures are usually much lower than clinic pressures has been confirmed in a number of studies, the results of some of which [2–15] are plotted in Fig. 8.1. In patients with severe hypertension Corcoran *et al.* [16] reported that clinic pressures were on average 20/10 mmHg higher than home readings, and that these clinic readings were also higher than readings taken in hospital by a nurse. In mildly hypertensive subjects Laughlin *et al.* [11] found clinic pressures to be 11/5 mmHg higher than home pressures; in our own study [2] there was a similar difference, of 10/5 mmHg. Badskjaer and Nielsen [17] reported an average difference of 13/3 mmHg, but there was no correlation between the home and clinic pressures. In a second study Laughlin *et al.* [18] reported that home pressures showed a progressive decline with repeated measurement, which we did not find: in our subjects the average pressures measured during the first and third week of home recordings were the same. Kenny *et al.* [3] measured blood pressure by four different techniques on three occasions, separated by intervals of 2 weeks, in 19 patients with borderline hypertension. The techniques included conventional clinic measurement, basal blood pressure (measured after lying for 30 min in a quiet room), daytime ambulatory pressure, and self-recorded home pressure. None of the four measures showed any consistent change over the 3 study days, although there was an insignificant downward trend in all of them. For all 3 days, the clinic pressures were consis-

tently higher than any of the other measures, but there were no significant differences between any of the other three measures. The average difference between clinic and home pressures was 9/4 mmHg.

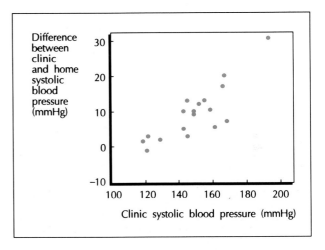

Fig. 8.1. Comparison of the average levels of clinic and self-monitored home systolic blood pressure. Data from 14 published studies, four of which included more than one group of subjects [2–15].

In another study comparing the reproducibility of home, clinic and ambulatory pressures we took two sets of each type of measurement separated by an interval of 2 weeks [4]. In hypertensive patients we found a significant decline in systolic pressure in the clinic over this period, but the home and ambulatory pressures showed no significant change. In normotensive subjects there was no consistent change in any of the three measures of blood pressure. These findings support the notion that the fall in clinic pressure on successive visits is largely spurious, and primarily due to habituation to the clinic setting or regression to the mean.

In normotensive subjects the differences between clinic and home pressures are much smaller than in hypertensive subjects (see Fig. 8.1). In an epidemiological population survey Welin *et al.* [5] found only minor differences. These investigators also reported that subjects who were most familiar with the clinic setting exhibited the smallest differences between the home and clinic readings. Similar results were reported by Beckman *et al.* [6], who found that subjects labelled mildly hypertensive had systolic pressures 15 mmHg higher in the clinic than at home, whereas in normotensive subjects this difference was only 2 mmHg. Finally, Julius *et al.* [7] reported a mean difference of 14/4 mmHg between clinic and home readings in a series of patients with borderline hypertension, but no difference (1/−3 mmHg) in normotensive subjects.

The discrepancy between home and clinic pressures raises the question: which is closer to the true pressure? To answer this we trained 93 patients, with a wide range of blood pressures, to take their own pressures; they did this over a 3-week period [2]. They also had measurements of clinic pressure, and wore an ambulatory monitor for 24 h. As shown in Fig. 8.2, the home pressures were closer to the 24-hour average than the clinic pressures. There were also reasonably close correlations (r = 0.69 for systolic pressure and r = 0.71 for diastolic pressure) between the self-monitored and automatically determined home readings. Figure 8.2 also demonstrates the phenomenon seen in Fig. 8.1, namely that there is a progressively greater discrepancy between the clinic and the true pressure at higher levels of blood pressure.

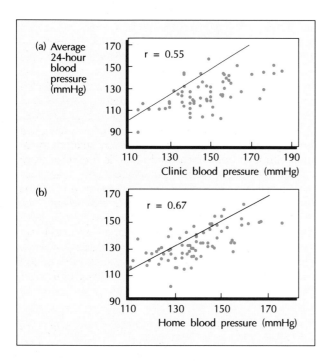

Fig. 8.2. (a) Comparison of clinic and average 24-hour pressure in 93 patients. (b) Corresponding comparison between home and 24-hour pressures. Lines of identity are shown. Reproduced with permission [2].

Reliability of home readings

Little information has been published on this question, but it is important. In our study comparing the reliability of home, clinic and ambulatory readings separated by an interval of 2 weeks [4], we found that the SDD for the home readings was 5.6/4.6 mmHg, which was similar to the SDD for ambulatory readings (5.3/5.4 mmHg), and lower than for clinic readings (9.7/6.76 mmHg). The correlation coefficients for all three sets of measurements were very close (0.96/0.94 mmHg for home, 0.93/0.87 mmHg for ambulatory, and 0.94/0.87 mmHg for

clinic readings). The superior reproducibility of home and ambulatory measurements may be largely explained by the greater number of readings.

Why are the differences between home and clinic pressures greater in hypertensive than in normotensive subjects?

Figure 8.1 shows that in normotensive subjects the difference between clinic and home blood pressure is usually rather small, while it becomes progressively greater in individuals with higher clinic pressures. Similar differences are seen when clinic pressures are compared with average daytime ambulatory pressures, as shown in Fig. 8.3, which is based on results of six studies [3,4,15,19–21]. One explanation for this is that blood pressure variability increases as a function of the severity of hypertension. As we have seen in Chapter 4, however, this increase is relatively modest. Furthermore, when the range of pressures occurring during ambulatory monitoring (expressed as the difference between the pressures during the day and night) is related to the average clinic pressure, as shown in Fig. 8.4, hypertensive subjects show only slightly greater changes than normotensive subjects. Thus, the greater difference between home and clinic pressures in the hypertensive subjects appears to be out of proportion to their overall level of blood pressure variability.

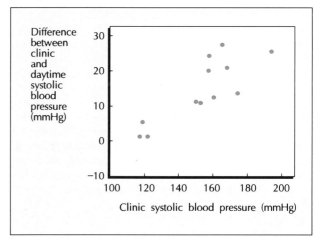

Fig. 8.3 Comparison of average levels of clinic and daytime ambulatory systolic blood pressure. Data from six published studies, three of which included more than one group of subjects [3,4,15,19–21].

It has been argued by Verdecchia *et al.* [26] that the difference between clinic and home blood pressures arises because the two measurements are taken at different times of day. They based this conclusion on a study in which clinic pressures were compared with home pressures recorded using an ambulatory monitor. They reported that clinic pressures were higher than the 24-hour average pressures, but not different from the home

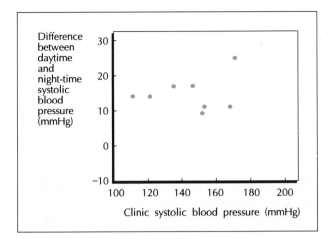

Fig. 8.4. Comparison of average levels of daytime and night-time systolic blood pressure measured during ambulatory monitoring. Data from five published studies, two of which included more than one group of subjects [10,22–25].

pressure recorded at the same time of day. It is incorrect, however, to equate ambulatory readings with self-recorded home readings, which by definition are taken with the subject seated and at rest.

An alternative explanation is that the higher clinic pressure occurs because some of the individuals with high clinic pressures have white coat hypertension. As with any other cardiovascular response, individuals must vary in the extent to which their blood pressure increases when it is checked in a clinic or physician's office. Therefore, if hypertension is initially diagnosed on the basis of a clinic reading above a certain cut-off point (as is virtually always the case), those individuals with the greatest pressor response to the clinic setting will be systematically selected out of the general population, and will be included with the 'true hypertensives'. Hence, the apparently greater difference between clinic and home pressures may be at least partly due to a selection bias occurring as a result of the way in which hypertension is diagnosed.

Factors influencing home blood pressure levels

As with any other measure of blood pressure, the level of pressure recorded during home monitoring shows considerable variability, and is likely to be influenced by a number of factors. The one that has received most attention is the time of day. In studies where morning and evening measurements were both taken, the evening readings tended to be higher for systolic pressure (by about 3 mmHg), but there were no consistent differences for diastolic pressure [5,18,26–28]. When pressures are recorded in the afternoon, they are likely to be the highest of the day [6,27].

There is relatively little information about whether pressures recorded on non-work days are the same as on work days. Welin *et al.* [5] concluded that there were no

differences, but in a study using ambulatory monitoring of blood pressure we found that the pressures at home in the evening were consistently higher if the patient had gone to work earlier in the day [29].

Diastolic blood pressure tends to fall after a meal, but the change is usually relatively small (around 3–5 mmHg), and systolic pressure is not affected [30]. If the subject has recently smoked a cigarette or drunk coffee, higher readings will be recorded [31]. Conversely, if the readings are taken soon after a period of heavy exercise, they are likely to be lower.

Technique of home blood pressure monitoring

Patients can be taught to record home blood pressures with reasonable accuracy. Gould *et al.* [32] compared self-recorded blood pressure taken with an aneroid sphygmomanometer with simultaneously determined intra-arterial pressure taken with an ambulatory monitor. There was no consistent difference in systolic pressure measured by the two techniques, and only 3 mmHg difference in diastolic pressure. There was also a reasonably good correlation between the self-monitored and intra-arterial pressure. Furthermore, the average home readings for systolic pressure were in good agreement with the average daytime ambulatory pressures, although home-measured diastolic pressures were less reliable. The act of inflating one's own sphygmomanometer cuff produces a transient elevation in blood pressure of around 12 mmHg, which lasts about 10 s; therefore, by the time the cuff is deflated to systolic pressure, the pressure may or may not have returned to baseline [33]. As shown in Fig. 8.5, this increase in blood pressure is due to the muscular activity involved in cuff inflation rather than to the compressing effects of the cuff on the arm.

If the cuff is deflated too quickly, however, it is possible that the pressure will not have returned to baseline, so that spuriously high systolic pressures may be recorded [34]. Patients should, therefore, be instructed to inflate the cuff more than 30 mmHg above the expected systolic pressure, and to deflate it slowly.

The different types of monitor available for home use have been described in Chapter 3. The most accurate is undoubtedly the mercury sphygmomanometer, but we usually recommend an aneroid sphygmomanometer as first choice. Such devices are reasonably accurate, and can very easily be checked by connecting the gauge to a mercury column with a Y-connector. Furthermore, they are the cheapest, and there is relatively little to go wrong. They do, however, require a certain degree of manual dexterity and hearing acuity. Models which have a D-ring cuff are easiest to operate. They can almost always be managed without problems by younger patients, but may cause problems in the elderly.

For patients who cannot use an aneroid or mercury recorder, one of the electronic devices may be prefer-

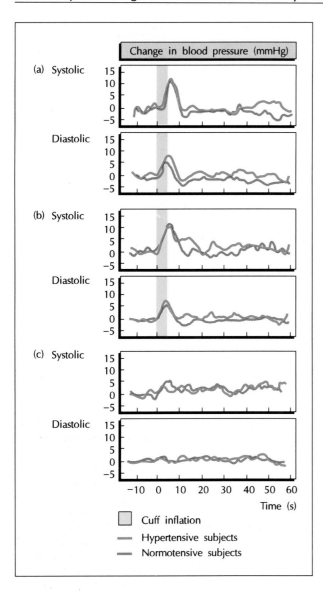

Fig. 8.5. Continuous non-invasive recording of systolic and diastolic pressures from a Finapres monitor. Pressure changes are relative to baseline levels 10 s before manoeuvre. (a) Effects of self-inflation of cuff worn on the opposite arm; (b) effects of self-inflation of cuff not worn by the subject; (c) effects of inflation of cuff by someone else. Reproduced with permission [33].

able. These are certainly easier to use, but, as reviewed above, are unpredictable in their accuracy. Hence it is essential to check the patient's machine on the patient, comparing it with simultaneously recorded auscultatory readings. Another potential advantage of such recorders is that they eliminate observer bias, particularly if they have a printer in addition to a visual display. It is worth noting that in a study of diabetic patients who monitored their blood glucose levels at home there was a tendency to report lower values than the machine displayed [35]; this was shown by inserting a memory chip in the machine without the patient's knowledge. It has not been established whether the same occurs with blood pressure monitoring, but it almost certainly does.

We generally instruct our patients to take two readings in both the morning and the evening and to measure their pressure 3 days a week for at least 2 weeks.

Home monitoring for the diagnosis of hypertension

In principle, the prediction of individual risk could be improved by using additional measures of pressure taken outside the clinic setting, such as home or ambulatory readings. Unfortunately, at present there are too few prospective data to allow determination of whether this is in fact the case. By providing a cheap and convenient method for increasing the number of readings, home monitoring has the potential of reducing the error in assessing the patient's true blood pressure, which is likely to be large if only a few clinic readings are used. It has been demonstrated that a better estimate of the true blood pressure can be obtained by taking a few readings on several different occasions than by taking a larger number on a single occasion (see Chapter 7).

No study has compared the prognostic values of home versus clinic pressure, and very few have related home pressures to the severity of target organ damage. Two studies that have done so [2,36] found that echocardiographically determined left ventricular mass correlated more closely with home pressure than with clinic pressure, as shown in Fig. 8.6. It should also be pointed out that many of the blood pressure readings recorded during the ambulatory monitoring studies cited above were taken while the patient was at home. In another study [37], however, we found that the correlation between ambulatory blood pressure and left ventricular hypertrophy was closer if the patient went to work during the day of recording than if he or she stayed at home.

Reference	N	Clinic		Home	
		SBP	DBP	SBP	DBP
Kleinert et al. [2]	45	0.22	0.07	0.45	0.40
Verdecchia et al. [36]	34	0.30	–	0.41	–

Fig. 8.6. Correlation between left ventricular mass and blood pressure measured either at home by self-monitoring or in the clinic. SBP, systolic blood pressure; DBP, diastolic blood pressure.

The other problem with home pressures is that they usually represent the level of pressure at the lower end of the waking range, when the patient is relatively relaxed. Thus, they do not necessarily provide a good guide to what happens to the patient's pressure when undergoing the stresses of daily life, such as during work. The pressure at work tends to be higher than the pressure at home, and is similar to the clinic pressure, although the latter is not necessarily a good guide to the level of pressure at work. In patients with mild hypertension we found only a moderate correlation between home and work blood pressures (r = 0.55 for systolic pressure and r = 0.65 for diastolic pressure) [2]. While the majority of subjects do show a higher pressure at work than at home [22], we have encountered others whose pressure is the same or even higher at home. This is particularly true of women with children [38].

A potential concern with the use of self-monitoring of blood pressure is that it will increase the patient's anxiety about his or her condition. In practice, however, this is not usually the case: in one study 70% of patients found the technique reassuring [28]. Nevertheless, there are some patients who become so obsessed with their blood pressure readings that self-monitoring becomes counter-productive.

As discussed above, clinic pressure tends to decrease with repeated visits. In a study by Padfield *et al.* [39] clinic blood pressure was measured on three occasions over a period of 4 weeks. At the first visit the patients were instructed in the use of home monitors, and asked to measure their pressure over 3 days. The pressure at the first clinic visit was higher than the home pressure, but there was no consistent difference between the final clinic pressure and the home pressure. The authors concluded that home blood pressure can be used to predict the results of repeated clinic measurements, and hence may be of use in making therapeutic decisions.

A practical schema for using home and ambulatory monitoring is shown in Fig. 8.7. Although this was originally derived for the evaluation of patients with apparently refractory hypertension [40], it can apply equally well to patients with mild hypertension. In the first step, if there is evidence of target organ damage attributable to the blood pressure from the clinical examination or laboratory tests, treatment can be started without any further evaluation of the severity of hypertension. If target organ damage is not detected, however, home monitoring is appropriate. If this reveals high readings, such as 140/90 mmHg or more, treatment may again be appropriate. If the pressures are less than this, however, an ambulatory recording will help to decide whether the clinic or the home pressures are closer to the true pressure.

Home monitoring for the evaluation of antihypertensive treatment

When patients are having their antihypertensive medication initiated or changed it is necessary to measure their blood pressure on repeated occasions. Home monitoring is ideal for this purpose, because it can obviate the need for many clinic visits. It has the additional advantage of avoiding the biases inherent in clinic pressure measurements.

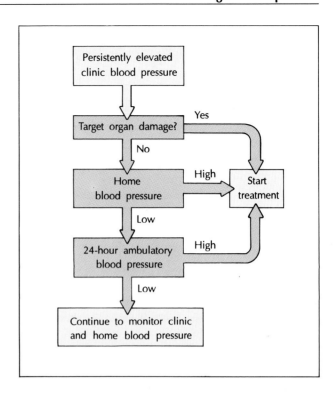

Fig. 8.7. Schema for the evaluation of hypertensive patients using clinic, home and ambulatory monitoring of blood pressure.

The greater statistical power inherent in the use of home recordings rather than clinic recordings for the evaluation of antihypertensive medications was well illustrated in a study by Ménard *et al.* [41]. They used a double-blind, within-patient crossover study, with 2-week periods of three different treatments (a diuretic, a beta blocker, and both together) separated by 2-week placebo periods. Blood pressure was measured in the clinic at the end of each treatment period, and patients also recorded their blood pressures at home using a semi-automatic machine. The effectiveness of all three treatment modes was similar for both measures of blood pressure. The greater number of home readings increased the sensitivity of the study to detect a difference in blood pressure between the treatment modalities. It was estimated that in order to detect a treatment effect of 5 mmHg, 27 patients would be needed if clinic blood pressures were used for the evaluation, but only 20 patients would be required if home pressures were used.

The validity of using home readings for monitoring the effects of treatment on blood pressure is well established. Cottier *et al.* [42] used small doses of clonidine and propranolol interspersed with blinded placebo periods, and found that home pressure was consistently lower during the periods of active treatment. Gould *et al.* [43] compared clinic, ambulatory (intra-arterial) and home pressures in two trials, one using verapamil, the other prazosin. For both agents, clinic pressure showed a greater change than home or ambulatory pressure as a result of treatment. However, there was no placebo phase, and so the greater fall in clinic pressure may have been partly due to a placebo response. The changes recorded by intra-arterial monitoring and by home monitoring were generally similar. In a study of 50 patients whose response to antihypertensive medication was monitored both at home and in the clinic, Ibrahim *et al.* [8] found that when there was a discrepancy between the two measures of blood pressure, ECG changes of LVH correlated most closely with the home pressure.

Effects on compliance

There is some evidence that the use of self-monitoring may improve patients' compliance with medication. Carnahan and Nugent [44] randomized 100 hypertensive subjects to two groups, one of which was trained in self-measurement of blood pressure while the other was not. Despite being prescribed the same medications, the clinic pressures decreased by 7/1 mmHg more in the self-monitoring group. Whether this was due to improved compliance or to a greater suppression of the white coat effect was not determined. A second study was performed by Haynes *et al.* [45], who selected 38 hypertensive patients who had complied poorly with prescribed medication. Half were asked to chart the number of pills they took every day and were also trained in self-measurement of blood pressure; the other half received no special instructions or training. Both blood pressure control and compliance (assessed by pill counts) improved significantly in the intervention group, but not in the other group.

Home blood pressures, target organ damage and prognosis

These subjects are reviewed in Chapter 13.

Official recommendations on the use of self-monitoring

Several national and international organizations have issued position papers on the use of home blood pressure monitoring. The National High Blood Pressure Education Program of the United States published one such paper in 1985 [46]. They concluded that all three types of device (mercury, aneroid and electronic) were reasonably accurate for home use, provided that they were properly calibrated and that the individual using them was appropriately trained. In addition, they suggested that self-monitoring might improve compliance, lead to a simplification of treatment programmes, and result in fewer office visits. They also expressed concern that some patients might become overly anxious about their blood pressure, or that they might regulate their own medication.

Similar recommendations have been issued by the World Hypertension League [47], who suggested applications

for both the diagnosis of hypertension and its treatment. For the former, they suggested an upper limit of normal for home readings of 140/90 mmHg. For the latter, a target pressure of less than 90 mmHg diastolic pressure was proposed. Their main concern was the possibility of inaccurate readings, as a result either of inadequate training or of inaccurate machines.

Summary and conclusions

Self-monitoring of blood pressure, usually carried out at home, is a practical and economical way of avoiding some of the pitfalls of relying exclusively on readings taken in the clinic. The number of readings can be much greater with self-monitoring, and they are also taken in a more natural environment. In hypertensive patients home pressure is almost always lower than clinic pressure, while in normotensive subjects they are about the same. This difference may be due in part to the white coat effect, because individuals who show a pressor response to the clinic setting will be selected out and labelled as hypertensive.

The readings obtained during home monitoring are usually representative of the generally relaxed home environment, and may be influenced by the time of day and by activities immediately preceding the reading, such as eating, smoking and exercise. They may not necessarily provide a good guide to the level of pressure at work. Patients can be taught to record home blood pressure with reasonable accuracy, although erroneous readings may be obtained if, for example, the cuff is deflated too rapidly. An aneroid or mercury sphygmomanometer is generally recommended, and in trained hands these are more accurate than electronic devices, many of which can give grossly inaccurate readings. However, electronic devices have two potential advantages: they can be used by patients whose hearing or manual dexterity is impaired, and they are immune to observer bias, particularly if they print out the readings.

Home monitoring may be useful both for the initial evaluation of hypertension and for following the response to treatment. However, very little information about the prognostic value of home monitoring is available. Most patients find that the use of home monitoring is reassuring, and compliance with prescribed treatment is generally improved.

While there is some overlap between the information obtained with home and ambulatory monitoring, there are also important differences. Home monitoring provides repeated measurements in the same situation over prolonged periods of time, and hence is ideally suited for monitoring changes in blood pressure induced by treatment or the progression of disease. Ambulatory monitoring, on the other hand, provides information about the diurnal profile of blood pressure, and hence may be more suited for the initial evaluation of the patient. The two techniques are therefore complementary.

References

1. AYMAN D, GOLDSHINE AD: Blood pressure determinations by patients with essential hypertension: the difference between clinic and home readings before treatment. *Am J Med Sci* 1940, 200:465–470.

2. KLEINERT HD, HARSHFIELD GA, PICKERING TG, ET AL: What is the value of home blood pressure measurement in patients with mild hypertension? *Hypertension* 1984, 6:574–578.

3. KENNY RA, BRENNAN M, O'MALLEY K, O'BRIEN E: Blood pressure measurements in borderline hypertension. *J Hypertens* 1987, 5 (suppl 5):483–485.

4. JAMES GD, PICKERING TG, YEE LS, HARSHFIELD GA, RIVA S, LARAGH JH: The reproducibility of average ambulatory, home, and clinic pressures. *Hypertension* 1988, 11:545–549.

5. WELIN L, SVARDSUDD K, TIBBLIN G: Home blood pressure measurements — feasibility and results compared to office measurements. *Acta Med Scand* 1982, 211:275–279.

6. BECKMAN M, PANFILOV V, SIVERTSSON R, SANNERSTEDT R, ANDERSON O: Blood pressure and heart rate recordings at home and at the clinic. *Acta Med Scand* 1981, 210:97–102.

7. JULIUS S, ELLIS CN, PASCUAL AV, ET AL: Home blood pressure determination. Value in borderline ('labile') hypertension. *JAMA* 1974, 229:663–666.

8. IBRAHIM MM, TARAZI RC, DUSTAN HP, GIFFORD RW: Electrocardiogram in evaluation of resistance to antihypertensive therapy. *Arch Intern Med* 1977, 137:1125–1129.

9. JULIUS S, MCGINN NF, HARBURG E, HOOBLER SW: Comparison of various clinical measurements of blood pressure with the self-determination technique in normotensive college males. *J Chron Dis* 1964, 17:391–396.

10. FLAPAN AD, STEWART SE, MCDOUGAL F, PADFIELD PL: Is self home-monitoring of blood pressure as good as 24-hour ambulatory monitoring? *J Hypertens* 1987, 5 (suppl 5):S491–S493.

11. LAUGHLIN KD, SHERRARD DH, FISHER L: Comparison of clinic and home blood pressure levels in essential hypertension and variables associated with clinic-home differences. *J Chron Dis* 1979, 33:197–206.

12. BIALY GB, RUDDY MC, MALKA ES, SILVAY LA, KAMALAKANNAN N: Comparison of office, home, and 24-hour ambulatory blood pressures in borderline and mild hypertension. *Angiology* 1988, 39:752–760.

13. BÄTTIG B, STEINER A, JECK T, VETTER W: Blood pressure self-monitoring in normotensive and hypertensive patients. *J Hypertens* 1989, 7 (suppl 3):S59–S63.

14. ABE H, YOKOUCHI M, SAITOH F, ET AL: Hypertensive complications and home blood pressure: comparison with blood pressure measured in the doctor's office. *J Clin Hypertens* 1987, 3:661–669.

15. O'BRIEN E, FITZGERALD D, O'MALLEY K: Comparison of clinic, home and ambulatory blood pressure measurements. *J Amb Mon* 1988, 1:285–291.

16. CORCORAN AC, DUSTAN HP, PAGE IH: The evaluation of antihypertensive procedures, with particular reference to their effects on blood pressure. *Ann Intern Med* 1955, 43:1161–1177.

17. BADSKJAER J, NIELSEN PE: Clinical experience using home readings in hypertensive subjects (indirect technique). *Acta Med Scand* 1982, (suppl 670):89–95.

18. LAUGHLIN KD, FISHER L, SHERRARD DJ: Blood pressure reductions during self-recording of home blood pressure. *Am Heart J* 1979, 98:629–634.

19. PICKERING TG, JAMES GD, BODDIE C, HARSHFIELD GA, BLANK S, LARAGH JH: How common is white coat hypertension? *JAMA* 1988, 259:225–228.

20. DUPONT AG, VANDERNIEPEN P, VOLCHAERT A, FINNE E, SIX RO: Noninvasive ambulatory monitoring of blood pressure in essential hypertension. Effect of age on variability and disparity. *J Clin Hypertens* 1986, 3:278–284.

21. DRAYER JIM, WEBER MA, HOEGER WJ: Whole-day BP monitoring in ambulatory normotensive men. *Arch Intern Med* 1985, 145:271–274.

22. PICKERING TG, HARSHFIELD GA, KLEINERT HD, BLANK S, LARAGH JH: Blood pressure during normal daily activities, sleep, and exercise. *JAMA* 1982, 247:992–996.

23. DRAYER JIM, WEBER MA: Definition of normalcy in whole-day ambulatory blood pressure monitoring. *Clin Exp Hypertens* [A] 1985, 7:195–204.

24. ZACHARIAH PK, SHEPS SG, SCHWARTZ GL, ET AL: Antihypertensive efficacy of lisinopril. Ambulatory blood pressure monitoring. *Am J Hypertens* 1988, 1 (suppl):274S–279S.

25. GOULD BA, MANN S, DAVIES AV, ALTMAN DG, RAFTERY EB: Does placebo lower blood-pressure? *Lancet* 1981, ii:1377–1381.

26. VERDECCHIA P, GATTESCHI DC, BENEMIO G, BOLDRINI F, GUERRERI M, PORCELLATI C: Home ambulatory blood pressure readings do not differ from clinic readings taken at the same time of day. *J Human Hypertens* 1988, 2:235–240.

27. ENGEL BT, BAARDER KR, GLASGOW MS: Behavioral treatment of high blood pressure. 1. Analyses of intra- and interdaily variations of blood pressure during a one-month, baseline period. *Psychosom Med* 1981, 43:255–270.

28. BURNS-COX CJ, RUSSELL REES J, WILSON RSE: Pilot study of home measurement of blood pressure by hypertensive patients. *Br Med J* 1975, 3:80.

29. PIEPER C, SCHNALL PL, WARREN K, PICKERING TG: Comparison of ambulatory blood pressure and heart rate on a work day and a non-work day: evidence of a 'carry-over effect'. (in press).

30. FAGAN TC, KONRAD KA, MAR JH, NELSON L: Effects of meals on hemodynamics: implications for antihypertensive drug studies. *Clin Pharmacol Ther* 1986, 39:255–260.

31. FREESTONE S, RAMSEY LE: Effect of coffee and cigarette smoking on the blood pressure of untreated and diuretic-treated hypertensive patients. *Am J Med* 1982, 73:348–353.

32. GOULD GA, KIESO HA, HORNUNG R, ALTMAN DG, CASHMAN PMM, RAFTERY EB: Assessment of the accuracy and role of self-recorded blood pressure in the management of hypertension. *Br Med J* 1982, 285:1691–1694.

33. VEERMAN D, VAN MONTFRANS GA, KAREMAKER J, WIELING W: Inflating one's own cuff does not increase self-recorded blood pressure. *J Hypertens* 1988, 6 (suppl 4):S77–S78.

34. VEERMAN D, VAN MONTFRANS GA, WIELING W: Effects of cuff inflation on self-recorded blood pressure. *Lancet* 1990, 335:451–453.

35. MAZZE RS, SHAMOON H, RASMANTIER R, ET AL: Reliability of blood glucose monitoring by patients with diabetes mellitus. *Am J Med* 1984, 77:211–217.

36. VERDECCHIA P, BENTIVOGLIO M, PROVVIDENZA M, SAVINO K, COREA L: Reliability of self-recorded arterial pressure in essential hypertension in relation to the stage of the disease. In *Blood Pressure Recording in the Clinical Management of Hypertension* edited by Germano G. Rome: Edizioni L. Pozzi, 1985, pp 40–42.

37. DEVEREUX RB, PICKERING TG, HARSHFIELD GA, ET AL: Left ventricular hypertrophy in patients with hypertension: importance of blood pressure response to regularly recurrent stress. *Circulation* 1983, 68:470–476.

38. JAMES GD, CATES EM, PICKERING TG, LARAGH JH: Parity and perceived job stress elevated blood pressure in young normotensive working women. *Am J Hypertens* 1988, 1:54A.

39. PADFIELD PL, LINDSAY BA, MCLAREN JA, PIRIE A, RADEMAKER M: Changing relation between home and clinic blood-pressure measurements: do home measurements predict clinic hypertension? *Lancet* 1987, ii:322–324.

40. PICKERING TG: Blood pressure monitoring outside the office for the evaluation of patients with resistant hypertension. *Hypertension* 1988, 11:96–100.

41. MÉNARD J, SERRURIER D, BAUTIER P, PLOUIN P-F, CORVOL P: Crossover design to test antihypertensive drugs with self-recorded blood pressure. *Hypertension* 1988, 11:153–159.

42. COTTIER C, JULIUS S, GAJENDRAGADLEAR SV, SCHORK MA: Usefulness of home BP determination in treating borderline hypertension. *JAMA* 1978, 248:535–558.

43. GOULD BA, HORNUNG RS, KIESO H, CASHMAN PMM, RAFTERY EB: An evaluation of self-recorded blood pressure during drug trials. *Hypertension* 1986, 8:267–271.

44. CARNAHAN JE, NUGENT CA: The effects of self-monitoring by patients on the control of hypertension. *Am J Med Sci* 1975, 269:69–73.

45. HAYNES RB, SACKETT DL, GIBSON ES, *ET AL.*: Improvement of medication compliance in uncontrolled hypertension. *Lancet* 1971, i:1265–1268.

46. HUNT JC, FROHLICH ED, MOSER M, ROCCELLA EJ, KEIGHLEY EA: Devices used for self-measurement of blood pressure. Revised statement of the National High Blood Pressure Education Program. *Arch Intern Med* 1985, 145:2231–2234.

47. Self-measurement of blood pressure: A statement by the World Hypertension League. *J Hypertens* 1988, 6:257–261.

9 Clinical aspects of ambulatory monitoring and determinants of normal ambulatory blood pressure

In this chapter some of the practical aspects of ambulatory monitoring that should be of particular help to the clinician will be reviewed. If a technique is to become clinically acceptable, it must satisfy a number of criteria, which are discussed below. Most importantly, it should be easy to perform, the data should be easy to interpret and the results should be reproducible. Blood pressure values obtained by ambulatory monitoring will be different from those obtained either by clinic measurement or by self-monitoring, and it is important to understand how the results obtained using the three techniques relate to each other. The diagnosis of hypertension has always rested on a dividing line separating 'normal' from 'abnormal', and the limits of normal ambulatory blood pressure need to be established. This chapter also reviews how normal ambulatory blood pressure values may vary according to demographic factors, such as age, race, obesity, and so forth. Finally, the potential clinical indications for ambulatory monitoring are reviewed.

The cost-effectiveness of ambulatory monitoring as a clinical diagnostic procedure and its potential impact on the health care system are discussed in Chapter 15.

Techniques of ambulatory monitoring

The original non-invasive ambulatory monitors were unreliable and bulky, and made a flatus-like noise when the cuff was being inflated. Times have changed, and the latest monitors are reliable, unobtrusive and virtually silent. An example (the Spacelabs 90207 recorder) is shown in Fig. 9.1. These developments have perfected the technique to the extent that it is suitable for routine clinical use.

Most of the commercially available non-invasive recorders are used in conjunction with an interface unit and personal computer. The latter is used both for pre-programming the recorder and for data storage and analysis. Before the subject is hooked up, new batteries are put in the recorder and the frequency of readings is programmed. In many cases this can be varied at different times of the day, for example in two periods corresponding roughly to waking hours and sleep (6.00 a.m. to 10.00 p.m. and 10.00 p.m. to 6.00 a.m.). In our centre, we prefer to have about 15 min between readings during the day and 30 min at night. This represents a compromise between what is scientifically desirable and what the subject finds tolerable. The subject is instructed to wear a loose-fitting shirt or blouse which buttons at the front, so that

the sleeve can go over the sphygmomanometer cuff and the connecting tube can be brought through the front of the shirt to connect with the recorder.

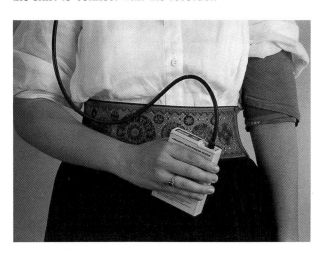

Fig. 9.1. The Spacelabs 90207 ambulatory monitor. The air hose is normally concealed under the subject's clothing, and the recorder is held in a carrying pouch.

When the subject arrives, the technician briefs him or her about the recording procedure. The cuff is usually applied to the non-dominant arm, and it is our custom first to measure the arm diameter so that the appropriate size of cuff can be used. For recorders that use the Korotkoff sound principle we palpate the brachial artery and then tape the microphone directly over it, about 5 cm above the elbow crease. Although some devices have a pouch for the microphone in the sphygmomanometer cuff, we believe that this increases the chance of the microphone being moved away from the brachial artery during the recording. The cuff is wrapped around the arm and taped down to maintain its position. A mercury column is then connected via a T-piece to the cuff, so that the cuff pressure can be monitored directly during the measurement process. The technician then takes three to five readings with the machine manually activated, while listening for Korotkoff sounds from a stethoscope placed distally to the cuff. Ideally, each of the two sets of readings should be within 5 mmHg of each other.

The subject is instructed to keep his or her arm still and in the neutral position during each cuff inflation, so that movement artefact is minimized and the cuff is always at heart level. Some recorders can be programmed to emit a tone just before the cuff is inflated, giving the subject time to position the arm correctly. We normally inform subjects that the recorder should be kept on for a full 24 h, although many investigators have used only daytime readings. When going to bed it is usually possible, and advisable, to take off the belt or strap holding the recorder and to place the recorder on the bedside table. With some types of recorder, such as those using the oscillometric technique, it is possible (though not necessarily desirable) for the subject to take off the recorder completely and re-attach it after showering or bathing. Subjects are also instructed about error codes, displayed by some recorders when it has not been possible to obtain a valid reading, for example because of arm movement or battery failure. It is also essential to give instructions about diary keeping, particularly for behavioural studies. Finally, we give our subjects a telephone number that they can use to speak to a technician or investigator if something goes wrong.

Ideally, the calibration procedure should be repeated when the subject returns to the laboratory 24 h later, but this may not always be practical. It is also helpful for the technician to review with the subject any problems that arose during the recording and the extent to which normal daily activities were interrupted, and also to go through the diary entries. Depending on the model, the recorder is then connected either directly or via an interface unit to the personal computer. The readings from the monitor are then downloaded into a data file where they can be edited and analysed using software provided by the equipment manufacturer. Most recorders can store

the data for a few days before they are transferred to computer files.

Evaluation of ambulatory recordings

One of the problems with 24-hour recorders is the large numbers of readings produced whose interpretation is not necessarily straightforward. Part of a typical printout of such data is shown in Fig. 9.2. As discussed in Chapters 4 and 5, the blood pressure may show substantial variations over 24 h, depending on the activity of the subject. A valid interpretation of such readings can only be made in the context of the circumstances in which they were recorded. Relatively little information is available about ambulatory blood pressures in normotensive people, although some norms have been proposed (and are discussed later). For the clinical evaluation of hypertensive patients, most physicians take the 24-hour or daytime average. The potential importance of including sleep readings is illustrated by the finding that in many conditions the blood pressure does not fall during the night (see Chapter 5).

Although the 24-hour average pressure is probably the most appropriate measure for establishing the diagnosis of hypertension, a number of caveats should be stated. First, the quality of the sleep readings varies considerably. In our experience, sleep may be interrupted by the inflation of the cuff, so that the variability of the blood pressure readings may be spuriously high. Consequently,

Reading #	Time	Systolic	Diastolic	MAP	Heart rate	Event code	Edit status	Diary activity
53	06:12	144	85	99	74	0		H,U,CH,H1,
54	06:27	130	71	84	70	0		H,U,W,H1,
55	06:42	129	61	78	55	0		H,S,R,H1,
56	06:57	181	93	124	69	0		H,U,CH,H1,
57	07:12	146	78	107	77	0		H,U,CH,H1,
58	07:27	148	72	87	60	0		H,S,E,H2,
59	07:42	145	74	96	79	0		H,U,CH,H1,
60	07:57	134	61	78	72	0		H,U,PH,H1,
61	08:12	132	67	90	72	0		H,U,W,H1,
62	08:27	134	55	72	56	0		H,S,MC,H2,
63	08:42	129	59	66	56	0		H,S,RD,H2,
64	08:57	120	63	77	55	0		SAME
66	09:14	135	65	85	65	0		H,U,BR,H1,
67	09:27	121	58	85	53	0		H,R,RD,H2,
68	09:42	126	67	78	58	0		SAME
69	09:57	122	63	74	56	0		H,R,R,H2,
70	10:12	124	62	79	53	0		H,R,R,H2,

Patient: AMY CHU — Ambulatory blood pressure data

Fig. 9.2. Part of a print-out of an ambulatory blood pressure report. All columns but the last are printed automatically. The last one requires manual data entry from the subject's diary, and the format can be varied by the user. The four items (H, U, CH, H1, etc.) are codes for location, position, activity and mood.

subjects disconnect the recorders at night. However, this problem is reduced significantly with the latest generation of recorders, which are quiet and unobtrusive. Another problem arises from the fact that the recorded blood pressure varies depending on which side the subject is lying (*see* Arm position, Chapter 2, p. 2.5). Second, the daytime level of blood pressure varies according to the activity of the subject during the recording period. Most important is the question whether the subject went to work or stayed at home: we have found that this variable alone may influence the average daytime pressure by 5 to 10 mmHg (see Chapter 11 and Fig. 11.2). Thus, we normally analyse the recordings in terms of the average 24-hour pressure, the average daytime pressure, and the pressures at work, at home and during sleep. It is also possible to analyse the effects of specific activities on blood pressure. The issues of data analysis are discussed further in Chapter 16.

How many readings are needed?

The interval between successive readings and the duration of the recording can be varied. It is important to develop some guidelines about what constitutes an adequate recording. Subjects frequently disconnect the recorder before the end of the full recording period, and readings are often missing as a result of, for example, movement artefact.

The question of the number of readings needed to characterize the blood pressure in a particular setting or situation has been examined by Llabre *et al.* [1], using generalizability (G) theory to study the reliability of blood pressure measurements. Based on a random-effect analysis of variance model [2], it allows for both systematic and random sources of variability; it is described in more detail in Chapter 16. For both normotensive and hypertensive individuals, Llabre's analysis indicated that five or six readings would provide an adequate representation (defined as a G* coefficient of 0.8 or higher) of the average pressure at work or at home.

Van Egeren [3] examined the effects of varying the frequency of readings by having subjects wear a monitor for two 24-hour periods, once with readings taken every 15 min during the day and 30 min at night, and once with readings every hour. The average levels of pressure at work, at home and during sleep were the same whichever sampling frequency was used, and the higher sampling frequency did not appear to alter the subjects' behaviour or activities. These results imply that if one is only interested in the average level of pressure during work, at home and during sleep, readings taken once an hour may suffice. However, when considered in the light of Llabre's results quoted above, the monitoring should last a minimum of 5 or 6 h for each period. From the other point of view, the results also show that more frequent readings (which we prefer) do not cause a major disruption of activities.

Di Rienzo *et al.* [4] came to similar conclusions using a different approach. They analysed continuous 24-hour intra-arterial recordings to investigate the effect of varying the intervals between readings on the estimates of the average level of pressure and its variability. Their analysis showed that the average level could be adequately characterized by readings every 60 min, but the variability (expressed as the standard deviation) required more frequent readings, taken every 5–15 min.

We recommend a minimum of 8 h (or 30 readings) for an adequate daytime recording and at least 3 h (or six readings) during sleep.

Reliability of ambulatory recordings

One of the rationales for making ambulatory recordings is that they will be more representative of an individual's true pressure than clinic measurements. A potential disadvantage is the likelihood of considerable variation in the individual's activities from one occasion to another. Therefore, it is very important to know how reliable (reproducible) such measurements are. This question was first addressed in one of the earliest papers on ambulatory monitoring, published by Sokolow's group in 1964 [5]. Subjects wore a Remler recorder for three successive days. The pressures on day 1 were significantly higher (by about 5 mmHg for systolic pressure and 3 mmHg for diastolic pressure) than on days 2 and 3, which were virtually identical. The differences were greater for the earlier part of the day than later on, by which time the subjects had presumably become habituated to the situation.

The results of 12 reliability studies are shown in Fig. 9.3. In each case, two 24-hour recordings were made without any intervention. All except one [6] used non-invasive ambulatory monitoring, and all except two [6,7] were made out of hospital in free-ranging subjects. The interval between the two recordings varied from 1 day [6] to 6 months [8]. The results are shown as the difference between the average daytime ambulatory pressure on the two occasions, the reliability (correlation) coefficient, and the SDD between them.

None of the studies showed any significant difference in the average ambulatory pressures between the two occasions over the short term (less than 6 months). The study with the longest interval (6 months) found a significant decrease in systolic pressure on the second occasion but no change in diastolic pressure. The finding of no consistent difference between recordings made on successive occasions does not in itself imply that there is good reliability but merely that there is no major order effect. However, five studies reported correlation coefficients between the two sets of readings ranging between 0.72 and 0.93 for systolic pressure and 0.53 and 0.87 for diastolic pressure (see Fig. 9.3). These results suggest that the reliability is acceptable and that a single recording can characterize an individual's average ambulatory pressure in the circumstance in which the recording was made. It has been argued, however, that product–moment (Pearson) correlations may not be the most appropriate method of evaluating the reproducibility of a test, as these are always expected to be high when

Authors	Subjects	Interval	Difference (T$_1$ − T$_2$) mmHg				Reliability	SDD (mmHg)
			Systolic	P	Diastolic	P		
Mann et al. [6]	17 HT	1 day	−	NS	−	NS	−	−
Marolf et al. [15]	31 HT	1 week	+ 1	NS	+ 2	NS	−	8/9
Prisant et al. (submitted)	73 HT	1 week	+ 0.4	NS	+ 0.5	NS	−	−
Drayer et al. [13]	6 HT	11 days	+ 2.0	NS	+ 1.0	NS	−	−
Weber et al. [7]	6 HT	2 weeks	− 3.0	NS	− 3.0	NS	0.72/0.76	−
James et al. [9]	14 HT/13 HT	2 weeks	+ 1.5	NS	+ 1.5	NS	0.93/0.87	5/5
Reeves et al. [16]	28 NT/HT	3 weeks	− 1.0	NS	− 1.0	NS	0.86/0.66	98
Fitzgerald et al. [12]	19 HT	4 weeks	+ 1.7	NS	+ 0.6	NS	−	−
Drayer and Weber [14]	56 HT	6 weeks	+ 1.0	NS	+ 1.0	NS	−	8/6*
Drayer et al. [13]	4 HT	9 weeks	0.0	NS	0.0	NS	−	−
Jacot des Combes et al. [10]	84 HT	3 months	0.0	NS	− 1.0	NS	0.82/0.78	−
Giaconi et al. [8]	22 HT	6 months	+ 4.0	< 0.005	+ 1.0	NS	0.81/0.53	−

NT, Normotensive; HT, hypertensive. *Estimated by Reeves [18].

Fig. 9.3. Studies of the reliability of daytime ambulatory blood pressure recordings.

the same variable is being measured [11]. A more appropriate technique may be one-way analysis of variance, which was used by Prisant *et al.* (submitted for publication).

The reliability of ambulatory blood pressure was recently reviewed by Reeves [17]. He concluded from six studies that it was not significantly better than the reliability of carefully measured clinic pressure, perhaps because the improved reliability resulting from the large number of ambulatory readings is offset by the poorer control compared with the clinic setting.

Four of the studies cited in Fig. 9.3 reported that, in contrast to the high reliability of the average levels of pressure, the within-subject variability of pressure (measured as the standard deviation or the coefficient of variation) showed poor reliability [7,9,10,12]. The reliability of the blood pressure variability can be improved if steps are taken to reduce the random error, for example by matching for equal numbers of readings on the two occasions and by using robust statistical techniques [18].

In marked contrast to the high level of reliability seen when the subjects' activities remain the same on the two recording days, we found that the blood pressure may be substantially lower on a non-work day than on a work day (by 7/6 mmHg in normotensive subjects) [19]. This is not an order effect, as subjects who wore the recorder on two work days separated by a non-work day still showed the lowest pressures on the non-work day (see Fig. 11.2).

The reliability of ambulatory blood pressures in children was studied by Langewitz *et al.* [20], who made 19 recordings in 86 children aged 10–12 years over a 2-year period. Each recording was made from 2.00 p.m. to 7.30 p.m., with readings taken every 30 min. The test–retest correlations for the average levels between successive recordings were 0.54 for systolic pressure and 0.36 for diastolic pressure. These relatively low correlations may be due to the relatively low range of pressures in this population and the relatively small number of readings taken per recording.

Studies comparing clinic, ambulatory and home pressures

Comparisons of the three methods of measuring blood pressure in the same patients have been reported in at least five studies [9,15,21–23]. In all of them, home blood pressures were recorded by the patients; two studies also included basal clinic pressures, measured after the patient had rested quietly for at least 30 min [22,23]. The average levels reported for clinic, home and ambulatory pressure are shown in Fig. 9.4. Several points can be made. First, in all five studies the differences between the three measures are greater for systolic pressure than for diastolic pressure. Second, the differences of systolic pressure between clinic and home readings are greater than between home and ambulatory readings; for the five hypertensive groups the average differences are 16 and 7 mmHg, respectively. Of the three measures of blood pressure, it is the clinic readings that are the 'odd man out'. Third, the situational differences in systolic pressure are greater in all the hypertensive groups than in the normotensive group (for which the corresponding values were 8 and − 3 mmHg).

One of the problems associated with clinic readings, which was particularly pronounced in the clinical trials of treatment of mild hypertension [24,25], is the tendency of blood pressure to fall with repeated visits. An important question concerns whether this change is a genuine one or merely a consequence of habituation to the clinic setting. We compared the reproducibility of three measures of blood pressure, clinic, ambulatory and home readings, taken on two occasions 2 weeks apart. Where possible, subjects went to work on both days during which they wore the ambulatory recorders [9]. The aver-

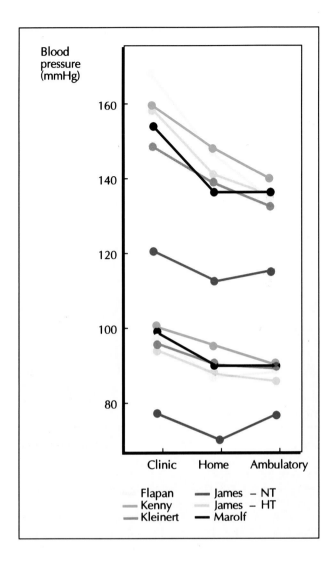

Fig. 9.4. Comparison of average values of clinic, home and daytime ambulatory pressures in five studies. Note that clinic readings are the highest, and that the difference is more pronounced for systolic than for diastolic pressure. NT, normotensive; HT, hypertensive.

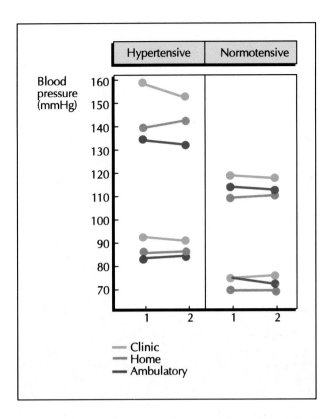

Fig. 9.5. Reproducibility of clinic, home and daytime ambulatory pressures measured on two occasions (1 and 2 in the figure) 2 weeks apart in hypertensive and normotensive subjects. Data from James *et al.* [9].

age levels of clinic systolic pressure decreased from the first to the second occasion in the hypertensives but not in the normotensives (Fig. 9.5). This change, however, was not associated with any change in either ambulatory or home pressures, both of which were highly reproducible. These findings indicate that the apparent fall in clinic pressures can be regarded as an artefact and is presumably an instance of regression to the mean. For all three measures of pressure, the correlation coefficients between the levels on the first and second occasion were high, ranging from 0.87 to 0.96.

A similar study was performed by Marolf *et al.* [15], who monitored 31 hypertensive patients over 7 days. Ambulatory pressures were recorded twice (on days 1 and 7), clinic pressures three times (on days 1, 4 and 7), and self-recorded home pressures every day. Like us, the authors found a significant decrease in clinic pressure (of 0/6 mmHg between day 1 and day 7), but no significant change in either of the other two measures. As shown in Fig. 9.5, the clinic pressures were the highest.

What is a normal ambulatory blood pressure?

Physicians who use ambulatory recordings for the diagnosis or evaluation of patients with mild hypertension are faced with the problem that there is no reason why any cut-off point based on clinic measurement of blood pressure should also be valid for ambulatory measurements. Therefore, some estimate of the range of ambulatory pressure in normotensive individuals is needed. Several issues here need to be resolved (Fig. 9.6). First, such data should be obtained from a representative sample of the population. Ideally, participants should be selected on a random basis, should include both sexes and a wide range of ages, and should be of different races. An important and as yet unresolved question is whether the subjects should be selected on the basis of their casual blood pressure (e.g. below 140/90 mmHg) or whether they should be selected randomly. Earlier studies have tended to use a high clinic pressure as an exclusionary criterion, but, given the unreliability of such measurements, it makes more sense to exclude only those individuals who either have known cardiovascular disease or are taking antihypertensive medication.

The second issue concerns the method of recording. Non-invasive recorders for which extensive validation data are available should be used. Subjects should be studied on a day that reflects their typical activities, which for most people is a work day. In addition, since sleep blood pressure may prove to have prognostic significance, the recordings should be carried out for a full 24 h.

Population studied
Selection criteria
Age, race, sex

Recording procedure
Type of recorder
Duration of recording (day or 24 hours)
Situation of recording (work day or non-work day)

Data analysis/summary statistics
Mean/median 24-hour average
Mean/median daytime average
Mesor/amplitude
Per cent readings above 140/90 mmHg (blood pressure load)

Definition of dividing line
Two standard deviations
90th percentile
Ambulatory blood pressure equivalent to clinic blood
     pressure of 140/90 mmHg
Cluster analysis

Fig. 9.6. Issues in defining normal ambulatory blood pressure.

The third issue concerns the way in which the data are analysed. As reviewed below, a number of summary statistics are currently being used, such as the average 24-hour level, mesor and amplitude, diastolic load, and so on.

Finally, some agreement needs to be reached on how the dividing line between normal and elevated pressures is determined. Some examples of measures that have been used include two standard deviations, the 90th percentile, and the ambulatory pressure equivalent to a clinic pressure of 140/90 mmHg. While several studies using non-invasive monitoring (including some from our own group) have included data from normotensive individuals, most are not very satisfactory. The average ambulatory blood pressures are shown in Fig. 9.7. The numbers of individuals studied are mostly quite small, and are not nec-

essarily representative of the general population. Most of the studies do not state how the subjects were selected; only one was based on a random population sample [32]. The upper limits of 24-hour ambulatory blood pressure shown in Fig. 9.7 are mostly two standard deviations above the average value, which is not necessarily the criterion used by the authors of these studies for defining the normal range. It is clear that the range in these numbers is considerable, and in many cases this particular criterion gives values that most people would consider unacceptably high. A study by Pomidossi et al. [34] used intra-arterial measurements and obtained somewhat lower values, but these are not included in the table because of the difference in recording techniques.

An alternative method of defining a normal 24-hour ambulatory blood pressure has been proposed by White and Morganroth [35], who suggested that the percentage of readings above 140/90 mmHg during waking hours and above 120/80 mmHg during sleep be used as a dividing line. They based this recommendation on a study of 20 normotensive and 20 hypertensive individuals (with clinic diastolic pressures of 94 mmHg or more) whose clinic and ambulatory pressures are shown in Fig. 9.8. On the basis of these data they proposed that 'mild' hypertension be defined by the presence of at least 50% of awake readings above 140/90 mmHg, and at least 50% of sleep readings above 120/80 mmHg.

The same concept has been used by Zachariah et al. [36]. They introduced the term 'blood pressure load', which they define as the percentage of 24-hour ambulatory systolic and diastolic pressure readings exceeding 140 and 90 mmHg, respectively. On the basis of two previous studies in normotensive subjects [27,37], they suggested that the upper limit of normal for the diastolic load should be 15%. However, although this corresponds to the average value reported in one of the studies [37], the range was very large (0–64%). This definition of normality brings back the old idea of the dividing line (discussed in Chapter 1). In the context of ambulatory recordings, it implies that there is a threshold phenomenon for the adverse effects of hypertension. With this type of analysis, two individuals may have the same percentage of readings above 140/90 mmHg but very different diurnal profiles and average 24-hour pressures.

The strongest argument in support of the use of systolic and diastolic loads rather than the average 24-hour level comes from a study by White et al. [38]. They related different measures of ambulatory pressure to three measures of cardiac structure and function (left ventricular mass index, peak left ventricular filling rate and left atrial index). Systolic load was defined as the percentage of readings above 140 mmHg during the day and above 120 mmHg at night; diastolic load was the percentage above 90 and 80 mmHg. In each case the correlation between blood pressure and the cardiac changes was closer for the load than for the average level of pressure.

A third method has been proposed by Baumgart et al. [39]. Its rationale is that we can, at present, only relate cardiovascular risk to clinic pressure, because this was used in all the epidemiological and actuarial stud-

| Author | Subjects | n | Average ambulatory blood pressure (mmHg) | | | Upper limit (mmHg) |
			Day	Night	24-hour	(24-hour)
Pickering et al. [26]	75% Men	25	117/80	98/64	114/77	138/91
Kennedy et al. [27]	Men < 30 years	19	119/67	108/58	115/64	133/72
	Men > 30 years	53	122/78	107/69	117/76	138/88
Wallace et al. [28]	Men < 30 years	25	120/74	105/62	115/70	130/82
	Men > 30 years	21	122/78	106/66	117/74	134/88
	Women < 30 years	25	110/77	97/64	106/73	123/85
	Women > 30 years	21	107/78	92/64	103/73	116/83
Drayer et al. [14]	Men	56	124/79	108/66	119/75	144/90
Pickering et al. [29]	70% Men	37	116/78	103/64	113/74	132/90*
Chau et al. [30]		72	125/69	108/60	119/65	140/78
O'Brien et al. [31]	Men/women	484	122/76	107/62	114/69	144/93
James et al. (submitted)	Women	121	119/75	105/61	115/72	131/84
						126/80*
Enstrom et al. [32]	Men	48	126/80	107/67	120/76	140/89
Lattuada et al. [33]	Men	131	–	–	121/74	141/88
	Women	115	–	–	116/74	138/88

*90th percentile.

Fig. 9.7. Ambulatory blood pressures in normal subjects.

| | Normotensives | | Hypertensives | |
	Systolic	Diastolic	Systolic	Diastolic
Clinic blood pressure	120 ± 9	79 ± 6	151 ± 10	101 ± 6
24-hour blood pressure	113 ± 9	72 ± 5	139 ± 12	87 ± 8
Awake blood pressure	118 ± 9	76 ± 5	149 ± 12	93 ± 9
% Readings > 140/90 mmHg	11 ± 2	10 ± 2	65 ± 7	59 ± 5
Sleep blood pressure	98 ± 9	60 ± 45	117 ± 9	77 ± 7
% Readings > 120/80 mmHg	5 ± 2	2 ± 1	52 ± 4	53 ± 6

Fig. 9.8. Office and ambulatory pressures in normotensive and hypertensive subjects. Data from White and Morganroth [35].

ies relating blood pressure to morbidity. Baumgart et al. derived a linear regression equation relating clinic pressure and ambulatory pressure from a large population of patients with varying degrees of hypertension in order to determine what level of daytime ambulatory pressure is equivalent to a generally accepted cut-off point for clinic pressure, such as 140/90 mmHg. For their data this was 135/84 mmHg; for a clinic pressure of 160/95 mmHg the corresponding value would be 146/87 mmHg. Similar regression equations have been published by Perloff et al. [40], which gave approximately the same ambulatory pressures for each clinic pressure. (For clinic pressures of 140/90 and 160/95 mmHg, the corresponding ambulatory pressures would be 133/83.5 and 145/87 mmHg.)

While superficially attractive, this type of approach has some limitations. First, it attempts to define the upper limit of 'normal' without studying normal subjects. The data from which the conventional clinic cut-off points

were derived were drawn from epidemiological surveys composed of unselected individuals (mostly normotensive), rather than patients referred to a clinic for evaluation of their blood pressure. In addition, this approach assumes that the association between clinic and ambulatory pressure is proportionally the same in normal and hypertensive subjects, whereas, as discussed in Chapter 8, we have reason to believe that there may be a selection bias favouring patients with white coat hypertension in referred populations. Nevertheless, it is of interest to note that estimated cut-off point (135/84 mmHg) is similar to the values estimated from the studies of normotensive subjects shown in Fig. 9.7.

Another method, proposed by Chau et al. [31], is based on cluster analysis, and uses both the clinic and ambulatory pressures to define the reference range. This technique has the advantage that it can allow for the fact that classification of subjects' pressures based on clinic readings may be quite inaccurate and permits the reallocation of individual subjects from one group to another. In a study of 72 normotensive subjects (clinic pressures below 140/90 mmHg) and 86 hypertensive patients (clinic pressures between 140/90 and 160/95 mmHg), Chau *et al.* reported daytime normal values of 126/73 mmHg before reallocation and 125/69 mmHg after reallocation. The corresponding night-time values were 111/63 and 108/60 mmHg. Although 49 of the 158 subjects were reallocated, the effects on the derived normal values were relatively modest.

The theoretically ideal way of defining the dividing line for a normal ambulatory pressure would be by relating it to morbidity, as was originally done for clinic pressure. In practice, this is unlikely to be achieved, but cross-sectional studies can be performed with target organ damage as the outcome measure in order to determine the upper limit of ambulatory pressure associated with an absence of target organ damage. This was attempted in the study by White *et al.* [38] referred to earlier, who concluded that patients with a systolic or diastolic load of less than 40% are unlikely to demonstrate any effects of hypertension on the heart.

Normal ambulatory blood pressure in special populations

When considering the definition of a normal ambulatory pressure it is important to recognize that a number of demographic variables may influence both the average level of blood pressure and its variations. Of these, the most important are age and sex, although once again the available data are relatively scarce. The factors known to influence ambulatory pressure in healthy individuals are discussed in the next sections.

Children

Relatively few studies of ambulatory monitoring have been reported in children. However, with the introduction of smaller and quieter recorders, this situation is likely to change. Studies using the earlier and bulkier recorders, such as the Avionics Pressurometer 3 [41–43] and the Spacelabs 5200 [44], found that the recorders were as reliable in children aged 10 years or more as in adults, and as well tolerated. Two studies have described diurnal blood pressure patterns in healthy normotensive children during a school day. In the first, by Egger *et al.* [44], 20 girls and 23 boys aged 10–16 years showed similar diurnal patterns, with a nocturnal decrease in blood pressure of 11% in the girls and 9% in the boys. Blood pressure was somewhat higher in the boys (see Fig. 9.9), but the boys were studied on a school day, while the girls were studied on a weekend day. Ambulatory blood pressure was positively correlated with the age, body weight and height of the children, confirming data obtained from casual readings [45].

In the second study, Wilson *et al.* [42] reported data from 178 adolescents aged 13–19 years (60% of whom were girls) during a school day. Subjects were classified

as cases if they had at least one hypertensive parent and as controls if both parents were normotensive. The main objective of the study was to investigate whether ambulatory pressure gave a better discrimination between cases and controls than casual pressure (measured as the average of four readings taken at the start of the ambulatory recording). There was also no significant difference in casual systolic pressure between the two groups, and a marginally ($P = 0.053$) significant difference in diastolic pressure (see Fig. 9.9). No significant difference was noted in the unadjusted ambulatory pressure between the two groups. However, when the influence of other variables was taken into account by using stepwise logistic regression analysis, the difference of the casual blood pressure was no longer significant, but ambulatory diastolic pressure was significantly ($P = 0.005$) higher in the cases than in the controls. The difference between the unadjusted and adjusted analyses was explained by the fact that the cases were significantly less active than the controls during the school hours.

		Daytime	Night-time	24-hour average
All	Systolic	123 ± 18	110 ± 12	118 ± 16
	Diastolic	71 ± 7	64 ± 10	68 ± 7
Boys	Systolic	130 ± 21	117 ± 14	126 ± 17
	Diastolic	74 ± 8	68 ± 12	72 ± 8
Girls	Systolic	113 ± 11	102 ± 7	109 ± 9
	Diastolic	68 ± 5	60 ± 6	64 ± 5
Boys were studied on a school day, girls at a weekend.				

Fig. 9.9. Twenty-four-hour blood pressure values in normal boys and girls. Data from Egger *et al.* [46].

A third study compared 10 hypertensive and nine normotensive adolescents [43]. The difference between the two groups was greatest during school hours (15/1 mmHg) and least during sleep (9/−5 mmHg). The authors recommended that measurements made at school were advisable for diagnosing hypertension, which is in agreement with our recommendation to monitor adults on a workday.

Finally, Harshfield *et al.* [46] reported a study of 199 adolescents with an average age of 13 years, but did not specify whether the recordings were made on a school day or not. The average daytime ambulatory pressure was 116/69 mmHg in both black and white children, although there was a different pattern in black and white boys during sleep, as described later.

Elderly

The diurnal rhythm of blood pressure does not appear to differ greatly between younger and older subjects [27,47]. This is somewhat unexpected, since older subjects tend to sleep less and have a more fragmented sleep pattern [48]. However, there may be some individuals whose pressure does not fall during the night: in a study of 21 elderly hypertensives (mean age 70 years) Kobrin *et al.* [49] found that 14 showed a normal diurnal rhythm of blood pressure but seven had similar levels of pressure throughout the 24 hour period. Interestingly, these patients all had evidence of cardiovascular disease, whereas this was true of fewer than half of the patients whose blood pressure showed a normal fall during the night. The variability of systolic pressure, but not necessarily of diastolic pressure, tends to increase with age [47,50].

The correlation between clinic and ambulatory 24-hour blood pressure may be less good in the elderly. Drayer *et al.* [47] reported correlations of 0.69 and 0.71 (systolic and diastolic pressure) in patients aged less than 55 years, and 0.42 and 0.43 in those aged over 55 years. Furthermore, the difference between clinic and ambulatory pressures may be greater in elderly than in young hypertensive individuals, according to some authors [50] but not others [51]. This, of course, may result in a greater misclassification of such patients: in one study 42% of elderly subjects classified as hypertensive on the basis of their clinic pressures were normotensive on ambulatory monitoring [52]. This study was described in more detail in Chapter 7.

Sex
Relatively little information is available concerning the difference in ambulatory blood pressure between men and women, but what there is indicates that pressure is lower in women, at any rate before the menopause. Adolescent boys have been reported to have slightly higher systolic ambulatory pressures than girls (by 4 mmHg) but similar diastolic pressures [46]. In the Allied Irish Bank study [31], of which only preliminary results are currently available, the average 24-hour pressure for men was 9/6 mmHg higher than for women; the difference was greatest between the ages of 17 and 45 years, and was not significant above the age of 45. The study reported by Wallace *et al.* [28] also found higher pressures in men. These studies were performed in whites, but it has also been shown that black men have higher ambulatory pressures than black women [53].

Pregnant women
The measurement of blood pressure during pregnancy is of particular importance because hypertension may put both the mother and the fetus at risk. As with hypertension in the non-pregnant state, the relationship between risk and blood pressure is a continual one [54]. The situation is complicated by the fact that blood pressure decreases during normal pregnancy, so that repeated and reliable monitoring is desirable[1]. In a normal pregnancy this decrease reaches 10–15 mmHg in systolic and diastolic pressure by 16–20 weeks with a slow return to non-pregnant levels thereafter [55]. In women with essential

hypertension this fall may be even larger, but if this does not occur the prognosis is poor [56].

As clinically significant changes of pressure may occur over a relatively short period of time, a good case can be made for supplementing the clinic measurements of blood pressure with home or ambulatory monitoring. A potential problem with automatic monitors is the difficulty of measuring diastolic pressure accurately by the auscultatory method during pregnancy. Phase 4 of the Korotkoff sound is usually recommended (see Chapter 2), although most of the automatic devices that use the Korotkoff sound method give readings based on phase 5. Whether or not this is a problem for the automatic monitoring of blood pressure during pregnancy remains to be established.

Surprisingly little use has been made of self-monitoring of blood pressure during pregnancy. Rayburn *et al.* [57] described their experience in an obstetric clinic where self-monitoring was standard practice for hypertensive women. Patients were trained to take readings in the morning and afternoon using an aneroid sphygmomanometer. As with other hypertensive patients (see Chapter 8), the home pressures were usually lower than the clinic pressures (in 52% of patients) and only rarely higher (in 20% of patients). Rayburn *et al.* concluded that patients with chronic hypertension cannot be managed effectively without home monitoring.

The role of ambulatory monitoring in pregnant women has also been relatively neglected. However, as described in Chapter 5, pre-eclamptic toxaemia is one of the numerous conditions in which the normal diurnal rhythm of blood pressure may be absent or even reversed [58–60]. Data for the range of ambulatory pressures in normotensive pregnant women are scanty, but in a small study of 11 women in their third trimester, Margulies *et al.* [61] quote values of 110 ± 7 mmHg during waking hours and 71 ± 5 mmHg during sleep, giving a nocturnal decrease in pressure of 12%. The highest pressures occurred between 7.00 p.m. and 10.00 p.m. This is in contrast to the normal diurnal patterns seen in normotensive pregnancy and in patients with essential hypertension. Ambulatory monitoring, therefore, has the potential to discriminate between patients with pre-eclampsia and essential hypertension. So far, only a few patients have been studied with this technique, and there is no prognostic information relating to these differences, but it is tempting to hypothesize that reversal of the normal diurnal rhythm is associated with a poor prognosis.

Race
In westernized societies the prevalence of hypertension is much higher in blacks than in whites [62], but despite extensive investigation the reason for this remains unexplained [63]. The finding of a difference in the diurnal pattern of blood pressure between blacks and whites is, therefore, of considerable interest. Harshfield *et al.* [46] performed ambulatory blood pressure recordings in 92 white and 107 black adolescents aged 10–15 years. The

---

[1]The unreliability of clinic readings in this context is dramatically illustrated in Fig. 2.8.

two groups had similar blood pressures while awake, but black boys had significantly higher systolic and diastolic pressure while asleep (by about 5 mmHg). The same differences were not seen for heart rate. In girls the nocturnal fall in blood pressure was the same for both races. A diminished nocturnal fall in blood pressure has been reported for adult blacks of both sexes in studies performed in the United States using non-invasive monitors [53,64]. However, another study performed in Europe, using invasive recordings, failed to find a difference in the diurnal patterns of black adults and white adults [65]. That these different findings are due to environmental factors rather than to the method of recording or genetic factors is suggested by the finding that blacks in Barbados, when studied using the same technique as in the United States, do show a normal nocturnal decline in blood pressure [66].

Should the normal range of ambulatory pressure be standardized to demographic variables?

It is clear from the previous section that the average ambulatory pressure in healthy individuals varies according to a number of demographic and other factors. Thus, pre-menopausal women have values 5–10 mmHg lower than men of the same age. This raises the question whether the dividing line for the upper limit of 'normal' ambulatory pressure should be lower for women than for men. Actually, this applies equally well to clinic pressures, where women also tend to have lower values than men [67]. In this case, however, such demographic factors are not normally taken into consideration when deciding what the dividing line should be, except in the case of children.

On balance, it would seem appropriate to follow the same policy for ambulatory as for clinic pressures. Thus, it is likely that the damage done by hypertension is determined more by the absolute level of pressure than by whether it is outside the 'normal' range for a particular subgroup of the population. Pre-menopausal women not only have lower clinic and ambulatory blood pressures than men but, for any given level of (clinic) blood pressure, are also at lower risk of morbidity, as shown by the Framingham Heart Study [67] and the Medical Research Council trial of the treatment of mild hypertension [68], to give but two examples. If the dividing line for ambulatory blood pressure is set lower for women than for men, it would mean that a woman with a blood pressure of, for example, 138/88 mmHg would be treated, whereas a man with the same absolute level of pressure would not. Clearly, this makes no sense.

The second reason for recommending a single dividing line is more practical. If we adopt a different dividing line for men and women, should we not logically also standardize it for age and race as well? The potential permutations and combinations are endless.

Other influences on ambulatory blood pressure

Family history
Since hypertension is probably about 50% genetically determined [69], an understanding of the effects of a positive family history on the pattern of ambulatory pressure would be of considerable interest. In their study of black and white adolescents, Harshfield *et al.* (submitted for publication) found that children with a positive family history had a slightly higher casual systolic pressure. Although family history appeared to influence the ambulatory blood pressure of boys, the findings were somewhat paradoxical. White boys with a positive family history had a slightly higher 24-hour systolic pressure (by 3 mmHg) than those without, but the opposite was true for black boys: systolic pressure was 6 mmHg lower in those with a positive family history. In this study, however, the black boys with normotensive parents tended to be a little older, taller and heavier, which might account for the differences in blood pressure. No differences were seen for girls of either race. It should be noted that adolescence is a period of rapid change, and differences in blood pressure may merely reflect differences in physical maturation.

The work of Wilson *et al.* [42], showing that children with a positive family history had higher daytime ambulatory pressures than those without, has been described earlier.

A recent study by Ravogli *et al.* [71] is of particular interest in this respect. Three groups of normotensive young adults (average age 22 years) with no, one or both parents who were hypertensive were studied by ambulatory monitoring and reactivity testing. Subjects with two hypertensive parents had higher casual and ambulatory pressures (both during the day and night) than subjects with a negative family history, but no difference was found in short-term variability or reactivity. This study suggests that a higher baseline pressure, rather than an increased reactivity, is inherited.

Renin status
Harshfield *et al.* [70] categorized 159 black and white adolescents according to their renin–sodium profile (low-, normal- or high-renin). They found that casual and ambulatory daytime blood pressures were similar in all three groups, but the high-renin group showed both a smaller fall in and a greater variability of blood pressure during sleep. Since renin secretion is typically highest at night (see Chapter 5), it is possible that the higher renin levels in the high-renin group were sufficient to lessen the nocturnal fall in blood pressure. It is, however, also possible that the greater variability of blood pressure during the night reflects a more disrupted sleep.

Physical fitness

Several studies have shown that fitness is associated with lower resting blood pressure [72]. In a study of black and white adolescent boys and girls Harshfield *et al.* [73] classified individuals as 'more fit' or 'less fit' according to their maximum oxygen consumption during exercise testing. In girls of both races and in black boys increased fitness was associated with lower ambulatory pressures both when awake and when asleep; no such association was found in white boys.

Obesity

The relationship between obesity and ambulatory pressure has received little attention. In a study of non-obese men, we used several measures of blood pressure, which included an initial screening casual reading, a subsequent reading taken by a nurse at the worksite, and ambulatory pressures [74]. Body fat and its distribution were evaluated by height, weight, body mass index, and waist and hip circumferences. In these subjects the highest blood pressures were the ambulatory work readings, while the home readings were higher than the screening or nurse readings. Body weight and both waist and hip circumferences were all significantly correlated with screening, nurse and sleep blood pressures, but not with home or work pressures. Our interpretation of this somewhat unexpected finding, which is in marked contrast with the associations reported between ambulatory pressure and target organ damage (see Chapter 13), is that in situations where the blood pressure is the dependent variable, correlations with other variables may be closest for 'basal' measures of pressure, and may be obscured by the effects of daily activities on blood pressure.

Clinical indications for ambulatory monitoring

While some would argue that there are, at present, no clearly defined clinical indications for ambulatory monitoring, there are a number of situations where a better knowledge of what is happening to a patient's blood pressure over 24 h might lead to different therapeutic decisions (see Fig. 9.10). The potential costs and benefits of performing ambulatory monitoring studies are analysed in detail in Chapter 15. Here, we shall focus on the more common clinical indications.

- Evaluation of newly diagnosed hypertensives without target organ damage
- Disparity between clinic and home pressures
- Resistant hypertension
- Intermittent symptoms possibly related to blood pressure changes
- Episodic hypertension
- Orthostatic hypotension/autonomic neuropathy
- Evaluation of treatment

Fig. 9.10. Clinical indications for ambulatory monitoring.

Evaluation of newly diagnosed hypertensives without target organ damage

In many patients, particularly those with mild hypertension, the only detectable abnormality is an elevated blood pressure, so that the therapeutic decisions that are finally reached will depend on how the blood pressure is evaluated. While the first approach should be to obtain clinic readings on more than one occasion, it may be helpful to supplement these with ambulatory recordings.

As shown schematically in Fig. 9.11, ambulatory monitoring may reveal a spectrum of diurnal patterns of blood pressure in patients with elevated clinic readings. First, some patients will have white coat hypertension (Fig. 9.11b), with normal ambulatory readings. Patients with persistently elevated ambulatory pressures, or sustained hypertension, may be subdivided into those who show a normal nocturnal fall in pressure, the 'dippers' (Fig. 9.11c), and those whose pressure remains high, the 'non-dippers' (Fig. 9.11d). While the pathological significance of these different patterns is poorly understood, it is reasonable to propose that the treatment of a non-dipper should be more aggressive than that of a patient with white coat hypertension. This issue is discussed in Chapter 10.

Disparity between clinic and home pressures

In any hypertensive patient, the finding of a major disparity between clinic and home readings (e.g. more than 15 mmHg) poses the question: which set of readings is closer to the true blood pressure? This can be resolved by an ambulatory recording.

Evaluation of 'resistant' hypertension

The patient whose clinic pressure remains high despite being prescribed multiple medications presents a not-uncommon clinical problem. Although in some cases this may be the result of a genuinely resistant hypertension, in others it may be due to non-compliance, or to an exaggerated white coat effect. Thus, the patient whose blood pressures are illustrated in Fig. 7.6 had clinic pressures that were persistently around 180/120 mmHg but normal ambulatory pressures. In one of the earliest clinical studies using intra-arterial ambulatory monitoring, Littler *et al.* [75] evaluated eight patients who had persistently elevated clinic pressures (averaging 191/114 mmHg) but no evidence of target organ damage. These patients were compared with eight unselected patients who also underwent ambulatory monitoring. The discrepancy between the clinic and ambulatory pressures was much greater in the former group (19/31 versus 8/12 mmHg). In a study of 15 patients with apparently resistant hypertension, Mejia *et al.* [76] found that six patients had an element of white coat hypertension, with a clinic systolic pressure at least 20 mmHg higher than the home pressures. Two others had 'cuff-inflation' hypertension, described in Chapter 7.

The best clue to this exaggerated white coat effect is a persistently elevated clinic pressure in the absence of target organ damage. Such patients can be evaluated either with ambulatory monitoring or initially with home monitoring.

Intermittent symptoms possibly related to blood pressure

Episodes of light-headedness, particularly in patients who are on antihypertensive medication, may be a manifestation of transient hypotension. This can readily be detected by ambulatory monitoring [77]. However, if such episodes are brief they may be missed if readings are taken every 15 min.

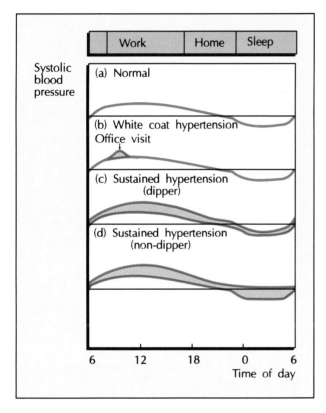

Fig. 9.11. Different diurnal blood pressure patterns which may be revealed by ambulatory monitoring in patients with hypertension suspected on the basis of clinic readings. The grey areas show the degree of elevation above normal.

Episodic hypertension

Episodic symptoms accompanied by transient elevations in blood pressure may occur in a variety of conditions. The use of ambulatory monitoring has been reported in patients with phaeochromocytoma [78] and panic attacks [79].

Orthostatic hypotension/autonomic neuropathy

In cases of orthostatic hypotension ambulatory monitoring may be extremely helpful, because supine hypertension is often also present, particularly during the night

(see Chapter 5). An example of this is shown in Fig. 9.12: there are huge swings of blood pressure during the day, depending to a large extent on changes in physical activity, and relatively stable but high pressures at night. In marked contrast, heart rate is relatively constant throughout the day and night.

Treatment of such patients usually involves administration of pressor drugs that, while alleviating the orthostatic hypotension, may exacerbate the nocturnal hypertension. Optimal treatment, therefore, requires a balance between the two, which can only be properly evaluated with ambulatory monitoring.

Patients with hypertension and diabetic autonomic neuropathy may also benefit from such an evaluation, which may demonstrate a paroxysmal elevation in pressure during the night.

Evaluation of treatment

Treatment evaluation is discussed in Chapter 10.

Summary and conclusions

Non-invasive ambulatory monitoring has now reached a level of technological development that makes it potentially applicable to routine clinical purposes; it can also provide better estimates of both the true blood pressure and its variability than conventional clinic measurements. A full 24-hour recording is recommended, with readings taken every 15–20 min, on a day that is representative of the patient's usual daily activities. Several studies have documented the reliability of ambulatory blood pressure recordings over intervals ranging from 1 day to 6 months. Studies comparing the three potential clinical methods of assessing blood pressure – clinic, home and ambulatory recordings – have shown that in hypertensive patients the clinic readings are consistently higher than readings obtained with the other two methods. The tendency for clinic readings to fall on successive occasions is not accompanied by similar changes in home or ambulatory readings.

No agreement has been reached about the upper limit of normal ambulatory blood pressure or about how it should be defined. The 95th percentile of the range in 'normotensive' subjects gives a value that is probably too high, which is perhaps not surprising since hypertension affects more than 5% of the population. More population-based studies are needed in this area. Although the normal values are affected by a number of factors such as age, sex, race, fitness and obesity, it is recommended that any definition of the normal range should be made independently of these variables.

The main clinical application of ambulatory monitoring is likely to be the evaluation of patients with mild hypertension who do not have evidence of target organ damage, and in whom there is often a disparity between the clinic and home readings. Other applications include the evaluation of resistant hypertension and of patients with intermittent symptoms which could be attributable

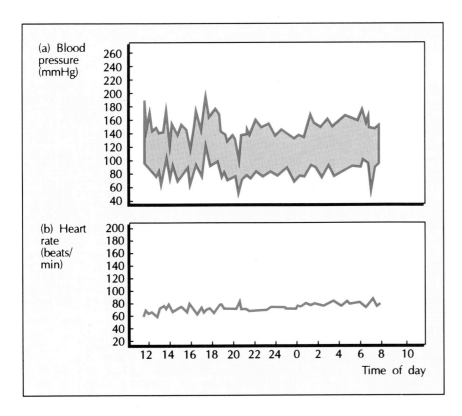

Fig. 9.12. Ambulatory recording of blood pressure (a) and heart rate (b) in a patient with idiopathic orthostatic hypotension.

to episodes of hypertension or hypotension. These are most marked in patients with autonomic neuropathy.

References

1. LLABRE MM, IRONSON GH, SPITZER SB, GELLMAN MD, WEIDLER DJ, SCHNEIDERMAN N: Blood pressure stability of normotensives and mild hypertensives in different settings. *Health Psychol* 1988, 7 (suppl):127–137.

2. CRONBACH LJ, GLASER GC, NANDA H, RAJARATRIAN N: *The Dependability of Behavioral Measurements.* New York: Wiley, 1972.

3. VAN EGEREN LF: Repeated measurements of ambulatory blood pressure. *J Hypertens* 1988, 6:753–755.

4. DI RIENZO M, GRASSI G, GREGORINI L, PEDOTTI A, MANCIA G: Continuous vs intermittent blood pressure measurements in estimating 24 hours average blood pressure. *Hypertension* 1983, 5:264–269.

5. KAIN HK, HINMAN AT, SOKOLOW M: Arterial blood pressure measurements with a portable recorder in hypertensive patients. I. Variability and correlation with 'casual' pressures. *Circulation* 1964, 30:882–892.

6. MANN S, MILLER-CRAIG WM, BALASUBRAMANIAN V, CASHMAN PMM, RAFTERY EB: Ambulant blood pressure: reproducibility and the assessment of interventions. *Clin Sci* 1980, 59:497–500.

7. WEBER MA, DRAYER JIM, WYLE GA, YOUNG JL: Reproducibility of the whole-day blood pressure pattern in essential hypertension. *Clin Exp Hypertens [A]* 1982, A4:1377–1390.

8. GIACONI S, PALOMBO C, GENOVESI-EBERT A, ET AL: Long-term reproducibility and evaluation of seasonal influences on blood pressure monitoring. *J Hypertens* 1988, 6 (suppl 4):S64–S66.

9. JAMES GD, PICKERING TG, YEE LS, ET AL: The reproducibility of average ambulatory, home, and clinic pressures. *Hypertension* 1988, 11:545–549.

10. JACOT DES COMBES B, PORCHET M, WAEBER G, BRUNNER HR: Ambulatory blood pressure recordings. Reproducibility and unpredictability. *Hypertension* 1984, 6:C110–C115.

11. BLAND JM, ALTMAN DG: Statistical methods for assessing agreement between two methods of clinic measurements. *Lancet* 1986, i:307–310.

12. FITZGERALD DJ, O'MALLEY K, O'BRIEN ET: Reproducibility of ambulatory blood pressure recordings. In *Ambulatory Blood Pressure Monitoring* edited by Weber MA, Drayer JIM. Darmstadt: Steinkopff, 1984, pp 71–74.

13. DRAYER JIM, WEBER MA, DEYOUNG JL, BREWER DD: Long-term BP monitoring in the evaluation of antihypertensive therapy. *Arch Intern Med* 1983, 143:898–901.

14. DRAYER JIM, WEBER MA: Reproducibility of blood pressure values in normotensive subjects. *Clin Exp Hypertens [A]* 1985, 7:417–422.

15. MAROLF AP, HANY S, BÄTTIG B, VETTER W: Comparison of casual, ambulatory and self-determined blood pressure measurement. *Nephron* 1987, 47 (suppl 1):142–145.

16. REEVES RA, LEENEN FHH, JOYNER CD: Reproducibility of office, exercise and ambulatory blood pressure and echocardiographic left ventricular mass in borderline hypertension. *Clin Invest Med* (in press).

17. REEVES RA: Stability of ambulatory blood pressure: implications for diagnosis of hypertension. *Clin Invest Med* (in press).

18. JAMES GD, PICKERING TG, SCHLUSSEL YR, ET AL: Measures of reproducibility of blood pressure variability measured by non-invasive ambulatory blood pressure monitors. *J Amb Mon* 1900, 3:139–147.

19. PIEPER C, SCHNALL P, WARREN K, PICKERING TG: Comparison of ambulatory blood pressure and heart rate on a work day and a non-work day: evidence of a 'carry-over effect'. *Am J Hypertens* (in press).

20. LANGEWITZ W, VON EIFF AW, GOGOLIN E ET AL: Reliability and validity of ambulatory blood pressure recording in children. *Clin Exp Hypertens [A]* 1985, 7:217–225.

21. KLEINERT HD, HARSHFIELD GA, PICKERING TG ET AL: **What is the value of home blood pressure measurement in patients with mild hypertension?** *Hypertension* 1984, 6:574–578.

22. KENNY RA, BRENNAN M, O'MALLEY K, O'BRIEN E. **Blood pressure measurements in borderline hypertension.** *J Hypertens* 1987, 5 (suppl 5):S483–S485.

23. FLAPAN AD, STEWART SE, MCDOUGAL F, PADFIELD PL: **Is self home-monitoring of blood pressure as good as 24-hour ambulatory monitoring?** *J Hypertens* 1987, 5 (suppl 5):S491–S493.

24. MANAGEMENT COMMITTEE OF THE AUSTRALIAN THERAPEUTIC TRIAL IN MILD HYPERTENSION: **Untreated mild hypertension.** *Lancet*, 1982, i:185–191.

25. MEDICAL RESEARCH COUNCIL WORKING PARTY: **MRC Trial of treatment of mild hypertension: principal results.** *Br Med J* 1985, 291:97–104.

26. PICKERING TG, HARSHFIELD GA, KLEINERT HD, BLANK S, LARAGH JH: **Blood pressure during normal daily activities, sleep, and exercise. Comparison of values in normal and hypertensive subjects.** *JAMA* 1982, 247:992–994.

27. KENNEDY HL, HORAN MJ, SPRAGUE MK, PADGETT NE, SHRIVER KK: **Ambulatory blood pressure in healthy normotensive males.** *Am Heart J* 1983, 106:717–722.

28. WALLACE JM, THORNTON WE, KENNEDY HL, ET AL: **Ambulatory blood pressure in 199 normal subjects, a collaborative study. In** *Ambulatory Blood Pressure Monitoring* edited by Weber MA, Drayer JIM. Darmstadt: Steinkopff, 1984, pp 117–128.

29. PICKERING TG, JAMES GD, BODDIE C ET AL: **How common is white coat hypertension?** *JAMA* 1988, 259:225–228.

30. CHAU NP, CHANUDET X, LARROQUE P: **A method to define reference profiles for ambulatory blood pressure, with application to blood pressure profiles in 158 young subjects.** *Clin Exp Hypertens [A]* 1988, 10:951–969.

31. O'BRIEN E, MURPHY J, TYNDALL A, ET AL: **Twenty-four hour ambulatory blood pressure in normotensive subjects.** *Am J Hypertens* 1990, 3:35A.

32. ENSTROM I, THULIN T, LINDHOLM L: **How good are standardized blood pressure recordings for diagnosing hypertension?** *J Hypertens* (in press).

33. LATTUADA S, ANTIVALLE M, RINDI M, ET AL: **24 h BP levels in normotensive subjects. A collaborative Italian Multicenter study.** *J Amb Mon* 1990, 3:41–45.

34. POMIDOSSI G, PARATI G, CASADEI R, ET AL: **Twenty-four hour ambulatory intra-arterial blood pressure in normotensive and borderline hypertensive subjects.** *J Hypertens* 1988, 6 (suppl 4):S67–S69.

35. WHITE WB, MORGANROTH J: **Usefulness of ambulatory monitoring of blood pressure in assessing antihypertensive therapy.** *Am J Cardiol* 1989, 63:94–98.

36. ZACHARIAH PK, SHEPS SG, ILSTRUP DM, ET AL: **Blood pressure load — a better determinant of hypertension.** *Mayo Clin Proc* 1988, 63:1085–1091.

37. DRAYER JIM, WEBER MA, NAKAMURA DK: **Automated ambulatory blood pressure monitoring: a study in age-matched normotensive and hypertensive men.** *Am Heart J* 1985, 109:1334–1338.

38. WHITE WB, DEY HM, SCHULMAN P: **Assessment of the daily blood pressure load as a determinant of cardiac function in patients with mild-to-moderate hypertension.** *Am Heart J* 1989, 118:782–795.

39. BAUMGART P, WALGER P, JÜRGENS U, RAHN KH: **Reference data for ambulatory blood pressure monitoring: what results are equivalent to the established limits of office blood pressure?** *Klin Wochenschr* 1990, 68:723–727.

40. PERLOFF D, SOKOLOW M, COWAN R: **The prognostic value of ambulatory blood pressure.** *JAMA* 1983, 249:2792–2798.

41. DANIELS SR, LOGGIE JMH, BURTON T, KAPLAN S: **Difficulties with ambulatory blood pressure monitoring in children and adolescents.** *J Pediatrics* 1987, 111:397–400.

42. WILSON PD, FERENCZ C, DISCHINGER P, BRENNER JI, ZEGER SL: **Twenty-four hour ambulatory blood pressure in normotensive adolescent children of hypertensive and normotensive parents.** *Am J Epidemiol* 1988, 127:946–954.

43. FIXLER DE, WALLACE JM, THORNTON WE, DIMMITT P: **Ambulatory blood pressure monitoring in hypertensive adolescents.** *Am J Hypertens* 1990, 3:288–292.

44. EGGER M, BIANCHETTI MG, GRANDINGER M, KOBELT R, OETLIKER O: **Twenty-four hour intermittent, ambulatory blood pressure monitoring.** *Arch Dis Child* 1987, 62:1130–1135.

45. OETLIKER O, BACHMANN E, FRAUCHIGER S, ET AL: **Blutdruckmessung bei Kindern: Normalwerte für eine bestimmte Altersklasse.** *Schweiz Med Wochenschr* 1978, 108:2033–2039.

46. HARSHFIELD GA, ALPERT BS, WILLEY ES, ET AL: **Race and gender influence ambulatory blood pressure patterns of adolescents.** *Hypertension* 1989, 14:598–603.

47. DRAYER JIM, WEBER MA, DEYOUNG JL, WYLE FA: **Circadian blood pressure patterns in ambulatory hypertensive patients. Effects of age.** *Am J Med* 1982, 73:493–499.

48. FEINBERG I, KORESKO RL, HELLER N: **EEG sleep patterns as a function of normal and pathological aging in man.** *J Psychiat Res* 1967, 5:107–144.

49. KOBRIN I, DUNN GF, OIGMAN W, ET AL: **Essential hypertension in the elderly: circadian variation of arterial pressure. In** *Ambulatory Blood Pressure Monitoring* edited by Weber MA, Drayer JIM. Darmstadt: Steinkopff, 1984, pp 81–185.

50. ROWLANDS DB, STALLARD TJ, LITTLER WA: **Continuous ambulatory monitoring of blood pressure and assessment of cardiovascular reflexes in the elderly hypertensive.** *J Hypertens* 1984, 2:615–622.

51. DUPONT AG, VANDERMIEPEN P, VOLCHAERT A, FINNE E, SIX RO: **Noninvasive ambulatory monitoring of blood pressure in essential hypertension. Effect of age on variability and disparity.** *J Clin Hypertens* 1986, 3:278–284.

52. RUDDY MC, BIALY GB, MALKA ES, LACY CR, KOSTIS JB: **The relationship of plasma renin activity to clinic and ambulatory blood pressure in elderly people with isolated systolic hypertension.** *J Hypertens* 1988, 6 (suppl 4):S412–S415.

53. HARSHFIELD GA, HWANG C, GRIM CE: **Circadian variation of blood pressure in blacks: influence of age, gender, and activity.** *J Hum Hypertens* 1990, 4:43–47.

54. PAGE EW, CHRISTIANSON R: **The impact of mean arterial pressure in the middle trimester upon the outcome of pregnancy.** *Am J Obstet Gynecol* 1976, 125:740–746.

55. MACGILLIVRAY I, ROSE GA, ROWE D: **Blood pressure survey in pregnancy.** *Clin Sci* 1969, 37:395–407.

56. CHESLEY LC, ANNITTO JE: **Pregnancy in the patient with hypertensive disease.** *Am J Obstet Gynecol* 1947, 53:372–381.

57. RAYBURN WF, ZUSPAN FP, PIEHL EJ: **Self-monitoring of blood pressure during pregnancy.** *Am J Obstet Gynecol* 1984, 148:159–162.

58. SELIGMAN SA: **Diurnal blood-pressure variation in pregnancy.** *J Obstet Gynaecol Br Commonwealth* 1971, 78:417–422.

59. REDMAN CWG, BEILIN LJ, BONNAR J: **Reversed diurnal blood pressure rhythm in hypertensive pregnancies.** *Clin Sci Mol Med* 1976, 51:687s–689s.

60. MURNAGHAN GA, MITCHELL RH, RUFF S: **Circadian variation of blood-pressure in pregnancy. In** *Pregnancy Hypertension, Proceedings of the First Congress of the International Society for the Study of Hypertension in Pregnancy* edited by Bonnar J, MacGillivray I, Symonds M. MTP Press, 1978, pp 107–112.

61. MARGULIES M, ZIN C, MARGULIES DC, VOTO LS: **Noninvasive ambulatory blood pressure control in normotensive pregnant women.** *Am J Hypertens* 1989, 2:924–926.

62. **The 1988 report of the Joint National Committee on detection, evaluation and treatment of high blood pressure.** *Arch Intern Med* 1988, 148:1023–1038.

63. ANDERSON NB, MYERS HF, PICKERING T, JACKSON JS: **Hypertension in blacks: psychosocial and biological perspectives.** *J Hypertens* 1989, 7:161–172.

64. MURPHY MB, NIELSON KS, ELLIOTT WJ: **Racial differences in diurnal blood pressure profile.** *Am J Hypertens* 1988, 1:55A [abstract].

65. ROWLANDS DB, DEGIOVANNI J, MCLEAY RAB, ET AL: **Cardiovascular responses in black and white hypertensives.** *Hypertension* 1982, 4:817–820.

66. WILSON TW, GRIM CM, WILSON DM ET AL: 24-hour blood pressure patterns in Barbadian blacks differ from US blacks. *Circulation* 1990, 81:726.

67. KANNEL WB: Hypertension and the risk of cardiovascular disease. In *Hypertension: Pathophysiology, Diagnosis, and Management* edited by Laragh JH, Brenner BM. New York: Raven, 1990, pp 101–107.

68. MEDICAL RESEARCH COUNCIL WORKING PARTY: Stroke and coronary heart disease in mild hypertension: risk factors and the value of treatment. *Br Med J* 1988, 197:1565–1570.

69. SCHIEKEN RM, EAVES LJ, HEWITT JK, ET AL. Univariate genetic analysis of blood pressure in children (the Medical College of Virginia Twin Study). *Am J Cardiol* 1989, 64:1333–1337.

70. RAVOGLI A, TRAZZI S, VITTANI A, ET AL: Early 24 hour blood pressure elevation in normotensive subjects with parental hypertension. *Hypertension* 1990, 16: 491–497.

71. HARSHFIELD GA, PULLIAM DA, ALPERT BS ET AL: Renin-sodium profiles of adolescents: influences on casual and ambulatory blood pressure. *Pediatrics* (in press).

72. PICKERING TG: Exercise and hypertension. *Cardiol Clin* 1988 5:311–318.

73. HARSHFIELD GA, DUPAUL LM, ALPERT BS, ET AL: Aerobic fitness plays a greater role in the circadian variation of blood pressure in black than white adolescents. *Hypertension* 1990, 15: 810–814.

74. GERBER LM, SCHNALL PL, PICKERING TG: Body fat and its distribution and its relation to casual and ambulatory pressure. *Hypertension* 1990, 15:508–513.

75. LITTLER WA, HONOUR AJ, PUGSLEY DJ, SLEIGHT P: Continuous recording of direct arterial pressure in unrestricted patients. Its role in the diagnosis and management of high blood pressure. *Circulation* 1975, 51:1101–1106.

76. MEJIA AD, EGAN BM, SCHORK NJ, ZWEIFLER AJ: Artifacts in measurement of blood pressure and lack of target organ involvement in the assessment of patients with treatment-resistant hypertension. *Ann Intern Med* 1990, 112:270–277.

77. WHITE WB: Hypertension with potential syncope secondary to the combination of chlorpromazine and captopril. *Arch Intern Med* 1986, 146:1833–1834.

78. IMAI Y, ABE K, MIURA Y, ET AL: Hypertensive episodes and circadian fluctuations of blood pressure in patients with pheochromocytoma: studies by long-term blood pressure monitoring based on a volume-oscillometric method. *J Hypertens* 1988, 6:9–15.

79. WHITE WB, BAKER HL: Episodic hypertension secondary to panic disorder. *Arch Intern Med* 1986, 146:1129–1130.

10 Evaluation of antihypertensive treatment by ambulatory monitoring

The effectiveness of antihypertensive treatment, whether pharmacological or non-pharmacological, is traditionally evaluated by blood pressure measurements made at regular intervals in the clinic. Ambulatory monitoring and self-monitoring by the patient offer a number of advantages, from the point of view both of the researcher attempting to assess a new form of treatment and of the clinician. The basis of this superiority rests on the unreliability of clinic measurements, not only because they may be unrepresentative of blood pressure levels outside the clinic, but also because of their relatively poor reproducibility from one occasion to another. Ambulatory monitoring also offers the possibility of evaluating the duration of efficacy of antihypertensive drug treatment. Some specific advantages of monitoring blood pressure away from the clinic are described below, and listed in Fig. 10.1. The disadvantages are relatively minor and are also reviewed below.

Advantages
Reduction of the placebo effect
Reduction in sample size
Avoidance of the unrepresentativeness of clinic
  pressures
Improved selection of patients
Evaluation of duration of effect
Evaluation of dose–response relationships
Evaluation of the effects of treatment on blood
  pressure variability
Evaluation of the effects of treatment on the diurnal
  blood pressure profile

Disadvantages
Inconvenience of multiple recordings
Uncontrolled conditions during recordings

Fig. 10.1. Advantages and disadvantages of ambulatory monitoring for evaluation of antihypertensive treatment.

Reduction of the placebo effect

A placebo has been defined as any therapeutic procedure, given either deliberately or unknowingly, which has an effect on a symptom or disease process without any specific activity for the condition being treated [1]. In hypertension research placebos are given for two reasons: first, to evaluate side effects of treatment, and, second, to control for non-specific effects on blood pressure. It is the latter which concerns us here.

When a placebo is administered chronically, blood pressure tends to fall gradually and progressively. In one study this fall was 46/16 mmHg in a group of patients with severe hypertension and 14/4 mmHg in a group with mild hypertension [2]. Most studies, however, report much smaller changes. In most cases it is not clear to what extent such changes in blood pressure are attributable to the placebo pill rather than to the tendency for blood pressure to decrease with repeated measurement. This may occur partly from habituation to the measurement procedure and partly from regression to the mean. That placebo effects can be explained by the latter has been most forcefully argued by McDonald *et al.* [3]. They estimated the apparent improvement that would be expected to follow the introduction of an inert treatment on the basis of the two factors which determine the degree of regression to the mean: the abnormality of the initial measure (in this case the height of the blood pressure) and the unreliability of the measure (in this case clinic measurements). They concluded that the size of the placebo effect reported in a number of trials (not all of which involved blood pressure) could be accounted for on the basis of regression to the mean. The important point about this phenomenon is that the abnormality for which the study population was originally chosen diminishes with time (or repeated measurement): its link with the placebo effect is explained by the fact that treatment is initiated after the abnormality has been detected.

The size of a placebo effect may also depend on the expectations of the patient. This was clearly illustrated by Shapiro *et al.* [4], who compared the response to *Veratrum* and a placebo in hypertensive patients. The study was (unintentionally) conducted in two phases, with a 6-week interval between them. In the first phase, the physician was highly enthusiastic about the potency of the treatment, but he became disillusioned during the second phase. The blood pressures he recorded were consistently higher (by 18/5 mmHg) during the second phase, regardless of whether the patients were on *Veratrum* or placebo.

When blood pressure is measured by a physician, another relevant factor may be the expectation of the physician. This was demonstrated in a study by Sassano *et al.* [5], who measured blood pressure with physician readings and with an automatic device (both in a clinic setting) in 200 patients being recruited for a drug study. There were two phases: in the first, patients were given placebo on a single-blind basis (i.e. the physician knew the patients were receiving placebo, but the patients did not); in the second, patients were given either placebo or active drug on a double-blind basis (when neither the patients nor the physician knew when they were taking placebo). During the single-blind period, the automatic device recorded a slight fall in pressure whereas the physician did not. During the double-blind period the automatic device recorded a similar fall (about 2 mmHg), but this time the physician recorded a greater fall (3 mmHg). The most plausible explanation for these findings is that the automatic device recorded the placebo component attributable to the patients' expectations (which should have been the same in both phases), while the differences in the physician's readings occurred because the physician was not expecting any change during the single-blind period (and recorded none), whereas he was expecting a change during the double-blind period, when half the patients were on active treatment.

The placebo response has presented a major problem for clinical trials investigating the effect of treating mild hypertension on cardiovascular morbidity. In the Australian trial [6], almost half the patients originally defined as having mild hypertension, on the basis of six clinic measurements spaced over 4 weeks, showed a decrease in pressure to normotensive levels during 3 years of placebo treatment. Similar findings have been reported in other trials [7], as shown in Fig. 10.2

An important consideration is whether these changes are confined to the clinic situation or also affect blood pressure at other times. As shown in Fig. 10.3, in a hypothetical patient whose blood pressure increases at the time of a clinic visit, a reduction in clinic pressure could occur either because the pressure response to the clinic situation (white coat effect) has diminished without any change in the pressure at other times, or because there has been a sustained decrease in blood pressure [8]. It seems reasonable to suppose that a placebo response might be of the first type (Fig. 10.3, treatment A), whereas a genuine therapeutic response would require a sustained reduction (treatment B). These two situations can, of course, be distinguished if blood pressure is measured outside the clinic.

Five studies have compared the effects of placebo therapy on clinic and ambulatory blood pressure. In the first, by Gould *et al.* [9], blood pressure was measured in the clinic using a random-zero sphygmomanometer and by intra-arterial ambulatory monitoring in three therapeutic situations while on no treatment, placebo or indoramin (an alpha-blocking agent). Clinic blood pressure showed a significant decrease in response to placebo (15/10 mmHg) but there was no significant decrease in

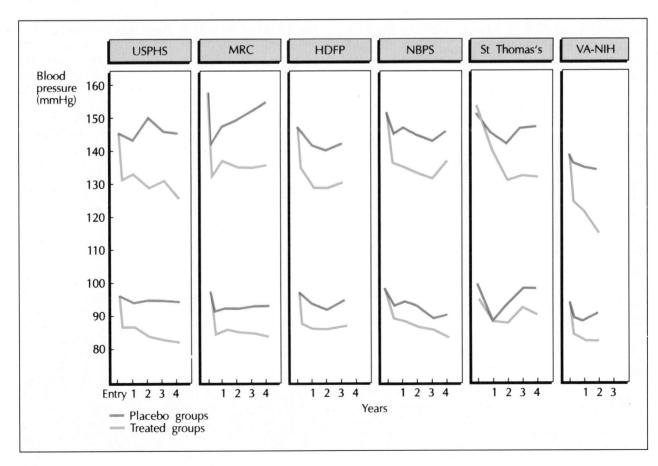

Fig. 10.2. Blood pressure changes in treated and placebo groups in six clinical trials of antihypertensive treatment. USPHS, US Public Health Service; MRC, Medical Research Council (UK); HDFP, Hypertension Detection and Follow-up Program; NBPS, Australian National Blood Pressure Study. Reproduced with permission [7].

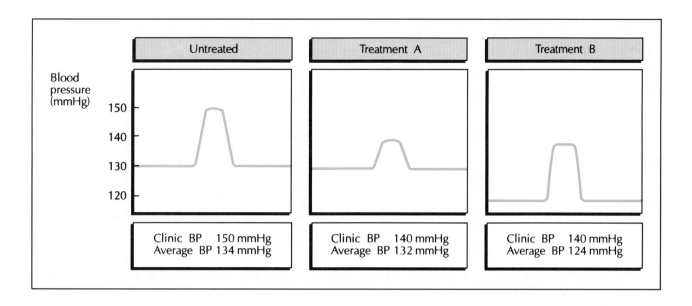

Fig. 10.3. Hypothetical blood pressure (BP) response to a clinic visit before and after treatment. In the untreated condition, the clinic visit provokes a pressor response. With treatment A, the clinic pressure is reduced without affecting pressure at other times; treatment B results in a similar reduction in clinic pressure without affecting the pressor response. Reproduced with permission [8].

the ambulatory pressures. In contrast, indoramin lowered clinic pressures (in comparison with placebo) by 6/8 mmHg and ambulatory pressure by a much greater amount (18/13 mmHg). In the second study, by Dupont et al. [10], non-invasive ambulatory monitoring was used in conjunction with clinic pressure measurement. Placebo treatment was associated with a significant reduction in clinic pressure (of 13/6 mmHg), but once again there was no significant effect on ambulatory pressure. In the third study, Parati et al. [11] carried out a randomized, double-blind, crossover study in which each of 15 patients had their blood pressure measured by clinic readings and by intra-arterial ambulatory monitoring on three occasions: while on no treatment, placebo or celiprolol (a beta blocker). The placebo had no significant effect on either measure of blood pressure, whereas celiprolol lowered both clinic and ambulatory pressures to a similar degree. Conway et al. [12] evaluated the effect of a placebo given for 1 month to 42 patients and observed no consistent change in ambulatory pressure. Finally, Bellet et al. [13] randomized hypertensive patients to receive either placebo or nicardipine (a calcium antagonist) for 3 weeks. The blood pressure response was evaluated with readings taken by a physician, a Sentron automatic (but non-ambulatory) recorder in the clinic, and non-invasive ambulatory monitoring. The placebo group showed insignificant decreases in pressure for the physician and Sentron readings, but a marginally significant decrease for ambulatory readings (of 4/3 mmHg). When plotted on an hourly basis, however, the placebo produced a significant effect on both systolic and diastolic pressure during the first hour of monitoring.

These findings, therefore, clearly indicate that the placebo effect is equivalent to situation A in Fig. 10.3 and has no therapeutic effect other than keeping the doctor (and

hence perhaps also the patient) happy. They also suggest that the continued decline in clinic blood pressure observed in the control groups of clinical trials (Fig. 10.2) may be an artefact of the clinic situation. Further support for this view is provided by our reproducibility study [14], in which we compared the reproducibility of clinic, home and ambulatory pressures in normotensive and hypertensive individuals over an interval of 2 weeks. In the hypertensive individuals clinic systolic pressure decreased significantly over this period, but this was not accompanied by any change in either home, or ambulatory, pressures. As discussed in Chapter 9, some reproducibility studies have shown modest decreases in ambulatory pressure on repeat measurement, which might explain any apparent placebo effects, such as those found by Bellet et al. [13].

Reduction in sample size

Any investigation into the effectiveness of an antihypertensive therapy has to take into consideration the fact that blood pressure is highly variable from one occasion to another. The requirements for estimating the sample size needed for a crossover or parallel group trial of antihypertensive therapy have been outlined by Hills and Armitage [15]. Three factors are predetermined by the investigator. These are the power of the study (usually 0.8 to 0.9), which is the probability of obtaining a significant result if there is a genuine difference between treatment conditions; the acceptable level of significance (usually $P < 0.05$); and the minimum difference between treatments to be detected. Given these requirements, which are independent of the method of measuring blood pressure, the determinant of the required sample size will be the variability of the blood pressure measurement itself, expressed as the SDD between measurements. It is clear, therefore, that the greater the variability of the blood pressure measurement, the more difficult it will be to detect an effect of treatment and the larger will be the sample size needed.

In a survey of 14 published trials of antihypertensive treatment, Freestone *et al.* [16] calculated that the SDD for single clinical measurements was 14 mmHg for systolic pressure and 9 mmHg for diastolic or mean pressure. The reliability of a variable measure such as blood pressure can be increased by combining a large number of observations. Therefore, on theoretical grounds alone, the use of home or ambulatory monitoring (with which it is easy to obtain multiple readings) should mean that smaller sample sizes are required. This has been demonstrated in a study of antihypertensive treatment where home and clinic pressures were used [17]. The greater reliability of home pressures enabled a difference between treatments of 5 mmHg to be detected in a sample of 20 patients, whereas 27 patients would have been required if clinic pressures were used. In a study comparing clinic and ambulatory (non-invasive daytime) readings, Coats *et al.* [18] estimated the SDD to be 20/14 mmHg for single clinic readings and 9/6 mmHg for average daytime pressures. On this basis they estimated that a crossover trial designed to detect a treatment effect of 8/5 mmHg would require 88 subjects if blood pressure were measured by single clinic readings, but only 16 subjects would be required if ambulatory readings were used.

In a subsequent analysis Conway and Coats [19] published a nomogram showing how the number of subjects required in a parallel group study (designed to detect a treatment effect of a given size) would be reduced by using ambulatory rather than clinic readings, on the assumption that the ambulatory recording included at least 20 readings (Fig. 10.4). For a 5 mmHg treatment effect 250 subjects would be required using clinic measure-

ments and 67 subjects using ambulatory recordings. For a crossover trial the number (n) would fall from 61 to 16, according to the equation:

$$n = 10 \times SDD^2/difference^2$$

where 'difference' is a 5 mmHg treatment effect.

Avoidance of the unrepresentativeness of clinic pressures

As the adverse effects of high blood pressure are assumed to depend on the average, or integrated, level of pressure over long periods of time, the goal of treatment should be to produce a sustained reduction in pressure. Several studies have compared clinic and ambulatory pressures [20,21], and although there is a reasonable overall correlation between clinic and ambulatory pressures (of the order of 0.6–0.7), in individual patients there may be a considerable variation between the two, reaching a maximum difference of 43/32 mmHg in one study [21]. In another study clinic blood pressure was measured both by a physician and by a nurse, and these readings were compared with the average ambulatory daytime pressures [22]. Again, there was poor agreement between either of the clinic measurements and the ambulatory pressures.

In the majority of studies where the effects of treatment on clinic and ambulatory pressures have been compared, there is reasonably good agreement between the two. Figure 10.5 shows the effects of six different classes of antihypertensive medication on clinic and daytime ambulatory pressures taken from 17 published studies [13,23–40]. For most types of medication the overall effects on the two measures of pressure are similar, but clinic pressures tend to overestimate the degree of blood pressure control during daily activities in studies using calcium antagonists and alpha blockers.

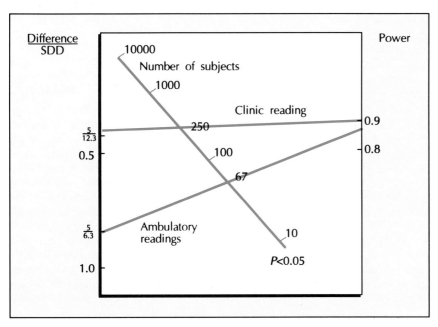

Fig. 10.4. Nomogram showing the numbers of patients required in a parallel group study to achieve a 90% chance of detecting a 5 mmHg treatment effect using either clinic readings (SDD 12.3 mmHg) or ambulatory readings (SDD 6.3 mmHg). Reproduced with permission [19].

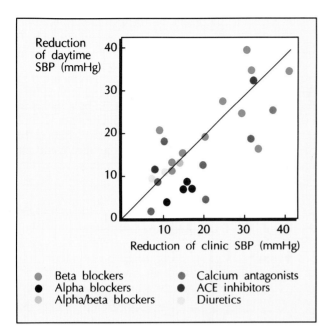

Fig. 10.5. Comparison of the effects of six classes of antihypertensive medication on clinic and ambulatory SBP. Each symbol represents the average changes for one type of medication for one study. The line is the line of identity.

The discrepancy between clinic and ambulatory pressures has been even more striking in other studies of antihypertensive treatment. In a trial of transdermal clonidine treatment, Schaller et al. [41] found no effect on clinic pressures, whereas the ambulatory pressures showed a significant decrease. In another study comparing the effects of labetalol and prazosin, Gray et al. [24] randomized patients to one or other drug after an initial placebo period. The dose of each drug was then titrated until the clinic blood pressure had reached the target level. Thus, for the clinic pressures the reductions in diastolic pressure for prazosin and labetalol were the same (13 mmHg for each). However, for the corresponding daytime ambulatory pressures they were not: for labetalol there was a 10 mmHg decline, whereas for prazosin the decline was only 5 mmHg. This study is quoted here not only because it provides another example of the discrepancy between clinic and ambulatory pressures, but also because it suggests that combined alpha and beta blockade may provide more effective control of blood pressure during daily life than alpha blockade alone. Enstrom et al. [23] compared enalapril and atenolol using both clinic and ambulatory recordings and found atenolol to be more effective when judged by clinic readings, as some patients appeared not to respond to enalapril. When these patients' 24-hour recordings were examined, however, they did show a satisfactory response similar to that of the atenolol-treated patients.

Despite this generally good agreement between the effects of medication on clinic and ambulatory pressure when analysed on a group basis, several studies have reported weak or insignificant correlations on an individual basis [27–33].

Although most drug studies have been of relatively short duration, for example 2–6 weeks for each treatment period, studies of longer duration have had to face the problem that clinic blood pressure tends to decrease over time. This has been most marked in studies in which cardiovascular morbidity has been the endpoint of treatment. However, it is also exemplified by studies investigating the effects of weight loss on blood pressure, which must, by necessity, have a long period of follow-up. Fortmann et al. [42] followed three groups of normotensive men for 1 year: a no-treatment control group, a weight-loss by diet group and an exercise group. After the study period there were similar decreases in clinic pressure in all three groups (of about 5/4 mmHg), but only the two intervention groups showed a significant fall in ambulatory pressure.

Improved selection of patients

As discussed in more detail in Chapter 7, a significant number of patients who are hypertensive in the clinic are found to have normal blood pressures at other times. Such patients may, therefore, not be ideal candidates for a trial of antihypertensive treatment. This point is well illustrated in a study conducted by Weber et al. [43], in which patients were randomly allocated to receive either placebo or diltiazem. The effectiveness of treatment was assessed by measuring both clinic and ambulatory blood pressures. Overall, the placebo had no effect on either set of blood pressures, while diltiazem lowered both. The patients who received diltiazem were divided into two groups, according to whether their ambulatory diastolic pressures were above or below 90 mmHg (all patients had clinic diastolic pressures above 95 mmHg). In the 'true hypertensives' (i.e. those whose pressure was high in both situations) diltiazem produced a significant reduction in ambulatory pressure (by 18/13 mmHg), whereas in the other white coat hypertensives it had no effect. Exactly the same phenomenon was reported by Lacourcière et al. [44] in a study of isradipine. They divided their patients into two groups: those with elevated ambulatory pressures and those with normal pressures (clinic pressure was similarly elevated in both groups). Isradipine lowered ambulatory pressure in the former group but not in the latter group, who might be classified as having white coat hypertension.

Gradman et al. [45] conducted a placebo-controlled double-blind study of an antihypertensive agent in which patients were selected in the conventional way: that is, the patients' antihypertensive drugs were replaced by a placebo for 4 weeks, during which time they made two clinic visits. Those with diastolic pressures above 95 mmHg (21 patients) were admitted to the protocol, while those with lower pressures (nine patients) were excluded. During this period ambulatory blood pressure was recorded; the average 24-hour levels were not significantly different (142/86 mmHg in the 'admitted' group and 137/82 mmHg in the 'excluded' group), as shown in Fig. 10.6. The differences between clinical and 24-

hour pressures were thus greater in the 'admitted' group, showing that this selection procedure tends to favour patients with white coat hypertension.

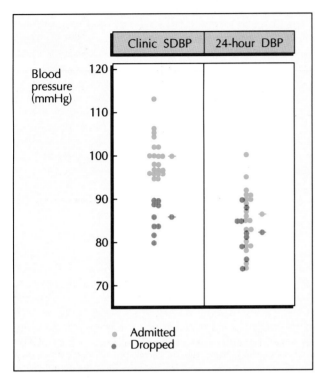

Fig. 10.6. Clinic supine diastolic blood pressures (SDBP) and 24-hour ambulatory diastolic pressures (DBP) in individual patients being evaluated for inclusion in a drug trial. Reproduced with permission [45].

As a result of such studies it might be argued that ambulatory monitoring should not only be used to evaluate the effects of treatment but also to select patients for clinical trials who are hypertensive both in the clinic and during ambulatory monitoring. This has not so far been done.

Evaluation of duration of effect: peak and trough effects

If a medication is taken as a once-daily dose it is important to know whether it is producing a sustained reduction in pressure throughout the day and night. Information about peak and trough effects has become a standard requirement for approval of a new antihypertensive drug by the Food and Drug Administration (FDA) in the United States. The procedure is designed to establish the most appropriate dosing interval. The peak represents the point of maximum blood pressure reduction and the trough the residual effect just before the next dose is given. In both cases the blood pressure changes with the active drug and placebo are compared, as shown in Figure 10.7. The calculation of trough to peak ratio has been described by Rose and McMahon [46]. The process is normally carried out by making repeated measurements

of blood pressure in a standardized clinic setting, which is relatively inconvenient and also means that this information is rarely gained from employed people. Thus, not only may the studied population be unrepresentative, but the effects of the drug may not be the same at rest as during activity. Ambulatory monitoring is clearly an ideal way to evaluate peak and trough effects; Whelton *et al.* [47], for example, were able to identify one trough time for lisinopril and two for captopril in a study comparing once-daily lisinopril with twice-daily captopril using ambulatory monitoring.

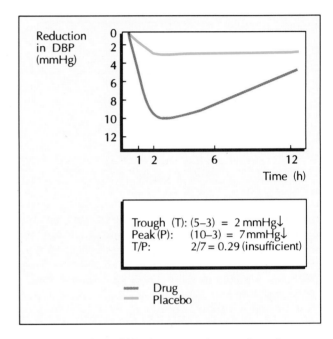

Fig. 10.7. Hypothetical blood pressure changes after administration of active drug and placebo, from which trough to peak ratio can be estimated. Reproduced with permission [46].

Hornung *et al.* [26] used intra-arterial ambulatory monitoring to determine whether nadolol, which has the longest half-life of all beta blockers (approximately 24 h), does in fact lower blood pressure for a full 24 h. They found that the entire blood pressure profile was shifted downwards by the drug. Furthermore, the patients were instructed to take the drug at 8.00 a.m., but in the hours immediately following this (between 9.00 a.m. and 12 noon) the reductions were not significant. Floras *et al.* [25] compared four beta blockers (atenolol, metoprolol, pindolol and slow-release propranolol), all given in once-daily dosage. Atenolol lowered the pressure for 24 h, propranolol for 22 h, pindolol for 15 h, and metoprolol for 12 h. Of particular interest was the finding that pindolol, which was the only drug with intrinsic sympathomimetic activity, did not lower blood pressure, and actually increased heart rate, during sleep. Thus, the difference between daytime and night-time blood pressure was attenuated.

Another example comes from a study by Conway *et al.* [48], who evaluated the effects of three different dose regimens of captopril on ambulatory pressure. Each patient had six ambulatory recordings, with, placebo and captopril administered alternately. The dose of captopril was fixed at 75 mg daily, given as either a single daily dose, or 37.5 mg twice daily or 25 mg three times daily. For the group as a whole (13 patients) the reduction in the average daytime blood pressure and the reduction 1 h after the morning dose (representing the maximum reduction after captopril administration) were the same for all three regimens. In three patients with very high renin levels, blood pressure control was not maintained for a full 24 h. Although the authors did not specifically state whether the hour-by-hour reduction in pressure was the same, they concluded that in the majority of patients captopril was effective when taken as a once-daily dosage.

Although prolonged monitoring is clearly essential to establish the duration of the antihypertensive effect of a new medication, it may be appropriate to restrict the patients' activity during the monitoring period. This would be particularly appropriate for initial dose-ranging studies, so that the variance of blood pressure produced by the medication can be more clearly distinguished from the variance occurring as a result of changes in activity. This was carried out in a study by Murdoch et al. [49], in which patients receiving captopril (25 mg twice daily) were admitted to an investigation unit for 7 h, which included the last hour of one dosage interval and the first 6 h of the next. Measurement of blood pressure was made every hour by a semi-automatic device. It was concluded that a twice-daily dose of captopril was not effective throughout each 12-hour interval, in contrast to the findings of Conway et al. cited above [48] using ambulatory monitoring.

Evaluation of dose–response relationships

The establishment of the minimum effective dose of any antihypertensive agent is clearly an important objective, from the point of view of reducing both the costs and the side effects of treatment. When captopril was first introduced, it was given three times daily, up to a maximum daily dose of 600 mg [50]. While it was certainly very effective at this dose, there was an unacceptably high prevalence of side effects, including proteinuria, neutropenia and skin rash [51]. It was not realized for some years that much smaller doses, such as 37.5 mg daily, would be effective in many patients [52]. Had ambulatory monitoring been used initially to evaluate the minimum effective dose, as in several subsequent studies [48,53], it is quite probable that these side effects could have been avoided.

Ambulatory monitoring was used to evaluate dose-response relationships study by Berglund et al. [36], who investigated the efficacy of two doses of a new long-acting beta blocker, pafenolol. When evaluated by the effect on casual blood pressure (measured 24 h after taking the medication), the efficacy of the two doses was the same, but the larger dose was significantly more effective at lowering daytime and night-time ambulatory pressures (Fig. 10.8).

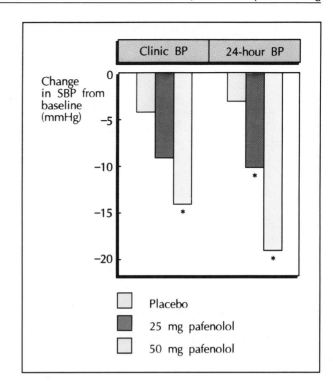

Fig. 10.8. The effects of placebo and two doses of pafenolol (25 and 50 mg daily) evaluated by clinic and 24-hour (ambulatory) blood pressure measurements. Asterisks show significant difference from placebo. Data from Berglund et al. [36].

Conway and Coats [19] have also pointed out that the conventional method of assessing the dose–response relationship of antihypertensive medications, by progressively increasing the dose until a desired reduction in clinic pressure is reached, will lead to an inevitable overestimation of the effective dose. This would occur because of the unreliability (high SDD) of clinic pressures. Even if the medication had no effect on blood pressure the high variability of the clinic pressures would lead to a significant number of patients being classified as responders on the second visit; a similar proportion would be classified as non-responders, because their clinic pressures would be higher. If the non-responders are given a larger dose, a similar proportion of them will be classified as non-responders on the next visit, leading to a further escalation of the dose. Conway and Coats suggested that a more reliable estimate of the dose–response relationship of a medication could be obtained by using more reliable measures of blood pressure (e.g. ambulatory monitoring) and by exposing all patients to all doses.

Evaluation of the effects of treatment on blood pressure variability

Blood pressure can be regarded as a steady-state or 'true' pressure, about which phasic variations occur. This variability can be measured either in absolute terms, for example by the standard deviation, or in relative (percentage) terms, for example by the coefficient of variation. As shown in Fig. 10.9, antihypertensive treatment can affect the tonic and phasic components of blood pressure in three ways. First, the tonic level of blood pressure may be lowered without any reduction in variability (Fig. 10.9b); second, there could be a proportional reduction in the tonic level of blood pressure and the variability, in which case the absolute, but not the relative, measures of variability would be reduced (Fig. 10.9c); third, the tonic level of blood pressure and all measures of variability might be lowered (Fig. 10.9d). This last effect would be regarded as a true reduction in blood pressure variability as a result of treatment.

One of the undoubted functions of the sympathetic nervous system is to produce short-term increases in blood pressure, such as those which occur during physical and mental arousal. It might be thought, therefore, that antihypertensive drugs which interfere with the functioning of the sympathetic nervous system (e.g. alpha or beta blockers) would reduce blood pressure variability over 24 h (as shown by Fig. 10.9d), whereas those that act independently of it (e.g. diuretics or angiotensin converting enzyme inhibitors) would not. The first study to address this question was conducted by West *et al.* [54] with tolamolol (a now-defunct beta blocker), using intra-arterial blood pressure monitoring. They found, somewhat surprisingly, that although the average level of blood pressure was reduced, there was no effect on its variability. Their findings have subsequently been confirmed for other beta blockers, including propranolol and nadolol [55,56]. Mancia *et al.* [56] found that with nadolol the standard deviation of mean arterial pressure within successive half-hour periods (i.e. short-term variability) was reduced, while the changes between half-hour periods (i.e. longer-term variability) was not. When variability was expressed as the variation coefficients (i.e. normalized for the level of pressure), neither short- nor long-term variability was affected. This was in marked contrast with heart rate, where all measures of variability were reduced. The same investigators reported identical findings for another beta blocker, celiprolol [11], and for a combined alpha/beta blocker, labetalol [57]. Floras *et al.* [58] studied patients before and after treatment with one of four beta blockers (atenolol, metoprolol, pindolol or propranolol). They found that although the awake mean arterial pressure was reduced (from 126 to 106 mmHg), there was absolutely no effect on blood pressure variability, which they measured as the standard deviation (the actual values were 14.6 mmHg before treatment and 14.9 mmHg after treatment). Clonidine, a centrally acting antihypertensive agent, lowers blood pressure without any significant effect on the standard deviation of mean arterial pressure either within or between successive half-hour periods [59].

Antihypertensive agents which act independently of the autonomic nervous system also fail to alter blood pressure variability. Agents that have been studied in this respect include nifedipine [31] (a calcium antagonist) and captopril [53] (an angiotensin converting enzyme inhibitor).

However, one study of the effects of verapamil [60], using non-invasive monitoring, reported a significant decrease of three different measures of variability as a result of treatment: the difference between the maximum and minimum values, the standard deviation, and the coefficient

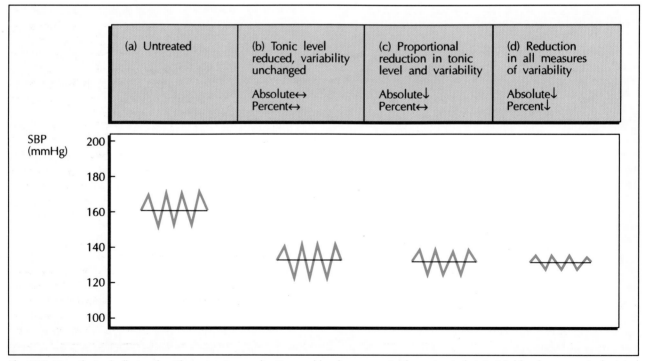

Fig. 10.9. Hypothetical effects of antihypertensive medication on blood pressure. In the untreated state (a), blood pressure is depicted as oscillations around a steady-state level. (b,c,d) Different treatment effects which produce the same reduction in average pressure but different effects on variability.

of variability. Variability was less pronounced during the night and was unaffected by treatment.

Evaluation of the effects of treatment on blood pressure reactivity

This topic, which is evaluated by laboratory testing rather than by ambulatory monitoring, is discussed in Chapter 12. It is concluded that reactivity, like other measures of blood pressure variability, is not significantly affected by treatment.

Evaluation of the effects of treatment on white coat hypertension

This is a neglected but potentially important area of study. If pharmacological treatment lowers blood pressure by the same amount in all situations, it could result in an excessive reduction of pressure outside the clinic setting in patients with white coat hypertension, who by definition are normotensive to begin with, except in the clinic. Alternatively, the blood-pressure-lowering effects might be more pronounced in the clinic setting, which would be equivalent to a placebo effect.

A limited amount of evidence supports the latter possibility. Two studies cited above [43,44] found that the calcium antagonists under investigation had relatively little effect on ambulatory pressure in patients who might be classified as white coat hypertensives, while they did lower ambulatory pressure in patients with more sustained hypertension. No study has so far systematically compared the responses to drug treatment in patients with white coat and sustained hypertension.

Evaluation of the effects of treatment on the diurnal blood pressure profile

It has been observed that the diurnal blood pressure profile is generally unaffected by treatment, but there may be different effects with different types of medication.

Alpha blockers

In a study of prazosin given twice daily (mean daily dose 13.8 mg) Gould et al. [32] found an insignificant change in the diurnal blood pressure profile, except for a reduction during 2 out of 24 hours. However, using a different alpha blocker, indoramin, they found a generally similar reduction in blood pressure throughout the day and night without any clear change in the diurnal profile [9]. Drayer et al. [35] found that terazosin, a long-acting alpha blocker, also shifted the diurnal profile of blood pressure downwards.

Beta blockers

Numerous studies have examined the effect of beta blockers on the diurnal blood pressure profile. Except in those instances where the pharmacological effects of the drugs did not persist for a full 24 h [25], the general trend has been a reduction in pressure to a similar extent throughout the day and night [25,26,30,61,62], as shown for propranolol in Fig. 10.10. In some cases, however, the effect during the night has been less marked [56]. White et al. [40] found that cetamolol, a cardioselective beta blocker, had the greatest antihypertensive effect during work, with a lesser effect at home, and an insignificant effect during sleep.

Third-generation beta blockers such as celiprolol, which combine beta$_1$ antagonism with beta$_2$ agonism, have interesting differences in comparison with other agents. They cause no decrease in resting heart rate and have little effect on blood pressure at night [11]. As a result, the diurnal profile is flattened.

Alpha/beta blockers

When an alpha/beta blocker such as labetalol is used it has been observed that the diurnal profile is significantly flattened: when given twice daily to patients with isolated systolic hypertension, there was a marked reduction in the peak of systolic pressure occurring between 8.00 a.m. and 12 noon, but it had relatively little effect on the pressure at night [63] (Fig. 10.11). This actually confirmed, but did not acknowledge, the findings of an earlier study by Balasubramanian and colleagues [64], who concluded that the pre-waking rise in systolic pressure was not affected by the drug, whereas the increase that occurred at the time of waking was greatly attenuated. However, another study [57] found no significant change in the diurnal profile.

Calcium antagonists

All the calcium antagonists investigated with 24-hour monitoring, including verapamil [27,65,66], nifedipine [65,67], diltiazem [43] and isradipine [44], have been found to lower blood pressure without much change in the diurnal profile.

Angiotensin converting enzyme inhibitors

Both the long-acting agents, such as ramipril [68], lisinopril [47,69,70] and perindopril [71], and the shorter-acting captopril [47,53,72] have been reported to lower blood pressure without altering the diurnal profile.

Centrally acting agents

Although several different centrally acting agents exist, relatively little information is available regarding their effects on the circadian rhythm of blood pressure. Gould et al. [73] studied the effects of methyldopa given three times daily and found that it lowered blood pressure effectively during the day. However, methyldopa had no significant effect on blood pressure during the night, hence flattening the diurnal profile.

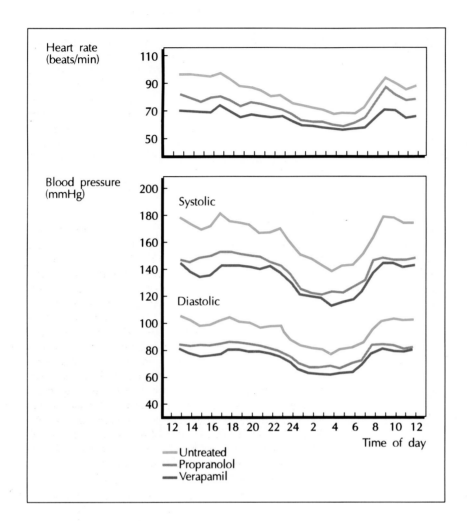

Fig. 10.10. The effects of propranolol and verapamil on the diurnal profile of blood pressure. Reproduced with permission [30].

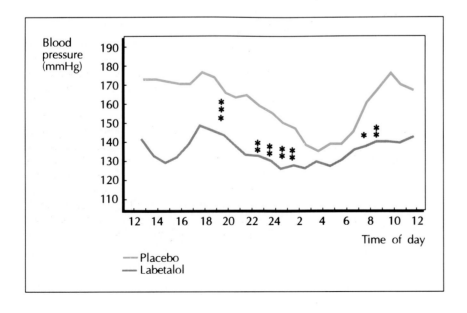

Fig. 10.11. The effects of labetalol on ambulatory pressure. Asterisks show significant reduction. Reproduced with permission [63].

Diuretics

Although diuretics continue to rank among the most widely prescribed antihypertensives, there is a serious lack of information concerning how long they affect blood pressure. The reason for this is not hard to find: studies of the effects of antihypertensives using ambulatory monitoring are almost always financed by pharmaceutical companies, and most of the currently used diuretics were introduced before ambulatory monitoring became fashionable. Thus, the only published study used xipamide, a long-acting, non-thiazide diuretic currently unavailable [74]. Blood pressure was reduced to an equal extent throughout the day and night.

Combination treatments

A few studies have also examined the effects of giving combinations of two different medications. An example is a study by Fogari et al. [75] of a fixed combination of captopril and hydrochlorothiazide given in a one-daily dosage. They showed that giving the medication in the evening (8.00 p.m.) produced a somewhat better control of 24-hour pressure than giving it in the morning (9.00 a.m.)

Implication of the different effects on the diurnal profile

It is clear that the majority of antihypertensive agents have relatively little effect on the diurnal rhythm of blood pressure, although there is a tendency to lower pressure a little more during the day. Raftery and Carrageta [76] proposed that the conspicuous lack of effect of beta blockers may mean that the increase in pressure during the morning is mediated by alpha-adrenergic vasoconstriction. This is not supported by their own data, however, since they have also reported that neither of two alpha blockers tested, prazosin and indoramin, flattened the curve.

The two agents that do appear to have a preferential effect on the increase in blood pressure during the day are labetalol and methyldopa. The former blocks both alpha- and beta-adrenergic receptors, and the latter inhibits central sympathetic outflow. The increased pressure during the day is almost certainly largely mediated by the sympathetic nervous system, and the fact that both limbs (alpha and beta) have to be blocked to impair this increase may be another example of the principle that the central nervous system will increase pressure by whatever mechanism is available, as discussed in Chapter 4. These findings also imply that the renin–angiotensin system does not play a major role in regulating the diurnal rhythm of blood pressure.

Evaluation of the effects of non-pharmacological treatment

In view of the expense and side effects associated with pharmacological treatment of hypertension, interest has grown in the use of non-pharmacological methods. These have taken a variety of forms, but may be loosely classified into three major groups: dietary, exercise and relaxation. A common feature of all non-pharmacological methods is that they require an active and sustained behavioural change by the patient. A potential concern with all three groups is therefore the possibility of placebo effects.

Dietary treatment

The effects of weight loss by dietary calorie restriction were compared with the effects of exercise in normotensive men by Fortmann et al. [42], using both clinic and ambulatory pressures. The former decreased to the same extent in the two treatment groups and a control group, while small but significant decreases in ambulatory pressure were seen only in the treatment groups. A study by Richards et al. [77] reported the effects of a combined dietary manipulation — sodium restriction and potassium supplementation — in a small group of patients evaluated by both clinic and ambulatory pressures. Neither measure of blood pressure showed any significant change, perhaps because the number of patients was too small, or the sodium restriction was inadequate. We have also conducted a study (submitted for publication) which showed that sodium depletion produced similar reductions in clinic and ambulatory pressures.

Another study evaluated the effects of sodium restriction in normotensive subjects [78] who remained supine throughout the 24-hour period of study. Systolic pressure was 10 mmHg lower on the low-sodium diet, but diastolic pressure was unchanged. The diurnal profile was hardly affected.

Exercise

Several studies have shown that a programme of aerobic exercise training can lower blood pressure both at rest [79] and during exercise [80], but few have used either ambulatory or self-monitoring to assess the duration of the effect over a 24-hour period. Van Hoof et al. [80] studied 25 men before and after 4 months of exercise training using non-invasive ambulatory monitoring. Resting blood pressure measured in the laboratory decreased by 4/5 mmHg, but only the change in diastolic pressure was significant. However, there was a significant decrease in systolic pressure of 7 mmHg during exercise. Twenty-four-hour monitoring showed a significant decrease in diastolic pressure (5 mmHg) during the day but no effect at night. There was no significant change in systolic pressure, although heart rate was reduced throughout the day and night. These effects would be consistent with a reduction in sympathetic activity during the day.

How should the effects of treatment be analysed?

The previous discussion clearly indicates that ambulatory monitoring permits much more detailed information to be acquired about the effects of an antihypertensive agent than clinic measurements. However, there is as yet no standard method for analysing or expressing the results. A number of methods have been used, as shown in Fig. 10.12. These are reviewed below, and the techniques are described in more detail in Chapter 16.

Effects on overall or average level of blood pressure
Average 24-hour blood pressure
Average daytime blood pressure
Per cent readings above 140/90 mmHg (blood
    pressure load)

Peak and trough effects
Consecutive hourly averages

Effects on diurnal profile (long-term variability)
Awake–sleep blood pressure
Cosinor analysis
Area under the curve

Effects on short-term variability
Standard deviation, etc.
Histogram
Response to standard challenges

Fig. 10.12. Methods for analysing effects of antihypertensive treatment on ambulatory blood pressure.

Effects on average pressure
The most widely used method has been to express the effects of the drug on the average 24-hour or daytime ambulatory pressure [33,48]. This has the advantage of being both simple and relevant.

Another method entails describing the effects on the percentage of readings above an arbitrary value, for example 140/90 mmHg for daytime values and 120/80 mmHg for sleep values. These have been proposed as criteria for normality by White and Morganroth [81]. As discussed in Chapter 9, we believe that this method may be more misleading than enlightening.

Peak and trough effects
In principle, analysis of peak and trough effects using serial measurements of blood pressure before and after

each dose of the drug should be quite simple. With ambulatory blood pressure recordings, several workers have analysed consecutive hourly averages (e.g. by multiple t-tests) to evaluate the duration of effect [25,36]. This approach has several problems. First, the use of multiple t-tests is inappropriate in data which are not independent of each other. Second, with non-invasive recorders it is usual to obtain between two and four readings per hour, so that the reliability of an hourly average may be quite low.

The fact that there is a consistent diurnal variation in blood pressure adds a significant complication to this analysis. It may be more difficult to detect a subtle effect on blood pressure during the working day, when blood pressure is relatively labile, than during the evening, when it is more stable. This may explain why White *et al.* [39] found that nitrendipine lowered pressure at home but not at work. Furthermore, it cannot be assumed that a medication given at 8.00 a.m. will have the same peak and trough effect as when it is given at 8.00 p.m. Indeed, there is evidence that at least one drug (verapamil) may have an absorption rate of only half as much in the afternoon as in the morning [37].

Area under the curve (AUC)
This traditional method of quantifying the effects of a drug on blood pressure compares the area of the plot of blood pressure against time with and without the drug. It has been used recently in a study of ambulatory monitoring comparing lisinopril with captopril [47]. It gives much the same information as the average pressure and is an insufficient description on its own, because two drugs with similar AUCs may have quite different time courses of action. Its use is not encouraged by the FDA.

Effects on diurnal profile
Many studies have concluded that antihypertensive medications have little effect on the diurnal profile (see above). In general, however, such studies have not used any formal analysis to justify this statement. One simple way of evaluating diurnal profile would be to compare the difference between the average pressure while awake and during sleep before and after treatment.

Cosine analysis has also been used for this purpose. This technique was described in Chapter 5 and, while mathematically appealing, presupposes that the diurnal rhythm is basically a sine (or cosine) wave, which clearly it is not.

Effects on short-term variability
The most widely used measures of blood pressure variability have been the standard deviation and coefficient of variation. As discussed in Chapter 4, short-term variability cannot be reliably evaluated with non-invasive recorders. It is, however, possible to examine the effects of specific activities on blood pressure and to see how these changes are affected by treatment.

A popular technique has been to combine ambulatory recordings with standardized laboratory tests, such as exercise, cold pressor test and tilt. These are reviewed in Chapter 12.

Disadvantages of ambulatory monitoring

The main limitation of ambulatory monitoring for the evaluation of treatment is the number of recordings that can be carried out in any one patient. Two or three recordings is usually the limit, and patient compliance falls off sharply if more are attempted. Thus, it may not be easy to determine how quickly a drug takes effect, and self-monitoring may be preferable.

The second potential problem is the variability in blood pressure on different recording days. The more 'ambulatory' the patients, the more variability (and also artefact) is likely to occur, which may confound the analysis of the effects of the drug. An extreme example of this would occur if one recording was made on a work day and another on a non-work day. Thus, the activities of the patients should be standardized as much as possible from one recording to another.

These disadvantages are relatively minor compared with the advantages.

Should blood pressure be reduced throughout the day and night?

The official view of the FDA is that blood pressure should be lowered throughout the day and night, on the grounds that the agents which have been shown to reduce cardiovascular morbidity do produce such a sustained reduction of blood pressure. Although this is certainly logical, it is not necessarily the optimum form of control. An alternative approach would be to attempt to reduce the peaks in pressure that occur during the day, with a lesser reduction during the night. As we have seen in Chapter 6, there is a marked circadian rhythm of many cardiovascular morbid events, with a peak incidence in the morning hours between 6.00 a.m. and 12 noon, when blood pressure is also at its highest. Although a direct causal link between the two cannot be drawn, the data suggest that a link might exist.

Floras [82] has recently argued that excessive reduction in blood pressure during the night may actually be harmful. In a study of hypertensive patients without overt CHD who underwent 24-hour intra-arterial pressure monitoring, diastolic pressures of 30–40 mmHg were common while on treatment with beta blockers but not before treatment. He suggested that coronary perfusion might be impaired at such low pressures in patients with CHD. General support for this view comes from several studies which have shown that the absence of consistent prevention of myocardial infarction as a result of treating hypertension could be the net result of two opposing ef-

fects: a moderate reduction in pressure lowers morbidity, but a more severe reduction raises it [83–88]. Thus, the relationship between blood pressure and morbidity from CHD in treated patients takes the form of a J-shaped curve. The level of minimal morbidity has been estimated to occur at a diastolic pressure of about 87 mmHg [89]. Other studies have, however, suggested that the phenomenon is more a function of the extent of blood pressure reduction than the absolute level [90,91]. More direct supportive evidence is provided by a study of diltiazem, which was found to exacerbate silent myocardial ischaemia in hypertensive patients but not in normotensive people [92]. In subjects treated with beta blockers the normal circadian rhythm of myocardial infarction and sudden cardiac death is not seen (see Chapter 6), but this appears to be due to a reduced incidence of events during the day rather than an increased incidence at night.

A counter-argument in favour of lowering blood pressure during the night could be put forward. Myocardial oxygen demand is lower during the night, and in many patients the lower perfusion pressure may therefore be appropriate. As we have seen in Chapter 6, most patients show less myocardial ischaemia during the night than during the day. The phenomenon of the J-shaped curve has been criticized on the grounds that the number of patients representing the shorter arm of the J has been very small. There are also many patients whose blood pressure does not fall at night. Although the pathological significance of this has not been established there is evidence that such patients are at increased risk of LVH, and it could be argued that a sustained reduction in pressure would be beneficial.

Summary and conclusions

Ambulatory monitoring offers many advantages over conventional clinic measurements for evaluating the effectiveness of antihypertensive medications; these clearly outweigh the disadvantages. The elimination of the placebo effect and the greater reproducibility of ambulatory measurements mean that smaller sample sizes are required in drug studies. Furthermore, the fact that clinic pressures frequently misrepresent the true blood pressure becomes unimportant when ambulatory recording is used, in terms of both the selection of patients and the evaluation of drug effects. The efficiency of drug studies is likely to be improved when patients are selected on the basis of their ambulatory rather than clinic pressures, which so far has not been done. The effects of drug treatment on white coat hypertension are not well understood and warrant further study. The duration of the effects of treatment over the 24-hour period can be assessed, and hence the appropriate frequency of dosing. Ambulatory monitoring studies will enable new questions to be addressed, such as whether treatment should be equally effective throughout the day and night or should be focused on times when the pressure is highest. An interesting and somewhat surprising finding is that most forms of pharmacological treatment lower the tonic component of blood pressure but have little effect on its phasic variations. Ambulatory monitoring is also ideally suited to the evaluation of non-pharmacological treatment, in which placebo effects may confound the changes in clinic pressure.

References

1. SHAPIRO AK: Etiological factors in placebo effect. *JAMA* 1964, 187:712–714.
2. GRENFELL RF, BRIGGS AH, HOLLAND WC: Antihypertensive drugs evaluated in a controlled double-blind study. *South Med J* 1963, 56:1410–1415.
3. MCDONALD CJ, MAZZUCA SA, MCCABE GP: How much of the placebo 'effect' is really statistical regression? *Stat Med* 1983, 2:417–427.
4. SHAPIRO AP, MYERS T, REISER MF, FERRIS EB: Comparison of blood pressure response to veriloid and to the doctor. *Psychosom Med* 1954, 16:478–488.
5. SASSANO P, CHATELLIER G, CORVOL P, MÉNARD J: Influence of observer's expectation on the placebo effect in blood pressure trials. *Curr Ther Res* 1987, 41:305–312.
6. DOYLE AE: Response to placebo treatment in hypertension. *Hypertension* 1983, 5 (suppl III):III3–III4.
7. MIALL WE, BRENNAN PJ: Observations on the natural history of mild hypertension in the control groups of therapeutic trials. In *Mild Hypertension, Natural History and Management* edited by Gross F, Strasser T. Chicago: Pitman, Year Book Medical Publishers, 1979, pp 38–46.
8. PICKERING TG, HARSHFIELD GA, DEVEREUX RB, LARAGH JH: What is the role of ambulatory blood pressure monitoring in the management of hypertensive patients? *Hypertension* 1985, 7:171–177.
9. GOULD BA, MANN S, DAVIES AB, ALTMAN DG, RAFTERY EB: Does placebo lower blood-pressure? *Lancet* 1981, ii:1377–1381.
10. DUPONT AG, VAN DER NIEPEN P, SIX RO: Placebo does not lower ambulatory blood pressure. *Br J Clin Pharmacol* 1987, 24:106–109.
11. PARATI G, POMIDOSSI G, CASADEI R, ET AL.: Evaluation of the antihypertensive effect of celiprolol by ambulatory blood pressure monitoring. *Am J Cardiol* 1988, 61:27c–33c.
12. CONWAY J, JOHNSTON J, COATS A, SOMERS V, SLEIGHT P: The use of ambulatory blood pressure monitoring to improve the accuracy and reduce the numbers of subjects in clinical trials of antihypertensive agents. *J Hypertens* 1988, 6:111–116.
13. BELLET M, PAGNY J-Y, CHATELLIER G, CORVOL P, MÉNARD J: Evaluation of slow release nicardipine in essential hypertension by casual and ambulatory blood pressure measurements. Effects of acute versus chronic administration. *J Hypertens* 1987, 5:599–604.
14. JAMES GD, PICKERING TG, YEE LS, HARSHFIELD GA, RIVAS L, LARAGH JH: The reproducibility of average ambulatory, home, and clinic pressures. *Hypertension* 1988, 11:545–549.
15. HILLS M, ARMITAGE P: The two-period cross-over clinical trial. *Br J Clin Pharmacol* 1979, 7:7–20.
16. FREESTONE S, SILAS JH, RAMSAY LE: Sample size for short-term trials of antihypertensive drugs. *Br J Clin Pharmacol* 1982, 14:265–268.
17. MÉNARD J, SERRURIER D, BAUTIER P, PLOVIN P-F, CORVOL P: Crossover design to test antihypertensive drugs with self-recorded blood pressures. *Hypertension* 1988, 11:153–159.
18. COATS AJS, CONWAY J, SOMERS K, ISEA JE, SLEIGHT P: Ambulatory pressure monitoring in the assessment of antihypertensive therapy. *Cardiovasc Drug Ther* 1989, 3:303–311.
19. CONWAY J, COATS A: Value of ambulatory blood pressure monitoring in clinical pharmacology. *J Hypertens* 1989, 7 (suppl 3):29–32.
20. HARSHFIELD GA, PICKERING TG, BLANK S, LARAGH JH: How well do casual blood pressures reflect ambulatory blood pressures? In *Blood Pressure Recordings in the Clinical Manage-*
21. *ment of Hypertension* edited by Gemano G. Rome: Edizioni Pozzi, 1985, pp 50–53.
21. JACOT DES COMBES B, PORCHET M, WAEBER B, BRUNNER HR: Ambulatory blood pressure recordings. Reproducibility and unpredictibility. *Hypertension* 1984, 6:C110–C114.
22. PORCHET M, BUSSIN JP, WAEBER B, NUSSBERGER J, BRUNNER HR: Unpredictability of blood pressure recorded outside the clinic in the treated hypertensive patient. *J Cardiovasc Pharmacol* 1986, 8:332–335.
23. ENSTROM I, THULIN T, LINDHOLM L: A plea for more comprehensive blood pressure measurements when evaluating drug treatment of hypertension. *J Hypertens* 1988, 6:959–964.
24. GRAY JM, SILVERMAN HM, GORWIT JI: Comparison of labetalol and prazosin in hypertensive patients using automated ambulatory monitoriong. *Am J Med* 1988, 84:904–910.
25. FLORAS JS, JONES JV, HASSAN MO, SLEIGHT P: Ambulatory blood pressure during once-daily randomized double-blind administration of atenolol, metoprolol, pindolol, and slow-release propranolol. *Br Med J* 1982, 285:1387–1392.
26. HORNUNG RS, GOULD BA, KIESO H, RAFTERY EB: A study of nadolol to determine its effect on ambulatory blood pressure over 24 hours, and during exercise testing. *Br J Clin Pharmacol* 1982, 14:83–88.
27. CARDILLO C, SARI L, MUSUMECI V ET AL.: Casual versus 24-hour ambulatory blood pressure recording in the evaluation of chronic administration of sustained-release verapamil. *J Hum Hypertens* 1988, 2:281–285.
28. WHITE WB, SCHULMAN P, KARIMEDDINI MK, SMITH V-E: Regression of left ventricular mass is accompanied by improvement in rapid left ventricular filling following antihypertensive therapy with metoprolol. *Am Heart J* 1989, 117:145–150.
29. WAEBER G, BECK G, WAEBER B, BIDIVILLE J, NUSSBERGER J, BRUNNER HR: Comparison of betaxolol with verapamil in hypertensive patients: discrepancy between office and ambulatory blood pressure. *J Hypertens* 1988, 6:239–245.
30. HORNUNG RS, JONES RI, GOULD BA, SONECHA T, RAFTERY EB: Twice-daily verapamil for hypertension: a comparison with propranolol. *Am J Cardiol* 1986, 57:89D–93D.
31. MCLEAY R, STALLARD TJ, WATSON RDS, LITTLER WA: The effect of nifedipine on arterial pressure and reflex cardiac control. *Circulation* 1983, 67:1084–1089.
32. GOULD BA, HORNUNG RS, KIESO HA, CASHMAN PMM, RAFTERY EB: Prazosin alone and combined with a β-adrenoreceptor blocker in treatment of hypertension. *J Cardiovasc Pharmacol* 1983, 5:678–684.
33. RION F, WAEBER B, GRAF HG, JAUSSI A, PORCHET M, BRUNNER HR: Blood pressure response to antihypertensive therapy: ambulatory versus office blood pressure readings. *J Hypertens* 1985, 3:139–143.
34. COX JP, O'BOYLE CA, MEE F ET AL.: The antihypertensive efficacy of verapamil in the elderly evaluated by ambulatory blood pressure measurement. *J Hum Hypertens* 1988, 2:41–47.
35. DRAYER HIM, WEBER MA, DEYOUNG JL, BREWER DD: Long-term BP monitoring in the evaluation of antihypertensive therapy. *Arch Intern Med* 1983, 143:898–901.
36. BERGLUND G, DEFAIRE U, CASTENFORS J ET AL.: Monitoring 24-hour blood pressure in a drug trial. Evaluation of a noninvasive device. *Hypertension* 1985, 7:688–694.
37. ELDON MA, BATTLE MM, VOIGTMAN RE, COLBURN WA: Differences in oral verapamil absorption as a function of time of day. *J Hypertens* 1989, 29:989–993.
38. O'BRIEN E, COX JP, FITZGERALD DJ, O'MALLEY K: Discrepancy between clinic and ambulatory blood pressure measurement in the evaluation of two antihypertensive agents. *J Hum Hypertens* 1989, 3:259–262.
39. WHITE WB, SMITH V-E, MCCABE EJ, MEERAN MK: Effects of chronic nitrendipine on casual (office) and 24-hour ambulatory blood pressure. *Clin Pharmacol Ther* 1985, 38:60–64.
40. WHITE WB, SCHULMAN P, MCCABE EJ, HAGER WD: Effects of chronic cetamolol therapy on resting, ambulatory, and exercise blood pressure and heart rate. *Clin Pharmacol Ther* 1986, 39:664–668.

41. SCHALLER MD, NUSSBERGER J, WAEBER B, PORCHET M, BRUNNER HR: Transdermal clonidine in hypertensive patients: effect on office and ambulatory recorded blood pressures. *JAMA* 1985, 253:233–236.
42. FORTMANN SP, HASKELL WL, WOOD PD: Effects of weight loss on clinic and ambulatory blood pressure in normotensive men. *Am J Cardiol* 1988, 52:89–93.
43. WEBER MA, CHEUNG DG, GRAETTINGER WF, LIPSON JL: Characterization of antihypertensive therapy by whole-day blood pressure monitoring. *JAMA* 1988, 259:3281–3285.
44. LACOURCIÈRE Y, POIRIER L, DION D, PROVENCHER P: Antihypertensive effect of isradipine administered once or twice daily on ambulatory blood pressure. *Am J Cardiol* 1990, 65:467–472.
45. GRADMAN AH, PANGAN P, GERMAIN M: Lack of correlation between clinic and 24 hour ambulatory blood pressure in subjects participating in a therapeutic drug trial. *J Clin Epidemiol* 1989, 42:1049–1054.
46. ROSE M, MCMAHON FG: Some problems with antihypertensive drug studies in the context of the new guidelines. *Am J Hypertens* 1990, 3:151–155.
47. WHELTON A, MILLER WE, DUNNE B, HAIT HI, TRESZNEWSKY ON: Once-daily lisinopril compared with twice-daily captopril in the treatment of mild to moderate hypertension. Assessment of offfice and ambulatory blood pressures. *Ann Intern Med* (in press).
48. CONWAY J, WAY B, BOON N, SOMERS V: Is the antihypertensive effect of captopril influenced by the dosage frequency? A study with ambulatory monitoring. *J Hum Hypertens* 1988, 2:123–126.
49. MURDOCH DL, GILLEN GJ, MORTON JJ ET AL.: Twice-daily low-dose captopril in diuretic-treated hypertensives. *J Hum Hypertens* 1989, 3:29–33.
50. CASE DB, ATLAS SA, LARAGH JH, SULLIVAN PA, SEALEY JE: Use of first-dose response on plasma renin activity to predict the long-term effect of captopril: identification of triphasic response pattern of blood pressure response. *J Cardiovasc Pharmacol* 1980, 2:339–346.
51. BRUNNER HR, GAVRAS H, WAEBER B ET AL.: Oral angiotensin converting-enzyme inhibitor in long-term treatment of hypertensive patients. *Ann Intern Med* 1979, 90:19–23.
52. VETERANS ADMINISTRATION COOPERATIVE STUDY GROUP ON ANTIHYPERTENSIVE AGENTS. Low-dose captopril for the treatment of mild to moderate hypertension. I. Results of a 14-week trial. *Arch Intern Med* 1984, 144:1947–1953.
53. MANCIA G, PARATI G, POMIDOSSI G ET AL.: Evaluation of the antihypertensive effect of once-a-day captopril by 24-hour ambulatory blood pressure monitoring. *J Hypertens* 1987 (suppl 5):S591–S593.
54. WEST MJ, SLEIGHT P, HONOUR AJ: Clinical trial of the beta-adrenoreceptor-blocking agent tolamolol with the use of 24 hour blood pressure recordings. *Clin Sci Mol Med* 1976, 51:545s–547s.
55. DE LEEUW PW, FALKE HE, KHO TL, VANDONGEN R, WESLER A, BIRKENHAGER WA: Effects of beta-adrenergic blockade on diurnal variability of blood pressure and plasma noradrenaline levels. *Acta Med Scand* 1977, 202:389–392.
56. MANCIA G, FERRARI A, POMIDOSSI G ET AL.: Twenty-four-hour hemodynamic profile during treatment of essential hypertension by once-a-day nadolol. *Hypertension* 1983, 5:573–578.
57. MANCIA G, POMIDOSSI G, PARATI G ET AL.: Blood pressure response to labetalol in twice and three times daily administration during a 24-hour period. *Br J Clin Pharmacol* 1982, 13 (suppl):27–34.
58. FLORAS JS, HASSAN O, VANN JONES J, OSIKOWSKA BA, SEVER PS, SLEIGHT P: Factors influencing blood pressure and heart rate variability in hypertensive humans. *Hypertension* 1988, 11:273–281.
59. MANCIA S, FERRARI A, GREGORINI L, ET AL.: Evaluation of a slow-release clonidine preparation by direct continuous blood pressure recording in essential hypertensive patients. *J Cardiovasc Pharmacol* 1981, 3:1193–1202.

60. NOVO S, ALAIMO G, ABRIGNANI MG, LONGO B, MURATORE G, STRANO A: Noninvasive blood pressure monitoring evaluation of verapamil slow-release 240-mg antihypertensive effectiveness. *J Cardiovasc Pharmacol* 1989, 13 (suppl 4):38–41.
61. MANN S, MILLAR-CRAIG MW, ALTMAN DG, MELVILLE DI, RAFTERY EB: The effects of metoprolol on ambulatory blood pressure. *Clin Sci* 1979, 57:375S–377S.
62. FAVRE L, ADAMEC R, BOXHO G: Effect of bopindolol on the circadian blood pressure profile in essential hypertension. *J Cardiovasc Pharmacol* 1986, 8 (suppl 6):60–63.
63. DE QUATTRO V, DE-PING LEE D, ALLEN J, SIRGO M, PLACHETKA J: Labetalol blunts morning pressor surge in systolic hypertension. *Hypertension* 1988, 11 (suppl I):I198–I201.
64. BALASUBRAMANIAN V, MANN S, RAFTERY EB, MILLAR-CRAIG MW, ALTMAN D: Effect of labetalol on continuous ambulatory blood pressure. *Br J Clin Pharmacol* 1979, 8:119S–123S.
65. GOULD BA, HORNUNG RS, MANN S, BALASUBRAMANIAN V, RAFTERY EB: Slow channel inhibitors verapamil and nifedipine in the management of hypertension. *J Cardiovasc Pharmacol* 1982, 4:S269–S373.
66. CARDILLO C, MUSUMECI V, MORES N, FOLLI G: Effects of sustained-release verapamil on 24-hour ambulatory blood pressure and on pressor response to isometric exertion in hypertensive patients. *J Cardiovasc Pharmacol* 1989, 13 (suppl 4):31–33.
67. HORNUNG RS, GOULD BA, JONES RI, SONECHA T, RAFTERY EB: Nifedipine tablets for hypertension: a study using continuous ambulatory intra-arterial monitoring. *Postgrad Med J* 1983, 59 (suppl 2):95–107.
68. HEBER MA, BRIGDEN GS, CARVANA MP, LAHIRI A, RAFTERY EB: First dose response and 24-hour antihypertensive efficacy of the new once-daily angiotensin converting enzyme inhibitor, ramipril. *Am J Cardiol* 1988, 62:239–245.
69. ZACHARIAH PK, SHEPS SG, SCHWARTZ GL, ET AL.: Antihypertensive efficacy of lisinopril. Ambulatory blood pressure monitoring. *Am J Hypertens* 1988, 1 (suppl):274S–279S.
70. HERPIN D, CONTE D: Assessment of the antihypertensive effect of lisinopril using 24-hour ambulatory monitoring. *J Hum Hypertens* 1989, 3:11–15.
71. WEST HJNW, SMITH SA, STALLARD THJ, LITTLER WA: Effects of perindopril on ambulatory intra-arterial blood pressure, cardiovascular reflexes, and forearm blood flow in essential hypertension. *J Hypertens* 1989, 7:97–104.
72. MEIJER JL, ARDESCH HG, VAN ROOIJEN JC, DEBRUIJN JHB: Low dose captopril twice daily lowers blood pressure without disturbance of the normal circadian rhythm. *Postgrad Med J* 1986, 62 (suppl 1):1091–1095.
73. GOULD BA, HORNUNG RS, KIESO HA, CASHMAN PMM, RAFTERY EB: An intra-arterial profile of methyldopa. *Clin Pharmacol Ther* 1983, 33:438–444.
74. RAFTERY EB, MELVILLE DI, GOULD BA, MANN S, WHITTINGTON JR: A study of the antihypertensive action of xipamide using ambulatory intra-arterial monitoring. *Br J Clin Pharmacol* 1981, 12:381–385.
75. FOGARI R, TETTAMANTI F, ZOPPI A, POLETTI L, BUTTA GF: Evaluation of the efficacy of once-daily administration of captopril plus hydrochlorothiazide by 24-hour ambulatory blood pressure monitoring. *Curr Ther Res* 1988, 44:1050–1057.
76. RAFTERY EB, CARREGETA MO: Hypertension and beta blockers: are they all the same? *Int J Cardiol* 1985, 7:337–346.
77. RICHARDS AM, NICHOLLS MG, ESPINER EA, ET AL.: Blood-pressure response to moderate sodium restriction and to potassium supplementation in mild essential hypertension. *Lancet* 1984, i:757–761.
78. CUGINI P, DANESE D, BATTISTI P, DIPALMA L, LEONE G, KAWASAKI T: Usefulness of 24-hour blood pressure patterns and response to short-term sodium restriction in normotensive subjects in detecting a predisposition to systemic arterial hypertension. *Am J Cardiol* 1989, 64:604–608.
79. JENNINGS G, NELSON L, NESTEL P ET AL.: The effect of changes in physical activity on major cardiovascular risk factors, hemodynamics, sympathetic function, and glucose utiliza-

tion in man: a controlled study of four levels of activity. *Circulation* 1986, 73:30–40.

80.   VAN HOOF R, HESPEL P, FAGARD R, LIJNEN P, STAESSEN J, AMERY A: Effect of endurance training on blood pressure at rest, during exercise and during 24 hours in sedentary men. *Am J Cardiol* 1989, 63:945–949.

81.   WHITE WB, MORGANROTH J: Usefulness of ambulatory monitoring of blood pressure in assessing antihypertensive therapy. *Am J Cardiol* 1989, 63:94–98.

82.   FLORAS JS: Antihypertensive treatment, myocardial infarction, and nocturnal myocardial ischaemia. *Lancet* 1988, ii:994–996.

83.   CRUICKSHANK JM, THORP JM, ZACHARIAS FJ: Benefits and potential harm of lowering high blood pressure. *Lancet* 1987, ii:581–584.

84.   WILHELMSEN L, BERGLUND G, ELMFELDT D *ET AL*: Beta-blockers versus diuretics in hypertensive men. Main results from the HAPPHY trial. *J Hypertens* 1987, 5:561–572.

85.   SAMUELSSON O, WILHELMSEN L, ANDERSSON OK, PENNERT K, BERGLUND G: Cardiovascular morbidity in relation to change in blood pressure and serum cholesterol levels in treated hypertension: results from the primary prevention trial in Göteborg, Sweden. *JAMA* 1987, 258:1768–1776.

86.   COOPE J, WARRENDER TS: Randomized trial of treatment of hypertension in elderly patients in primary care. *Br Med J* 1986, 293:1145–1151.

87.   WALKER PC, ISLES CG, LEVER AF, MURRAY GD, MCINNES GT: Does therapeutic reduction of diastolic blood pressure cause death from coronary heart disease? *J Hum Hypertens* 1988, 2:7–10.

88.   FLETCHER AE, BEEVERS DG, BULPITT CT, *ET AL*: The relationship between a low treated blood pressure and IHD mortality: a report from the DHSS Hypertension Care Computing Project (DHCCP). *J Hum Hypertens* 1988, 2:11–15.

89.   CRUICKSHANK JM: Coronary flow reserve and the J curve relation between diastolic blood pressure and myocardial infarction. *Br Med J* 1988, 297:1227–1230.

90.   COOPER SP, HARDY RJ, LABARTHE CR, *ET AL*: The relation between degree of blood pressure reduction and mortality among hypertensives in the Hypertension Detection and Follow-Up Program. *Am J Epidemiol* 1988, 127:387–403.

91.   ALDERMAN MH, OOI WL, MADHAVAN S, COHEN H: Treatment-induced blood pressure reduction and the risk of myocardial infarction. *JAMA* 1989, 262:920–924.

92.   FELL D, GOODMAN J, MCLAUGHLIN PR, *ET AL*: Modification of silent and exercise-induced ischaemia by diltiazem in stable coronary disease. *Clin Invest Med* 1988, 5:D49.

11 Blood pressure monitoring for studying the role of behavioural factors in cardiovascular disease

The role of behavioural factors in hypertension may, at first sight, seem somewhat peripheral to the central theme of this book. However, ambulatory monitoring is proving to be an invaluable tool for its evaluation. The idea that stress[1] may be related to the development of hypertension is as old as the concept of hypertension itself [1], but supportive evidence is sparse. A huge amount of effort has been put into laboratory studies of cardiovascular reactivity, discussed in the next chapter, which have provided only limited insights into the role of behavioural factors. Ambulatory monitoring has opened a new field of inquiry and permits a more ethological or anthropological approach to the problem than was previously possible. Thus, we can now study people in their natural environments and evaluate the effects of the stresses of everyday life on blood pressure.

There is increasing evidence for a subtle over-activity of the sympathetic nervous system in the early stages of essential hypertension [2]: what is the 'prime mover' leading to such over-activity? Although it may be genetic, it is equally plausible that environmental stressors play a role. As discussed briefly in Chapters 1 and 4, it is relatively easy to show that stress can cause a transient elevation in blood pressure. However, this is of doubtful relevance to sustained hypertension, which appears to be primarily a disorder of the tonic regulation of blood pressure rather than of its short-term variability. This chapter therefore places particular emphasis on the time course of the effects of stress on blood pressure and the mechanisms by which the cardiovascular effects of a stressor may outlast the stimulus.

Conceptual issues

Psychological stress is a subjective experience. It can be regarded as the resultant of the individual's perceptions and of the environment in which he or she is placed. In other words, stress, like beauty, is 'in the eye of the beholder'. To take this analogy further, there are some things that virtually everyone considers beautiful, whereas others are more a matter of individual preference. In the case of stress, similarly, there are some things that everyone finds stressful (war, for example), but other situations (such as public speaking) may be regarded as very stressful by some individuals and not by others. The majority of the stresses of daily life come into the latter category. The physiological effects of the perceived

stress will, in turn, depend on the physiological constitution of the individual. Any number of factors could influence the blood pressure or cardiac response, including genetic predisposition, the state of sodium balance and a host of other factors. Thus, it would be naive to expect any simple relationship between stress and hypertension. Rather, we should look for a combination of factors which, when acting together, might contribute to a sustained elevation in pressure. The three types of factors that should be considered would be *psychological variables* (including both the individual's personality and previous experience), which interact with the *environmental stressors* to produce the perceived level of stress. The cardiovascular effects of this will, in turn, depend on the individual's *physiological susceptibility*. These interactions are shown in Fig. 11.1.

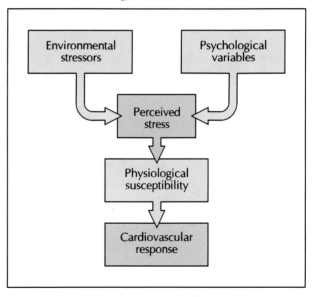

Fig. 11.1. Three major components mediating the effects of behavioural stress on cardiovascular disease.

There is considerable support from animal experiments for this multifactorial approach. Attempts to induce chronic hypertension have in general not been very successful. The most widely quoted animal model has been the CBA strain of mice [3,4]. The mice are housed in colonies consisting of a series of chambers connected by plastic tubes, only wide enough to fit one mouse. Mice reared in isolation and subsequently put in the colonies develop higher pressures than mice which are housed in the colonies from birth. In this model we can identify

---

[1]'Stress' is a useful but poorly defined term, having been used by various authors to describe a stimulus, a response, or an intervening process. In this chapter it refers to an individual's perception of an adverse environment, in which the stimuli are referred to as 'stressors'. The concept of stress as it relates to hypertension has been well reviewed by Krantz and Lazar [1].

the three factors described above. First, the psychological variable can be equated with the previous experience of the mouse (bred in isolation or in the colony); second, the environmental stressor is determined by the design of the colony: the narrowness of the tubes means that only one mouse can pass through at one time, so that a social hierarchy develops; and third, the importance of physiological susceptibility is shown by the finding that rats are immune to this type of hypertension [5]. Another example of the interaction of factors is provided by Anderson's work on dogs. He showed [6] that aversive conditioning (the environmental factor) does not, on its own, cause a sustained elevation in pressure, but if combined with a high sodium intake (the physiological factor), it can do so.

Studies of the role of behavioural factors in human cardiovascular disease have largely focused on the first of these two factors: the psychological variables. Considerable attention has been paid to the roles of suppressed anger and submissiveness in hypertension, and of the type A behaviour pattern in coronary heart disease. Physiological susceptibility has been studied in laboratory tests of cardiovascular reactivity (reviewed in Chapter 12), but environmental or psychosocial factors have received little attention. They form the chief focus of this chapter.

Blood pressure monitoring and personality variables

The idea that hypertension might be a psychosomatic disorder resulting from a particular personality type has been around for 50 years, since Alexander [7] and others proposed that hypertensives were characterized as individuals who were inhibited in their expression of anger and had a need to please others in their inter-personal relationships. Since then numerous studies have examined the relationships of self-reported levels of anger and anxiety with blood pressure [8–15]. In the vast majority of cases these studies have used clinic measures of pressure as the dependent variable.

As discussed in Chapter 7, clinic pressures may not be representative of an individual's true level of pressure. Therefore, it does not necessarily follow that any association observed between personality variables and clinic blood pressure would hold true for other, more valid measures of pressure. This is of particular concern because the differences between clinic and home or ambulatory pressures certainly have a behavioural origin, although at present there is no good evidence that white coat hypertension is the product of any specific personality type.

No published data yet relate personality traits to ambulatory blood pressure. However, Schneider *et al.* [16] compared measures of anger and anxiety in two groups of subjects with borderline hypertension and related them to home and clinic pressures. The group with elevated levels in both situations, whom we would classify as having true hypertension, scored significantly higher on

'Anger-In', that is inhibited anger, than the group whose pressure was high only in the clinic (i.e. white coat hypertension). There were no significant differences in measures of anxiety between the two groups. We [17] have collected data on personality variables (including measures of anger and anxiety) in more than 200 men studied with ambulatory monitoring, and found no associations with either clinic or ambulatory blood pressure.

The type A behaviour pattern has not traditionally been associated with high blood pressure. However, numerous studies have shown that type A individuals show a larger blood pressure response than type B individuals to behaviour challenges administered under controlled laboratory conditions [18]. A recent study by Van Egeren and Sparrow [19] using ambulatory blood pressure monitoring was designed to investigate whether these reactivity differences could also be seen during normal daily activities. The average levels of blood pressure were very similar in the two groups, but the type A people showed significantly greater increases in pressure during activities such as walking, drinking coffee or attending a meeting than the type B people.

Somewhat different results were obtained by Schneider *et al.* [20]. They studied 33 healthy men classified as either type A or type B, using both laboratory tests of reactivity and ambulatory monitoring. Type A men showed greater diastolic pressure responses to mental arithmetic, but not to isometric exercise, than type B men; ambulatory blood pressures were the same in the two groups.

Effects of environmental stressors on the diurnal profile of blood pressure

For most people, the day can be divided into three periods of approximately 8 h each, corresponding to the time spent at work, at home and asleep. When ambulatory blood pressure recordings were analysed in this way, we found that the pressure is, on average, about 5 mmHg higher at work than at home, with a further fall during sleep [21]. As our subjects had mostly sedentary jobs, we believe that the higher pressures are predominantly due to psychosocial influences rather than to more vigorous physical activity during work.

It is also possible that the difference between the work and home blood pressure is simply the effect of the time of day, since our subjects were working during the day and at home in the evening. However, as reviewed in Chapter 5, the diurnal rhythm of blood pressure in shift workers follows the sequence of work rather than the time of day. Furthermore, we have measured ambulatory blood pressure in the same individuals on a work day and a non-work day, and found that the pressure during the usual hours of work was higher on the work day than on the non-work day (submitted for publication), as shown in Fig. 11.2. This difference did not appear to be simply due to the effects of greater physical activity on the work day, because it persisted after statistically controlling for the effects of posture (evaluated from the subject's diaries). Frankenhaeuser *et al.* [22] have also observed that blood pressure is higher on a work day than on a non-work day.

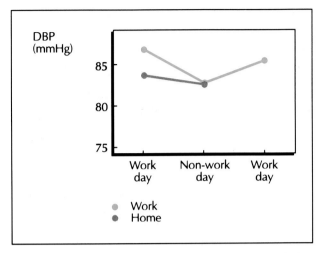

Fig. 11.2. Ambulatory blood pressure measured on two work days and one non-work day.

James *et al.* [23] made ambulatory blood pressure recordings and timed urine collections in 50 normotensive working women doing technical and clerical jobs who also kept diaries describing their activities, emotions and perceptions of stress. The average pressures were 116/78 mmHg at work, 113/74 mmHg at home and 102/63 mmHg during sleep. Urine collections were made for each of these three periods and were analysed for noradrenaline and adrenaline excretion.

The most powerful behavioural predictor of systolic pressure was the perception that one's job is stressful. This was associated with higher pressures in all three situations: at work, at home and during sleep (Fig. 11.3). The

perception that there was more stress at work than at home on the day of the study was associated with higher systolic pressures at work, but not at home or during sleep.

Potential sources of domestic stress were also related to blood pressure. Being married was associated with higher work diastolic pressures, and having children was associated with higher systolic and diastolic pressures both at work and at home. Women who reported higher levels of stress at home than at work also had relatively higher diastolic pressures at home than at work. Thus, single women whose main source of stress was at work showed a pattern similar to the one seen in men whereas married women with children, whose level of stress may be higher at home, did not show the typical decrease in blood pressure when they returned home, as shown in Fig. 11.4. In effect, such women have two full-time jobs. This finding is analogous to the observation made in the Framingham study that women employed in clerical jobs who also had children and were married to men with blue-collar jobs had the highest incidence of coronary heart disease [24].

Urine catecholamine excretion rates were also highest at work in the majority of subjects. The changes in urine noradrenaline and adrenaline were significantly correlated with the changes in systolic blood pressure and diastolic blood pressure from sleep to work, but only after adjusting for the level of stress at work relative to the level at home [25]. These results suggest that catecholamines have a more direct effect on blood pressure during periods of high stress.

The potential importance of the higher blood pressure at work has been shown in a study in which we related different measures of blood pressure to LVH in 100 patients. LVH was most strongly correlated with the pressure at work, which tended to be higher than the pressure at other times [26]. In fact, not all subjects went to work on the day of study, although virtually all were employed.

	Work		Home		Sleep	
	β	P	β	P	β	P
Systolic pressure						
Job stressful	3.66	0.01	4.34	0.0006	3.10	0.02
Stress difference	0.81	0.05	–	–	–	–
Boss unsupportive	− 2.56	0.05	–	–	–	–
Children	–	–	2.58	0.05	–	–
Diastolic pressure						
Stress difference	–	–	–	–	− 1.1	0.001
Home stress	− 0.72	0.05	–	–	–	–
Married	4.30	0.02	–	–	–	–
Children	–	–	3.09	0.005	2.58	0.01
β, Regression coefficients for stepwise regression analysis, with corresponding *P* values.						

Fig. 11.3. Psychosocial factors affecting ambulatory blood pressure in working women [23].

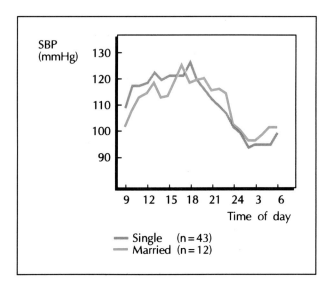

Fig. 11.4. Ambulatory blood pressure measured in single women and married women with children.

The better correlation with work pressure was found because the correlation between ambulatory blood pressure and LVH was higher for the subjects who went to work on the day of the recording than for those who stayed at home. For those who did go to work, the correlations were equally good whether the home or work pressures were taken. These results have since been confirmed by a Japanese group, in a very different cultural setting [27]. In this study, the difference between work and home blood pressures was much greater in the hypertensive subjects than in the normotensive subjects (8/10% versus 3/3% for systolic pressure and diastolic pressure). We interpreted these results as suggesting that the intermittent elevation in blood pressure associated with the regularly recurring stress of work may play a special role in contributing to the development of LVH (although, as discussed later, the effects of chronic occupational stress on blood pressure are not necessarily intermittent). The fact that LVH may develop as a result of intermittent stimulation seems reasonable because it readily occurs in athletes, who exercise for only a few hours a day [28,29]. Furthermore, Julius et al. [30] have shown that intermittent elevation in blood pressure produced for several hours a day by compression of the thighs can produce LVH.

Can intermittent elevations in blood pressure lead to sustained hypertension?

Folkow [31] has proposed that the intermittent elevations in blood pressure occurring in response to re-

peated exposure to environmental stressors could result in sustained hypertension. He argued that the crucial intervening variable is hypertrophy of the resistance vessels induced by the elevations in pressure, which would eventually raise peripheral resistance even in the absence of the stressors. Evidence supporting this hypothesis is fragmentary. Spontaneously hypertensive rats raised in isolation show an attenuated development of hypertension in comparison with rats reared in a more sociable environment [32], although the pattern of blood pressure change has not been studied by continuous monitoring. A much more direct test of this hypothesis has been carried out by Julius et al. [30]. They observed that compression of the thighs in dogs could produce an acute increase in blood pressure for as long as the compression was applied, but without causing any upward drift of the resting pressure, as shown in Fig. 11.5.

The 'carry-over effect' of stress on blood pressure

A puzzling aspect of our study [26] of LVH and ambulatory blood pressure was that although the correlation between the two was closest when studied on a work day, similar correlations were obtained whether the home or work pressures were used. We have subsequently performed another study (submitted for publication) in which ambulatory blood pressures measured on a work day and a non-work day were compared in the same subjects. As expected, the blood pressure was significantly higher on the work day, but, unexpectedly, the pressure was higher not only during the hours of work but also in the evening, when the subjects were at home (Fig. 11.6). This finding indicates that there may be a 'carry-over' of the effects of the work environment to the home setting, and may further explain why we found similar correlations between work and home pressures with LVH in subjects who were monitored on a work day [26].

Frankenhaeuser et al. [22] also compared blood pressures measured on a work day and a non-work day in male and female managers and clerical workers. They found that, for most people, the blood pressure was highest during working hours and decreased by about 5 mmHg when they returned home. As the subjects measured their own pressures in the seated position these differences cannot be explained by differences in physical activity. In female managers the pattern was different from that in male managers: the pressure did not fall on returning home and was higher in the evening on the work day than on the non-work day. This finding might be interpreted as a carry-over effect (Frankenhaeuser referred to it as a slower 'unwinding' in the female managers), but may also reflect a higher level of mental and physical activity during the evening in the female managers than in their male counterparts or in the clerical workers.

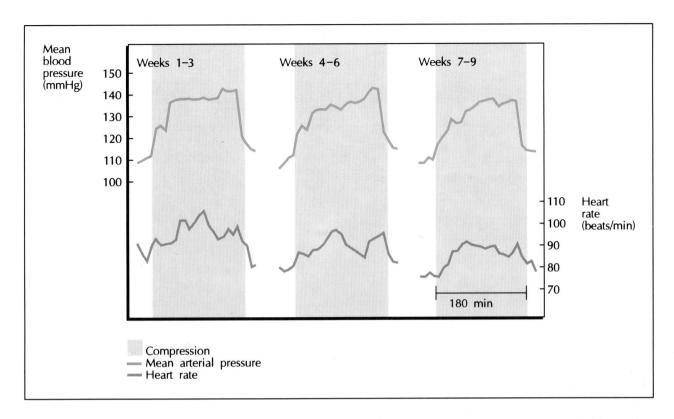

Fig. 11.5. Effect of repeated intermittent thigh compression on the mean blood pressure and heart rate of dogs. Note the absence of any change in the baseline (pre-compression) pressures. Reproduced with permission [30].

Self-monitoring for evaluating the effects of intermittent stress

Although ambulatory monitoring is ideal for examining the effects of stress on the diurnal profile of blood pressure, it is not so well suited to examining the changes that may occur over periods of days or weeks. We have recently been using self-monitoring with an Instromedix device (see Chapter 3) in a study of people exposed to cyclical stress in the form of deadlines at work. This type of monitor has the advantage of storing the blood pressure readings automatically in its memory and is, therefore, immune from observer error and bias. Subjects keep a monitor by their desk at work, so that it is possible to record changes in blood pressure over a 3-month period. Using this technique, we have found considerable variations between different subjects' susceptibility to deadline stress.

Two related models for evaluating the effects of chronic stress

The basic concept of psychological stress involves a combination of arousal and distress. This was formulated by Marianne Frankenhaeuser as the 'effort–distress model' [33]. This model has two orthogonal axes of effort and distress, providing four quadrants cor-

responding to high and low levels of the two factors (Fig. 11.7a). The physiological effects of these can be distinguished by measuring catecholamine and cortisol excretion. Effort on its own results in sympathetic arousal without increasing cortisol excretion, whereas effort with distress is characterized by an elevation in both catecholamines and cortisol. Frankenhaeuser suggested that the perceived level of personal control is a crucial modulating factor: effort without distress occurs when the subject is in control of the situation, whereas a lack of control is almost always associated with a feeling of distress.

This model has been used mostly for acute laboratory and field studies, but an analogous model has been developed for quantifying chronic occupational stress. This is the 'job strain model' developed by Karasek and Theorell and their colleagues [34,35]. This model has been shown to predict the prevalence of CHD, originally in a large Swedish study [34], but also subsequently in the United States [36]. In this model, job strain is defined by two orthogonal scales (Fig. 11.7b). The first measures psychological job demands, which is a subjective measure of the work load. The second measures decision latitude, which is equivalent to the degree of control which the subject perceives that he has over his job (the instrument was originally developed for men). Decision latitude is the combination of two subscales: decision authority and skill discretion. These scales are based on the subject's perception of his job, as evaluated by a questionnaire (the Job Content Survey). It is possible to construct a

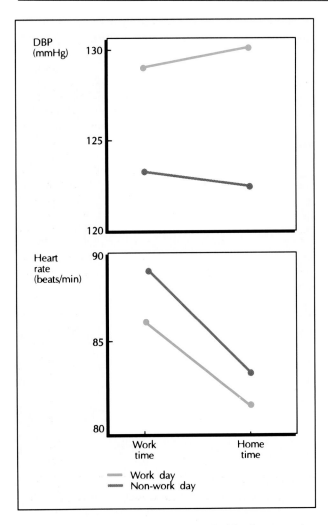

Fig. 11.6. Evidence of a 'carry-over effect' for blood pressure, but not heart rate, in normotensive subjects. (a) Diastolic pressure at home in the evening is higher on a work day than a non-work day; (b) heart rate shows no difference between the two days.

viduals doing the same job. Subjects whose score puts them in the 'high strain' quadrant (combining high demands with low decision latitude) are at the greatest risk for developing CHD symptoms and morbidity [34–36]. Most high-strain jobs are those that are traditionally regarded as blue collar jobs, whereas the professions (e.g. medicine, law and accounting) are in the quadrant defined by high work load and high control. Since different individuals with similar job descriptions may have very different perceptions of their level of job strain, the locations of particular types of jobs on this grid are only approximations. It is worth noting that several studies have shown that cardiovascular (and other) diseases are more prevalent in people with lower socio-economic status, many of whom work in high-strain jobs [37,38].

Can chronic exposure to low-grade stress lead to a re-setting of the diurnal profile of blood pressure?

If stress plays a role in the development of sustained hypertension, it should be possible to demonstrate an association between chronic stress and an upward re-setting of the diurnal profile of blood pressure to a hypertensive level; in other words, it should be possible to demonstrate that stress can raise the sleeping blood pressure. Although not originally designed with this in mind, our study of occupational stress and blood pressure, described in some detail later, has provided data compatible with this statement [39] (submitted for publication). This study was designed to evaluate the association between job strain and blood pressure, using a case–control design in which cases were defined as individuals who had an elevated diastolic pressure both on screening and at work (greater than 85 mmHg), and controls had normal pressures in both situations (less than 85 mmHg).

The hypothesis for the case–control study was that exposure to job strain would increase the likelihood of being a case. At seven worksites in New York, we studied 87 cases and 128 controls. Not surprisingly, the cases tended to

'map' of different jobs with the two scales as the axes (Fig. 11.7), based on the average scores of several indi-

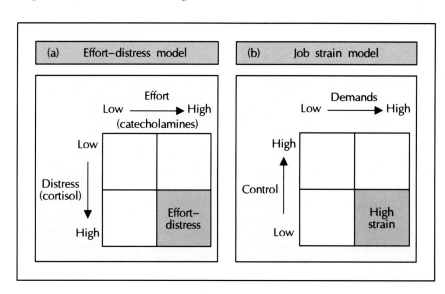

Fig. 11.7. Two related models for evaluating the effects of stress. (a) The effort–distress model of Frankenhaeuser; (b) the job strain model of Karasek and Theorell.

be older than the controls, but when the cases and controls were stratified by age, the odds ratio for the cases working in 'high-strain' jobs was 3.1 [39]. This association between job strain and blood pressure could not be accounted for by any of the known factors influencing blood pressure, such as sodium intake, obesity, alcohol intake, education level, smoking and level of physical activity. Neither of the two principal components of job strain — decision latitude and psychological demand — discriminated between cases and controls independently, indicating that the effects of job strain on blood pressure require the interaction of the two components. Furthermore, individuals in high-strain jobs had higher left ventricular mass than the others.

We had expected that the effects of job strain on blood pressure would be greatest during working hours, but when we compared the ambulatory pressures in subjects in high-strain jobs with those whose jobs were less stressful, we found that the pressures were elevated to a similar extent while at work (by 7.6/2.5 mmHg), at home (by 6.5/2.9 mmHg) and during sleep (by 7.8/1.7 mmHg) [41]. Thus, chronic exposure to high job strain appears to be associated with an upward re-setting of the diurnal blood pressure profile.

These data, therefore, strongly supported our original hypothesis that subjects with high job strain have higher blood pressures, and that this elevation in pressure may be sufficiently sustained to begin to lead to the development of LVH. Although it is difficult to draw definite conclusions about cause and effect from a cross-sectional study such as this, there seems to be no good reason why subjects with higher pressures should choose high-strain jobs, which would be the alternative explanation for our findings.

As shown in Fig. 11.3, women who perceive their job as being highly stressful also show a sustained elevation in pressure throughout the day and night.

Sex differences in the association between stress and blood pressure

Our study [39] of the associations between job strain and blood pressure has so far been confined to men, and it remains to be seen whether these findings can be extrapolated to women. Other work by our group suggests that there may be important sex differences in the interactions between psychosocial stress and blood pressure. In one study [40], the ambulatory blood pressure recordings of 137 men and 67 women were analysed to investigate whether factors such as changes of posture, location and emotion, all of which were recorded by the subjects in their diaries, had similar effects on blood pressure in men and women. The blood pressure readings corresponding to each diary entry were transformed into Z-scores to eliminate the influence of between-individual and between-sex differences in the average levels of blood pressure. In general, these three factors accounted for more of the overall blood pressure variance

in women than in men. Situation (at work, at home or elsewhere) was a highly significant determinant of systolic pressure in both men and women, but had less effect on diastolic pressure (Fig. 11.8). Posture (sitting, lying or standing) had a highly significant effect on both systolic and diastolic pressure in women, but surprisingly had no effect in men. Emotion (happiness, anger and anxiety) influenced both systolic and diastolic pressure in men, with the highest pressures occurring during anger. For systolic pressure in women, readings during emotional states were not a significant source of variation in the model, because all three emotions tended to elevate systolic pressure by about the same amount. For diastolic pressure, men again showed the biggest changes during anger, whereas in women the biggest changes occurred with anxiety. As shown in Fig. 11.9, the absolute effects of anger on blood pressure at work were twice as great in men as in women, whereas at home there was little difference.

		Men	Women
Posture	Systolic	NS	0.0001
	Diastolic	NS	0.0005
Location	Systolic	0.0001	0.0005
	Diastolic	0.07	NS
Emotion	Systolic	0.0001	NS
	Diastolic	0.001	0.0001

Fig. 11.8. Sources of variation of blood pressure in men and women (analysis of variance) [40]. Values are significance levels; NS, not significant.

		Work	Home
Men	Systolic	15.3	7.0
	Diastolic	13.1	8.4
Women	Systolic	5.0	9.6
	Diastolic	1.9	5.0

Fig. 11.9. Average effects of anger on blood pressure (mmHg) in men and women [40].

Slow pressor mechanisms which might mediate stress-induced hypertension

For any postulated mechanism linking the brain and blood pressure, the autonomic nervous system is the primary candidate. Evidence suggests that sympathetic nervous activity is subtly increased in many patients in the early stages of hypertension, and that structural changes in the resistance vessels play an increasing role in the later stages. It should be emphasized, however, that this increase in sympathetic activity is primarily tonic rather than phasic. There is abundant evidence that subjects with mild hypertension have an increased resting catecholamine excretion, heart rate and cardiac output [41–43], but, as reviewed in Chapter 12, there is some uncertainty whether the increase in sympathetic nervous activity during acute stress is the same as in normotensive subjects. If it is greater in hypertensives subjects, this may be merely a consequence of the higher basal level.

The sympathetic nervous system is normally regarded as being responsible primarily for the short-term regulation of blood pressure; other mechanisms, such as the role of the kidney [44] or structural changes in the resistance vessels [45,46], regulate the tonic level. This poses a problem for those who believe that stress may influence the development of hypertension. How is it that transient increases in sympathetic activity can lead to a sustained increase in blood pressure? There are, in fact, a number of possible mechanisms, which are reviewed below.

The adrenaline hypothesis

Recent pharmacological studies, predominantly conducted by Majewski and Rand [47–49], have identified a potential mechanism by which adrenaline may mediate stress-linked hypertension. It has been shown by studies both *in vitro* and *in vivo* that infusion of adrenaline in low doses (equivalent to the levels seen during naturally occurring stress) can enhance noradrenaline release from sympathetic nerve terminals [48]. This effect is thought to be mediated by pre-junctional beta$_2$ receptors, since it can be blocked by beta-blocking agents. Furthermore, circulating adrenaline may be taken up by the sympathetic nerve terminals, stored with noradrenaline as a co-transmitter, and released with it during sympathetic nerve stimulation. Two crucial components of this mechanism make it relevant to stress-induced hypertension. First, the release, re-uptake and pre-synaptic facilitation of noradrenaline release acts as a positive feedback loop; second, while the half-life of adrenaline in the plasma is only a few minutes, for adrenaline stored in the sympathetic nerves it may be many hours, providing the potential for producing sustained effects. This mechanism is illustrated schematically in Fig. 11.10.

Sustained experimental neurogenic hypertension has been quite hard to produce in practice, but has been achieved by Majewski *et al.* [50] in rats using a slow-release depot implantation of adrenaline. Blood pressure (but not heart rate) was elevated for 8 weeks, although by the eighth week no excess adrenaline could be detected in the plasma. This type of hypertension could be prevented by beta blockade.

Human studies have also implicated this mechanism. An acute infusion of adrenaline produces tachycardia, with an increased systolic pressure and slightly decreased di-

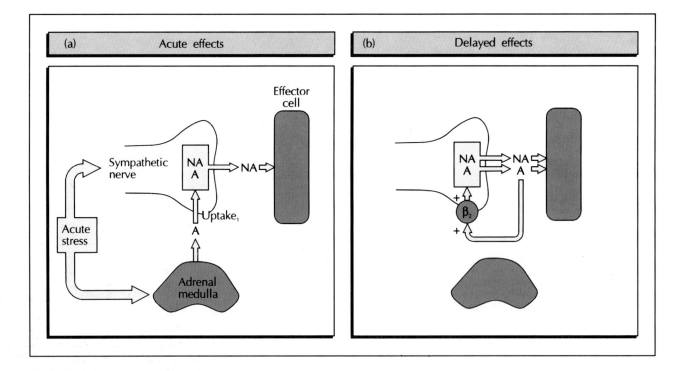

Fig. 11.10. Postulated mechanism for explaining the delayed pressor effects of adrenaline. (a) Adrenaline (A) released by the adrenal medulla in response to stress is taken up by sympathetic nerve terminals; (b) the delayed effect is explained by gradual release of adrenaline as a co-transmitter, which enhances noradrenaline (NA) release via stimulation of pre-synaptic beta$_2$ receptors.

astolic pressure. When the infusion is terminated, the plasma adrenaline level rapidly returns to normal, although the tachycardia and increased systolic pressure persist for an hour or two, and diastolic pressure rises to above baseline levels [51]. Adrenaline infusion can also enhance the pressor response to endogenous sympathetic stimulation, such as occurs during the cold pressor test or isometric exercise [52]. The mechanisms underlying this phenomenon have been investigated by Persson *et al* [53], who infused adrenaline into normotensive subjects and measured haemodynamic variables together with muscle sympathetic nerve activity (MSNA) and plasma catecholamines. During the infusion there was a modest decrease in diastolic pressure and central venous pressures (CVP) and a modest increase in MSNA and noradrenaline spill-over rate, which is thought to reflect sympathetic nerve traffic [54]. After the infusion was terminated both MSNA and spill-over rate increased dramatically (Fig. 11.11).

The reasons for this increase are not clear, but would be compatible either with pre-synaptic facilitation of noradrenaline release or with reflexly increased sympathetic nerve traffic, which may, for example, be mediated via the decreased CVP stimulating low-pressure baroreceptors [55]. The most impressive demonstration of the delayed pressor effect of adrenaline was provided by Blankenstijn *et al* [56], who infused adrenaline, noradrenaline or dextrose for 6 h in normal volunteers and monitored the effects on blood pressure over the next 16 h using intra-arterial monitoring. The infusion was given between 10.00 a.m. and 4.00 p.m., and the subjects were in bed from midnight to 8.00 a.m. Arterial pressure was at first reduced by the adrenaline but by the end of the infu-

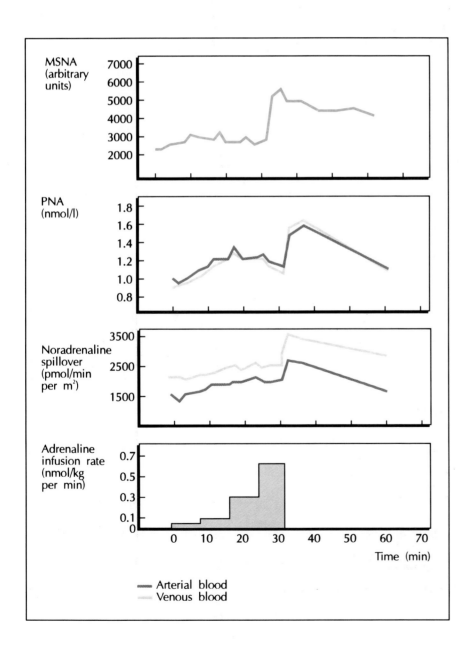

Fig. 11.11. Effects of intravenous infusion of adrenaline for 30 min on muscle sympathetic nerve activity (MSNA), plasma noradrenaline (PNA), and noradrenaline spill-over rate in arterial and venous blood. Reproduced with permission [53].

sion was above the baseline value, and remained elevated throughout the night (Fig. 11.12). Infusion of noradrenaline produced an initial elevation in pressure but no sustained effects. The pressor effect of adrenaline was most marked during periods of increased sympathetic activity, for example when the subjects were active, and not when they were at rest. The increased blood pressure following adrenaline infusion was not accompanied by any changes in heart rate.

Structural changes in the heart and resistance vessels

It is well recognized that the peripheral resistance is increased in most patients with sustained hypertension. That this is not wholly attributable to neurohumoral influences has been argued most forcefully by Folkow [45], on the basis of both anatomical and functional studies. Thus, even during maximal vasodilatation, such as occurs after a period of ischaemia, hypertensives still show an increased resistance to blood flow [45]. These changes are largely due to medial hypertrophy and can be regarded as an adaptive process in the presence of increased pressure and for flow. The extent to which stress can produce such changes is unclear, but there is evidence that the growth of vascular smooth muscle can be influenced by a number of stress-related factors, including angiotensin, catecholamines and corticosteroids (reviewed by Lever [46]).

Sodium retention and the kidney

The case for the dominant role of the kidneys in the long-term regulation of blood pressure has been put by Guy-

ton [44] on the basis of the phenomenon of pressure natriuresis: an increase in arterial pressure (by any mechanism) causes an increased sodium and water excretion, which tends to lower the blood volume and hence also the pressure. Sustained hypertension occurs only when the set point of the renal-volume mechanism for pressure control is re-set to a higher level of pressure. This could occur either because of sodium and volume retention, or because of a change occurring in the kidney (e.g. an increase in pre-renal resistance).

There is increasing evidence from animal experiments that environmental stress can cause sodium retention mediated via renal sympathetic nerve activity [57,58]. The same phenomenon has also been described in man [59].

In the borderline hypertensive rat, chronic exposure to conflict stress for 2 h a day can lead to sustained hypertension [60]. In the early stages of this process, however, exposure to the conflict situation produces only a slight increase in blood pressure. Analysis of the haemodynamic pattern shows that there is a profound renal and mesenteric vasoconstriction which is offset by skeletal muscle vasodilatation [61].

An analogous observation was made in humans by Wolf *et al.* [62] in 1955. They measured renal blood flow by para-aminohippurate clearance during stressful interviews and found that it decreased more in hypertensive subjects than in normotensive subjects. A more recent study by Hollenberg *et al.* [63] showed that the effects of a behavioural challenge on renal blood flow lasted much longer than the efffects on blood pressure.

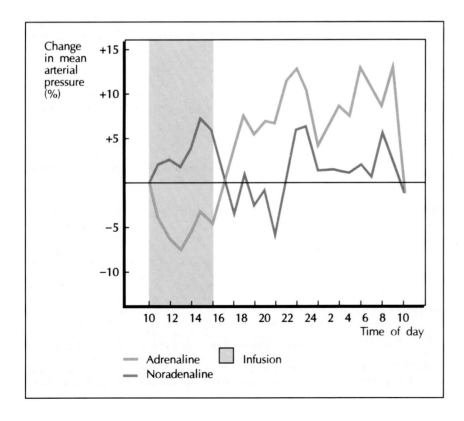

Fig. 11.12. Mean hourly values of percentage change of mean arterial pressure (relative to baseline levels) during and after a 6-hour infusion of adrenaline or noradrenaline. Baseline levels were obtained with a dextrose infusion. Reproduced with permission [58].

The role of glucocorticoids

An important physiological component of Franken-haeuser's effort–distress model is the increase in cortisol which occurs in the 'high effort – high distress' situation. Although most attention has been paid to the sympathetic nervous system as the prime mediator of stress-induced increases in blood pressure, there is also evidence to suggest that glucocorticoids may be involved. The effects of glucocorticoids on blood pressure are complex and not well understood, although there is agreement that they tend to have a pressor effect, as reviewed recently by Whitworth [64]. They may also increase the reactivity to adrenergic stimulation, particularly to adrenaline [65], although this effect is less certain in man [64,66]. Whitworth *et al.* [67] gave four different synthetic steroids to normal subjects for 5 days, at doses which had similar glucocorticoid activity but little or no mineralocorticoid effect. All four steroids raised blood pressure without any accompanying sodium retention. The effects on the diurnal profile of blood pressure were not evaluated but, as discussed in Chapter 5, it might be expected that the increase in pressure would be particularly pronounced at night.

Summary and conclusions

There is convincing evidence that sympathetic nervous system activity is increased in the early stages of hypertension, which makes an investigation of the role of stress, as one of the prime movers in this sequence, seem appropriate. It is proposed that any interaction between stress and blood pressure has at least three major components: the nature of the stressor, the psychological make-up of the individual exposed to it, and the individual's physiological susceptibility.

Previous investigations have paid little attention to a major problem in demonstrating an association between stress and hypertension, that is, the time course of the effects. Although it is easy to demonstrate a transient increase in blood pressure in response to an acute stressor, the relevance of this to sustained hypertension remains unclear. Ambulatory monitoring is ideally suited to resolving this issue, because it permits the study of the effects of the stresses of everyday life on the diurnal profile of blood pressure.

Individual differences in personality, such as the traits of anger, anxiety and the type A behaviour pattern, have not so far been shown to have any consistent effect on ambulatory blood pressure. However, it is clearly established that acute mood changes do affect ambulatory blood pressure.

That psychosocial factors can affect the shape of the diurnal profile of blood pressure has been demonstrated by comparing blood pressure measured at work and at home. Most people have higher pressures at work, which cannot be explained simply by the effects of time of day or physical activity. The pattern of diurnal activity may depend on the relative effects of occupational and domestic stress, as shown by the comparison of employed women who are single with those who have children. The latter have higher pressures in the evening.

There is also a limited amount of evidence for a 'carry-over effect', that is to say that the pressor effects of work may still be evident in the evening after returning home.

The chronic effects of low-grade stress on blood pressure and the heart may be investigated using the 'effort–distress' model of Frankenhaeuser or the 'job strain' model of Karasek and Theorell. In both cases there are two orthogonal components, roughly equivalent to demand and control. The most stressful situation appears to be one in which a high level of demand is coupled with a low level of control. With this model it has been shown that men employed in 'high-strain' jobs (high demand–low control) are more likely to be classified as hypertensive, and that this elevation in pressure is maintained throughout the day and night.

There are several potential mechanisms by which stress might induce a sustained increase in blood pressure. One such mechanism involves the 'adrenaline hypothesis', according to which adrenaline released during acute stress may be taken up by sympathetic nerve terminals and gradually released as a co-transmitter, with a delayed pressor effect. Structural changes in the heart and resistance vessels would also help to maintain a sustained increase in pressure. There is also evidence that stress may promote sodium retention by the kidney. Finally, the increased secretion of glucocorticoids may also raise blood pressure.

References

1. KRANTZ DS, LAZAR JD: **The stress concept: issues and measurement.** In *Handbook of Hypertension Vol. 9. Behavioral Factors in Hypertension* edited by Julius S, Bassett DR. Amsterdam: Elsevier, 1987, pp 43–58.

2. GOLDSTEIN DS, KOPIN IJ: **The autonomic nervous system and catecholamines in normal blood pressure control and in hypertension.** In *Hypertension: Pathophysiology, Diagnosis and Management* edited by Laragh JH, Brenner BM. New York: Raven Press, 1990, pp 711–747.

3. HENRY JP, STEPHENS PM, SANTISTEBAN GA: **A model of psychological hypertension showing reversibility and progression of cardiovascular complications.** *Circ Res* 1975, 36:156–164.

4. HENRY JP, MEEHAN WP, STEPHENS PM: **Role of subordination in nephritis of socially stressed mice.** *Clin Exp Hypertens [A]* 1982, 4:695–705.

5. HARRAP SB, LOUIS WJ, DOYLE AE: **Failure of psychosocial stress to induce chronic hypertension in the rat.** *J Hypertens* 1984, 2:653–662.

6. ANDERSON DE, KEARNS WD, BETTER WE: **Progressive hypertension in dogs by avoidance conditioning and saline infusion.** *Hypertension* 1983, 5:286–291.

7. ALEXANDER F: **Emotional factors in essential hypertension. Presentation of a tentative hypothesis.** *Psychosom Med* 1939, 1:173–179.

8. HARBURG E, JULIUS S, McGUIRE NF, McLEOD J, HOOBLER SW: **Personality traits and behavioral patterns associated with systolic blood pressure levels in college males.** *J Chron Dis* 1964, 17:405–414.

9. HARBURG E, ERFURT JE, HAUENSTEIN LS, *ET AL.*: **Socio-ecological stress, suppressed hostility, skin color, and black-**

white male blood pressure: Detroit. *Psychosom Med* 1973, 35:276–296.

10. HARBURG E, BLAKELOCK EH, ROEPER PJ: Resentful and reflective coping with arbitrary authority and blood pressure: Detroit. *Psychosom Med* 1979, 41:189–202.

11. ESLER M, JULIUS S, SZEIFLER A, *ET AL.*: Mild high-renin essential hypertension: neurogenic human hypertension? *N Engl J Med* 1977, 296:405–411.

12. KEENE TM, MARTIN JE, BERLER ES, *ET AL.*: Are hypertensives less assertive? A controlled evaluation. *J Consult Clin Psychol* 1982, 50:499–508.

13. SULLIVAN P, SCHOENTGER S, DEQUATTRO V, *ET AL.*: Anxiety, anger, and neurogenic tone at rest and in stress in patients with primary hypertension. *Hypertension* 1981, 3 (suppl II):II119–II123.

14. GOLDSTEIN HS, EDELBERG R, MEIER CF, DAVIS L: Relationship of resting blood pressure and heart rate to experienced anger and expressed anger. *Psychosom Med* 1988, 50:321–329.

15. DIMSDALE JE, PIERCE C, SCHOENFELD D, *ET AL.*: Suppressed anger and blood pressure: the effects of race, sex, social class, obesity, and age. *Psychosom Med* 1986, 48:430–435.

16. SCHNEIDER RH, BRENT ME, JOHNSON EH, BROBNY H, JULIUS S: Anger and anxiety in borderline hypertension. *Psychosom Med* 1986, 48:242–248.

17. FRIEDMAN R, SCHNALL P, PIEPER C, PICKERING T. Psychological variables in hypertension. *Psychosom Med* 1990, 52:232.

18. CONTRADA RJ, KRANTZ DS: Stress, reactivity, and type A behavior: current status and future directions. *Ann Behav Med* 1988, 10:64–70.

19. VAN EGEREN L, SPARROW AW: Ambulatory monitoring to assess real-life cardiovascular reactivity in type A and type B subjects. *Psychosom Med* 1990, 52:297–300

20. SCHNEIDER RH, JULIUS S, KARUNAS R: Ambulatory blood pressure monitoring and laboratory reactivity in type A behaviour and components. *Psychosom Med* 1989, 51:290–305.

21. PICKERING TG, HARSHFIELD GA, KLEINERT HD, BLANK S, LARAGH JH: Blood pressure during normal daily activities, sleep and exercise. Comparison of values in normal and hypertensive subjects. *JAMA* 1982, 247:992–996.

22. FRANKENHAEUSER M, LUNDBERG U, FREDRIKSON M, *ET AL.*: Stress on and off the job as related to sex and occupational status in white-collar workers. *J Organizational Behav* 1989, 10:321–346.

23. JAMES GD, CATES EM, PICKERING TG, LARAGH JH: Parity and perceived job stress elevate blood pressure in young normotensive working women. *Am J Hypertens* 1989, 2:637–639.

24. HAYNES SG, FEINLIEB M: Women, work and coronary heart disease: prospective findings from the Framingham Heart Study. *Am J Public Health* 1980, 70:133–141.

25. BROEGE P, JAMES GD: Cardiovascular adaptation to the urban environment. *Am J Phys Anthropol* 1990, 81:200.

26. DEVEREUX RB, PICKERING TG, HARSHFIELD GA, *ET AL.*: Left ventricular hypertrophy in patients with hypertension: importance of blood pressure response to regularly recurring stress. *Circulation* 1983, 68:470–476.

27. BABA S, OZAWA H, NAKAMOTO Y, UESHIMA H, OMAE T: Enhanced blood pressure response to regular daily stress in urban hypertensive men. *J Hypertens* 1990, 8:647–655.

28. COHEN JL, GUPTA PK, LICHSTEIN E, CHADDA KD: The heart of a dancer: non-invasive cardiac evaluation of professional ballet dancers. *Am J Cardiol* 1980, 45:949–965.

29. MORGANROTH J, MASON BJ, HENRY WL, EPSTEIN SE: Comparative left ventricular dimensions in trained athletes. *Ann Intern Med* 1975, 82:521–524.

30. JULIUS S, LI L, BRANT D, KRAUSE L, BUDA AJ: Neurogenic pressor episodes fail to cause hypertension, but do induce cardiac hypertrophy. *Hypertension* 1989, 13:422–429.

31. FOLKOW B: Sympathetic nervous control of blood pressure. Role in primary hypertension. *Am J Hypertens* 1989, 2:103S–111S.

32. HALLBÄCK M: Consequence of social isolation on blood pressure, cardiovascular reactivity and design in spontaneously hypertensive rats. *Acta Physiol Scand* 1975, 93:455–465.

33. FRANKENHAEUSER M: The sympathetic-adrenal and pituitary-adrenal response to challenge: comparison between the sexes. In *Biobehavioral Bases of Coronary Heart Disease* edited by Dembroski TM, Schmidt TH, Blumchen G. Basel: Karger, 1983, pp 91–105.

34. KARASEK R, BAKER D, MARXER F, AHLBOHM A, THEORELL T: Job decision latitude, job demands, and cardiovascular disease: a prospective study of Swedish men. *Am J Public Health* 1981, 75:694–705.

35. ALFREDSSON L, KARASEK R, THEORELL T: Myocardial infarction risk and psychosocial work environment: an analysis of the male Swedish working force. *Soc Sci Med* 1982, 16:463–467.

36. KARASEK RA, THEORELL T, SCHWARTZ JE, SCHNALL PL, PIEPER CF, MICHELA JL: Job characteristics in relation to the prevalence of myocardial infarction in the US Health Examination Survey (HES) and the Health and Nutrition Examination Survey (HANES). *Am J Public Health* 1988, 78:910–918.

37. BURING HJE, EVANS DA, FIORE M, ROSNER B, HENNEBERG CH: Occupation and risk of death from coronary heart disease. *JAMA* 1987, 258:791–792.

38. ROSE G, MARMOT MG: Social class and coronary heart disease. *Br Heart J* 1981, 45:13–19.

39. SCHNALL PL, PIEPER C, KARASEK RA, SHWARTZ JE, PICKERING TG: The relationship between job strain and diastolic blood pressure and left ventricular mass index: results of a case control study. *JAMA* 1990, 263:1929–1935.

40. JAMES GD, YEE LS, HARSHFIELD GA, PICKERING TG: Sex differences in factors affecting the daily variation of blood pressure. *Soc Sci Med* 1988, 26:1019–1023.

41. GOLDSTEIN DS: Plasma catecholamines in essential hypertension: an analytical review. *Hypertension* 1983, 5:86–89.

42. JULIUS S: Controversies in the resarch on hemodynamic mechanisms in the development of hypertension. In *Fundamental Fault in Hypertension* edited by Sambhi M. Boston: Martinus Nijhoff, 1984, pp 264–275.

43. PHILIPP T: Sympathetic nervous activity in essential hypertension. Activity and reactivity. *J Cardiovasc Pharmacol* 1987, 10 (suppl 4):S31–S36.

44. GUYTON AC: Dominant role of the kidneys and accessory role of whole-body autoregulation in the pathogenesis of hypertension. *Am J Hypertens* 1989, 2:575–585.

45. FOLKOW B: Cardiovascular structural adaptation: its role in the initiation and maintenance of primary hypertension. The Fourth Volhard Lecture. *Clin Sci Mol Med* 1978, 55 (suppl IV):3S–22S.

46. LEVER AF: Slow pressor mechanisms in hypertension: a role of hypertrophy of resistance vessels. *J Hypertens* 1986, 4:515–524.

47. MAJEWSKI H, RAND MJ: Prejunctional β-adrenoceptors as sites of action for adrenaline in stress-linked hypertension. *J Cardiovasc Pharmacol* 1987, 10 (suppl 4):S41–S44.

48. MAJEWSKI H, HEDLER L, STARKE X: The noradrenaline release rate in the anesthetized rabbit: facilitation by adrenaline. *Naunyn Schmiedebergs Arch Pharmacol* 1982, 321:20–27.

49. BROWN MJ, MACQUIN I: Is adrenaline the cause of essential hypertension? *Lancet* 1981, ii:1079–1081.

50. MAJEWSKI H, TUNG L-H, RAND MJ: Adrenaline-induced hypertension in rats. *J Cardiovasc Pharmacol* 1981, 3:1979–1985.

51. BROWN MJ, DOLLERY CT: Adrenaline and hypertension. *Clin Exp Hypertens [A]* 1984, 6:539–549.

52. VINCENT HH, BOOMSMA F, MAN IN'T VELD A, SCHALEKAMP MADH: Stress levels of adrenaline amplify the blood pressure reponse to sympathetic stimulation. *J Hypertens* 1986, 4:255–260.

53. PERSSON B, ANDERSSON OK, HJEMDAHL P, *ET AL.*: Adrenaline infusion in man increases muscle sympathetic nervous system activity from measurements of norepinephrine turnover. *J Hypertens* 1989, 7:747–756.

54. ESLER M, JENNINGS G, KORNER P, *ET AL.*: Assessment of human sympathetic nervous system activity from measurements of norepinephrine turnover. *Hypertension* 1988, 11:3–20.

55.   SUNDLÖF G, WALLIN BG: **Effect of lower body negative pressure on human muscle sympathetic nerve activity.** *J Physiol* 1978, **278**:525–532.

56.   BLANKENSTIJN PJ, MANN IN'T VELD A, TULEN J, *ET AL*: **Support for adrenaline-hypertension hypothesis: 18 hour pressor effect after 6 hours adrenaline infusion.** *Lancet* 1988, ii:1386–1389.

57.   KOEPKE JP, JONES S, DiBONA GF: **Stress increases renal nerve activity and decreases sodium excretion in Dahl rats.** *Hypertension* 1988, **11**:334–338.

58.   ANDERSON DE, DIETZ JR, MURPHY P: **Behavioral hypertension in sodium-loaded dogs is accompanied by sustained sodium retention.** *J Hypertens* 1987, **5**:99–105.

59.   LIGHT KC, KOEPKE JP, OBRIST PA, WILLIS PW: **Psychological stress induces sodium and fluid retention in men at high risk for hypertension.** *Science* 1983, **220**:429–431.

60.   LAWLER JE, BARKER GF, HUBBARD JW, ALLEN MT: **The effects of conflict on tonic levels of blood pressure in the genetically borderline hypertensive rat.** *Psychophysiology* 1980, **17**:363–370.

61.   KNARDAHL S, SANDERS BJ, JOHNSON AK: **Hemodynamic responses to conflict stress in borderline hypertensive rats.** *J Hypertens* 1989, **7**:585–593.

62.   WOLF S, CARDON PV, SHEPARD EM, WOLFF HG: *Life Stress and Essential Hypertension. A Study of Circulatory Adjustments in Man.* Baltimore: Williams and Wilkins, 1955.

63.   HOLLENBERG NK, WILLIAMS GH, ADAMS DF: **Essential hypertension: abnormal renal vascular and endocrine responses to a mild psychological stimulus.** *Hypertension* 1981, **3**:11–17.

64.   WHITWORTH JA: **Mechanisms of glucorcorticoid-induced hypertension.** *Kidney Int* 1987, **31**:1213–1224.

65.   KALSNER S: **Mechanism of hydrocortisone potentiation of respones to epinephrine and norepinephrine in rabbit aorta.** *Circ Res* 1969, **24**:383–395.

66.   SAMBHI MP, WEIL MH, UDHOJI VN: **Pressor responses to norepinephrine in humans before and after corticosteroids.** *Am J Physiol* 1962, **103**:961–963.

67.   WHITWORTH JA, GORDON D, ANDREWS J, SCOGGINS BA: **The hypertensive effect of synthetic glucocorticoids in man: role of sodium and volume.** *J Hypertens* 1989, **7**:535–549.

12 Comparison of blood pressure changes during laboratory testing and ambulatory monitoring: blood pressure reactivity

Cardiovascular reactivity testing has become a very popular method of examining the role of behavioural factors in the development of hypertension and CHD. It has an important application in blood pressure monitoring, both inside and outside the laboratory. In the previous chapter it was suggested that three critical factors are needed for stress to produce any sustained effects on blood pressure. These are the psychological constitution of the individual (personality and experience), the physiological constitution and the nature and chronicity of the stressors. Although field studies using ambulatory monitoring have the undoubted advantage of permitting the measurement of blood pressure during normal daily activities, the number of uncontrolled variables — different people are being compared in different circumstances — makes it hard to generalize about what is going on.

Laboratory testing offers the possibility of introducing some control into the situation. In particular, the environmental stressors can be standardized, so that any differences observed in the cardiovascular response can be attributed to individual differences in psychological or physiological susceptibility to those stressors.

If such laboratory measures of reactivity are made on their own, however, there are also problems. The choice of stressors may be critical, and many of those that have been used bear little or no resemblance to the stressors of everyday life. This chapter will address the issue of the generalizability or external validity of such reactivity testing. First, however, we shall briefly review the 'reactivity hypothesis', which provides the rationale for such studies.

The reactivity hypothesis

In its simplest form, this hypothesis states that individuals who show increased cardiovascular reactivity to psychologically stressful stimuli are at increased risk of developing cardiovascular disease. The latter is often taken to include hypertension and CHD as if they were a single entity, whereas of course they are not. Two forms of the hypothesis as it relates to hypertension have been proposed: in one, the 'recurrent activation model', the response to laboratory tests is assumed to be correlated with intermittent pressor responses to stress occurring in everyday life; in the other, the 'prevailing state model', the laboratory response predicts the average level of blood pressure [1]. It has also been suggested that stressors initially produce transient elevations in blood pressure

by neurohormonal mechanisms, and that these elevations may in turn induce structural changes in the arterial wall, which eventually result in a sustained increase in vascular resistance and hence in blood pressure [2]. It has been demonstrated recently, however, that neurogenically produced pressor episodes do not, on their own, lead to any sustained increase in the basal blood pressure level, although they can produce LVH [3].

We have reviewed elsewhere some of the criteria that the reactivity hypothesis must satisfy [4]. First, the degree of reactivity for an individual subject should be stable over time; second, it should, to some extent, be generalizable from one type of challenge to another; and third, it should be generalizable from the laboratory to the stresses of everyday life.

Evidence from animal studies

Animal studies of experimental hypertension have provided some support for the reactivity hypothesis. When compared with normotensive control rats, spontaneously hypertensive rats (SHR) show hyper-reactivity to some but not all stimuli. Therefore, their blood pressure response to a conditioned emotional stimulus is enhanced, as it is to drinking, but not to eating, grooming or general motor activity [5], as shown in Fig. 12.1. Over the long term, their blood pressure is also more sensitive to changes in the social environment [6].

There are at least two likely mechanisms for such hyper-reactivity. First, a central mechanism, possibly originating in the hypothalamus, can be postulated because young 'pre-hypertensive' SHR show an exaggerated heart rate and blood pressure response to noxious stimuli. Evidence that the heart rate response is centrally mediated rests on the observation that both sympathetic and vagal components are involved [7]. The fact that the hyper-reactivity is dependent on the nature of the stimulus is also most easily explained by a central mechanism.

The second likely mechanism is vascular hypertrophy, which is present even before the animals become hypertensive and may be genetically determined [2].

Techniques of measuring reactivity

Most studies of cardiovascular reactivity have used intermittent non-invasive measurement of blood pressure made by automatic non-invasive monitors such as the Di-

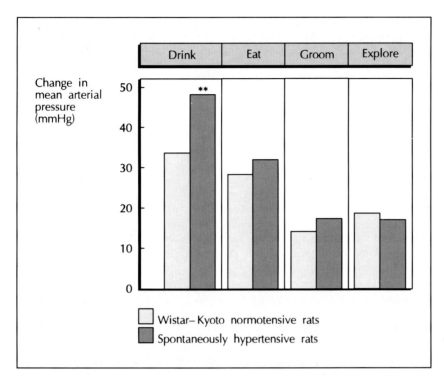

Fig. 12.1. Comparison of blood pressure reactivity (expressed as change in mean arterial pressure) in normotensive and spontaneously hypertension rats. Reproduced with permission [5].

namap (see Chapter 2). Typically, a number of different tasks are used, separated by baseline periods of 5 or 10 min. These tasks are commonly classified as active and passive. Active tasks (such as mental arithmetic and reaction time tasks) require an active response by the subject, whereas passive tasks (such as the cold pressor test[1]) do not. Reactivity is usually expressed as a change score: the difference between the peak or average level during the task and the baseline (which may be either the average baseline level immediately preceding the task or the average of the levels before and after). Although conceptually simple, this approach has some problems. First, the duration of the tasks is often quite short; as conventional non-invasive methods of recording blood pressure can only provide about one reading per minute, it may only be possible to obtain one or two readings of blood pressure during a test such as the cold pressor test (see Fig. 12.2). As a result, the error of such measurements is likely to be relatively large. However, as described in the next section, this error may be substantially reduced by using beat-to-beat monitoring of blood pressure. Another potential problem is that the tasks do not necessarily produce a steady-state or plateau level of blood pressure. With dynamic exercise testing it has been established that at least 3 min are needed to achieve this [8], but the pattern of change for many of the other commonly used tasks has not been studied systematically. Finally, one of the common goals of reactivity studies is to compare normotensive and hypertensive individuals. As reviewed below, evidence suggests that hypertensives show an increased reactivity. This evidence, however, is based on a greater absolute change in blood pressure. As hyper-

tensive people start from a higher baseline level, it does not necessarily follow that they would also show a greater percentage change, which might be a more appropriate way of expressing the results.

Reproducibility and generalizability of individual differences in reactivity

Several studies have investigated the test–retest reliability of blood pressure changes measured during reactivity testing [9–18]. Most have used non-invasive blood pressure measurements, as described above. The interval between tests ranged from 30 min to 4 years. Parati *et al.* [18] examined the short-term reproducibility of a number of tests, including isometric exercise and the cold pressor test, by performing each test at 30 min intervals during a single session. Their study was unique in that blood pressure was recorded intra-arterially. The variation coefficient of mean arterial pressure was quite large, being 22% for isometric exercise and 17% for the cold pressor test. Manuck and Schaefer [9] reported significant correlations between the blood pressure responses to a cognitive task repeated after 2 weeks, and also after 13 months. McKinney *et al.* [11] compared the response to three tasks (a video game, a reaction time test and the cold pressor test) over an interval of 3 months. They did not find good correlations between the change scores (the exact values of which were not reported), but did find significant correlations for the absolute values of pressure on the two occasions (ranging between

---

[1]This test is performed by placing the subject's hand or foot in iced water for 1–2 min.

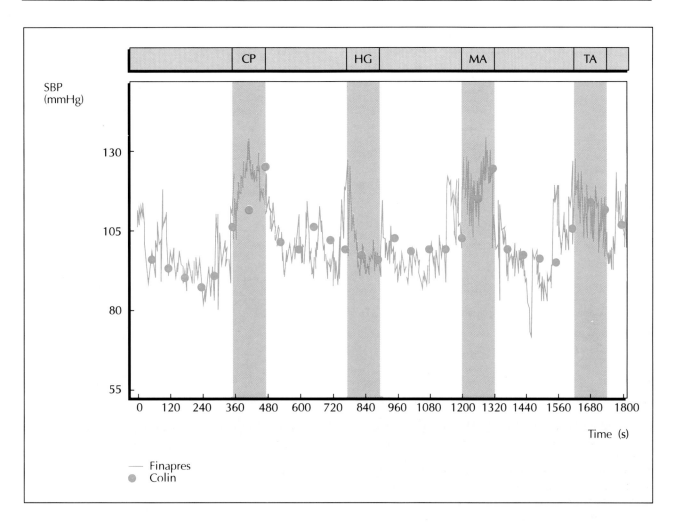

Fig. 12.2. Blood pressure changes during reactivity testing, measured intermittently using an ambulatory monitor (Colin), and continuously using a Finapres. CP, cold pressor test; HG, handgrip; MA, mental arithmetic; TA, talking. Reproduced with permission [16].

0.64 and 0.76, all $P<0.01$). Eich and Jacobsen [14] administered the cold pressor test twice over a 4-year period and categorized subjects according to whether or not they had a positive response, defined as a blood pressure rise of at least 20 mmHg. Only 60% of subjects with a positive response on the first occasion were still positive 4 years later.

The most comprehensive study to date was reported by Langewitz *et al.* [15], who performed reactivity testing (reaction time tasks and mental arithmetic) on four occasions at intervals of 4 weeks in 136 men. A feature of this study was that it was done under 'field conditions': that is, the place of testing and the people conducting the test varied from one occasion to another. One of their most interesting findings was that there was a progressive decrease from the first to the fourth occasion not only in the baseline pressure but also in the reactivity scores: for mental arithmetic the average response decreased from 13/8 to 6/5 mmHg. The test–retest correlations over the same period were similar in magnitude for baseline and reactivity tasks for systolic pressure (0.43 and 0.43, respectively), but for diastolic pressure were better for the baseline measures (0.51 and 0.27, respectively).

One of the problems with reactivity testing is the relatively brief exposure to the stimulus, so that the effect on blood pressure is a transient rise and fall without any steady-state or plateau level being reached. We have investigated the possibility that the poor reliability of reactivity testing may arise because the conventional intermittent measurements of blood pressure may not characterize these changes adequately [16]. We measured blood pressure using intermittent measurements with a Colin ABPM 630 monitor (see Chapter 3) and continuously with a Finapres monitor (see Chapter 2), as shown in Fig. 12.2. The reliability of the Colin measurements was good for the absolute levels of pressure but poor for the change scores, while the Finapres gave more reliable estimates of both measures.

These results make it clear that the relatively low reliability of reactivity measures is at least partly due to measurement error, and that this can be significantly diminished using continuous measurement of blood pressure.

Surprisingly few studies have systematically examined the extent to which an individual subject's response to one task will predict his or her response to another. Parati *et al.* [18] found that the responses to two predominantly mental tasks (mental arithmetic and mirror drawing) were quite well correlated with each other (r = 0.78, *P* < 0.01), as were the responses to two predominantly physical tasks (isometric exercise and the cold pressor test), but correlations between the mental and physical tasks were not significant. Fredrikson *et al.* [19] examined the correlation between the change scores for four tasks: an attentional demands task, mental arithmetic, the cold pressor test and isometric exercise. The only significant correlation for systolic pressure was between mental arithmetic and isometric exercise in normotensive subjects; for hypertensive subjects none of the correlations was significant.

These results suggest that there is very limited evidence for generalizability of reactivity across tasks, and that characterizing an individual as being generally 'hyper-reactive' has little validity at present.

Comparison of reactivity in normotensive and hypertensive subjects

Several studies have compared blood pressure reactivity in normotensive and hypertensive subjects. We [4] reviewed 39 of the studies that gave adequate details of the actual blood pressure levels and statistical comparison [19–57]. The two most extensively studied tests have been mental arithmetic and the cold pressor test. A more formal meta-analysis was undertaken by Fredrikson and Matthews [58]. They concluded that patients with essential hypertension (with blood pressures of at least 165/95 mmHg) showed an exaggerated systolic blood pressure response to passive stressors (including the cold pressor test) compared with normotensive controls, although this was seen in only 31 out of 63 studies. Overall, borderline hypertensive subjects showed a significantly greater response to active stressors (in eight out of 25 individual studies).

For mental arithmetic, which is predominantly a behavioural task, there is a fairly consistent tendency for hypertensive subjects to show an enhanced response, in contrast to predominantly physical tasks (cold pressor test and isometric or dynamic exercise), where there is less convincing evidence of any difference. For the cold pressor test and exercise (see Chapter 4) there is a trend for reactivity to be greater in patients with more severe hypertension. These findings would be consistent with increased reactivity being, at least in part, a consequence rather than a cause of the hypertension.

Genetic factors influencing differences in reactivity

Several studies have examined the influence of family history of hypertension on reactivity, and many have dealt with children. The meta-analysis by Fredrikson and

Matthews [58] concluded that 13 out of 30 studies demonstrated an increased blood pressure or heart rate reactivity in association with a positive family history of hypertension, and that overall this effect was significant in comparison with subjects without a family history. The difference was more reliable for active than for passive tasks. A more recent study of normotensive young adults found that subjects with a positive family history (either one or both parents hypertensive) had higher baseline pressures (measured both in the laboratory and during ambulatory monitoring) but no difference in the blood pressure response to four different stressors [59].

Physiological factors influencing differences in reactivity

Reactivity is normally defined as the size of a physiological response (usually blood pressure or heart rate) to a specific stimulus, which may be primarily physical (e.g. cold) or mental (e.g. mental arithmetic). It is often assumed that hyper-reactivity occurs as a result of a centrally mediated hyper-responsiveness. In fact, such a mechanism would be only one of a number of possible mediators, as shown in Fig. 12.3.

Relatively little attention has been paid to differences in perception or central nervous system processing as mediators of individual differences. Bohlin *et al.* [23] compared the responses of normotensive and borderline hypertensive subjects to a mental arithmetic task, but did not find any consistent differences in subjective ratings of task difficulty, irritation with the task or other subjective variables.

One way of localizing individual differences to the central nervous system would be to demonstrate differences in sympathetic nervous outflow, as manifested by changes in plasma catecholamine levels. Comparison of catecholamine release in normotensive and hypertensive individuals during reactivity testing has been made relatively rarely. Those comparisons that have been performed have for the most part not found any differences [19,23,40,44,52–63]. One study [63] reported a small but significantly higher increment of plasma noradrenaline in young hypertensive subjects during mental arithmetic but no difference in older subjects, and no difference at any age to the cold pressor test. Another study that reported a greater increment of noradrenaline during mental stress (in older but not in younger hypertensive subjects) exposed subjects to 30 min of continual stress, which is considerably longer than in most of the other studies [64]. Therefore, on the basis of plasma catecholamine measurements, there is no convincing evidence that the increased reactivity seen in hypertensive individuals in some studies is mediated centrally.

With dynamic exercise there is more evidence for an enhanced noradrenaline release in young hypertensive subjects, as shown by changes in venous plasma levels. Goldstein [65] reviewed eight studies and concluded

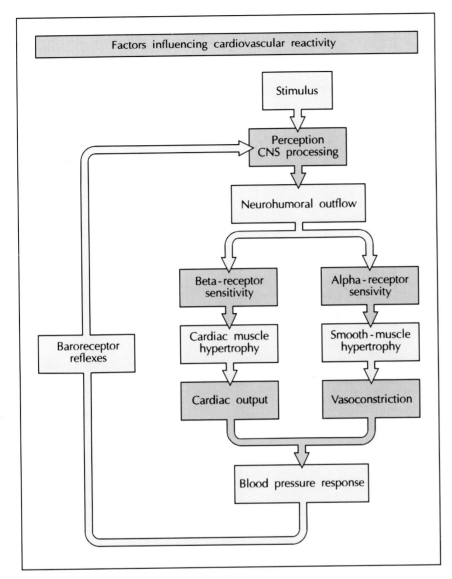

Fig. 12.3. Some of the psychological and physiological variables which may mediate individual differences in cardiovascular reactivity. Other potentially relevant factors (not shown) include sodium balance and membrane transport defects.

that seven of them showed a greater increment of noradrenaline during exercise in hypertensive compared with normotensive subjects, although this difference was not statistically significant. Two other studies not included in his analysis also showed a greater increment [66,67].

One explanation for this may be that conventional plasma catecholamine measurements may not adequately reflect the subtle differences in sympathetic activation which occur during brief exposure to mental stress. A more sophisticated measure is the noradrenaline spill-over rate, which is an index of the net release of noradrenaline into the circulation. Using this, Goldstein *et al.* have observed recently [68] that young patients with borderline hypertension show a normal forearm noradrenaline spill-over during mental challenge, but an exaggerated total body spill-over. In view of other work by Esler *et al.* [69], this probably originates in the heart and kidneys. However, in a study [70] in which sympathetic nerve activity was recorded directly (by microneurography from a tibial nerve), there was evidence of an exaggerated increase in blood pressure and MSNA during the

cold pressor test in borderline hypertensive individuals, whereas the response to isometric exercise was no different from normotensive subjects (Fig. 12.4). Interestingly, this same study found no group differences in the plasma catecholamine response.

Other factors which could influence reactivity are those which influence the responsiveness of the peripheral vasculature to a given change in sympathetic stimulation. A consistent body of evidence indicates that beta-adrenergic responsiveness is diminished in hypertension. This has been attributed to down-regulation of adrenergic receptors occurring in response to enhanced stimulation [71–74]. This finding seems to be at variance with reports of increased reactivity to mental stress in hypertensive subjects but can be reconciled with them if there is either an increased central sympathetic outflow during reactivity tasks in hypertensive subjects or an exaggerated end-organ response. Eisenhofer *et al.* [75] investigated the role of beta-adrenergic responsiveness in determining individual differences in cardiovascular reactivity to mental stress in normal subjects. Beta-adrenergic responsiveness

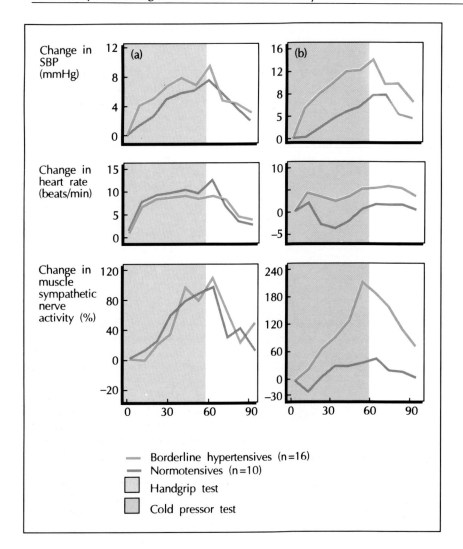

Change in SBP (mmHg)

Change in heart rate (beats/min)

Change in muscle sympathetic nerve activity (%)

—— Borderline hypertensives (n=16)
—— Normotensives (n=10)
▢ Handgrip test
▓ Cold pressor test

Fig. 12.4. Changes in systolic pressure, heart rate, and MSNA during (a) isometric exercise (handgrip) and (b) cold pressor test in normotensive and borderline hypertensive subjects. Reproduced with permission [70].

was evaluated by the effects of isoproterenol infusion on heart rate, and the responses to two mental stressors (a cognitive task and a video game) were also assessed. Significant correlations were found between heart rate responses to the mental stressors and to isoproterenol, indicating that heart rate reactivity was determined peripherally rather than centrally.

Changes in alpha-receptor sensitivity in hypertension are much more controversial [76–80]. A comprehensive study of this problem was undertaken by Egan *et al.* [81], who compared several components of alpha-adrenergic responsiveness in normotensive and hypertensive subjects. They measured plasma noradrenaline levels and the vasoconstrictor response to noradrenaline and angiotensin. They concluded that the increased alpha-mediated vascular tone in hypertensive subjects was best explained by a combination of increased sympathetic drive acting on a hypertrophied arterial system, with normal alpha-adrenergic sensitivity.

Another major factor influencing reactivity is hypertrophy of the arterial wall. As outlined theoretically by Folkow [2], and validated experimentally by Sivertsson [82], vascular hypertrophy results in an enhanced sensitivity to

vasoconstrictor influences without any change in the threshold.

The role of the baroreceptors has been discussed in Chapter 4. The sensitivity of the baroreflex (as manifested by its effects on heart rate) is actually diminished during reactivity tasks such as mental arithmetic [83] and isometric exercise [84]. Individuals with impaired baroreceptors are likely to show an exaggerated hyper-reactivity.

Psychological factors influencing differences in reactivity

As discussed earlier in Chapter 11, attempts to relate a specific personality type to hypertension have been disappointing. The picture is a little clearer with blood pressure reactivity: in a meta-analysis of 71 studies comparing cardiovascular reactivity in type A and type B individuals, Harbin [85] concluded that type A men showed a consistently greater reactivity of systolic (but not diastolic) pressure and heart rate to cognitive challenges. No differences could be detected between type A and type B women, which may simply mean that women found the task less challenging. In parallel with these findings, it has also been reported [86] that men and women scoring high on tests of hostility have a greater blood pressure reactivity when attempting a frustrating task.

With mental challenge tasks requiring an active response by the subject, it is to be expected that the subject's attitude to the task will affect the response. This has been neatly confirmed in a study by Smith et al. [87], who showed that the increase in blood pressure occurring during talking is much greater if the person talking is trying to persuade another person to change his or her opinion about something.

Does reactivity measured in the laboratory predict blood pressure changes during everyday life?

The rationale generally proposed for the use of laboratory tests of cardiovascular reactivity is that an individual's response to such a test may predict how he or she will respond to stressful situations in real life. Until quite recently, it was not possible to test this assumption, but with the introduction of ambulatory monitoring techniques a test can now be attempted.

Four studies have compared the response to laboratory stressors with blood pressure variability measured with the intra-arterial technique of ambulatory monitoring. Melville and Raftery [88] compared the response to two mental stressors, the Stroop test[2] and a stressful film, to blood pressure variability over 24 h, but found no significant correlations. Parati et al. [18] used four laboratory tasks (mental arithmetic, mirror drawing, the cold pressor test and isometric exercise) and also found no correlations between the reactivity to any of tasks and ambulatory blood pressure variability. Floras et al. [89] also used four tasks (mental arithmetic, a reaction time test, bicycle exercise and isometric exercise); they found that the blood pressure changes during all four tests gave significant correlations with daytime ambulatory blood pressure variability (ranging from $r = 0.26$ with mental arithmetic to $r = 0.53$ with the reaction time task). They suggested that the discrepancy between their findings and Parati's may have arisen because they used only daytime readings to express ambulatory blood pressure variability, whereas Parati et al. used the whole 24 h. Melville and Raftery, however, found no correlations with either measure. In a fourth study, Watson et al. [90] found that the systolic pressure response to the cold pressor test predicted daytime ambulatory pressure variability, whereas bicycle and isometric exercise did not.

Several studies have used non-invasive ambulatory monitoring techniques. McKinney et al. [11] used a video game task, a reaction time task and the cold pressor test, and found significant correlations between the absolute levels of blood pressure during the tasks and the average levels during different periods of ambulatory monitoring. They did not report any correlations between change scores during the laboratory testing and blood pressure changes during the ambulatory monitoring. In our own study [91] we used three laboratory tests (a video game, mental arithmetic and treadmill exercise) and also found correlations between the absolute levels of pressure during the laboratory tasks and ambulatory monitoring, but these were no better for the pressures measured during the tasks than at baseline, and no measure of blood pressure reactivity (i.e. change scores) showed any correlation with ambulatory blood pressure variability.

Van Egeren and Sparrow [17] examined the correlations between laboratory and ambulatory reactivity and found weak relationships between the two, the strongest relationship being between the diastolic pressure response to the cold pressor test and ambulatory blood pressure variability ($r = 0.43$, $P < 0.01$). In this study, laboratory reactivity was assessed on the same day that an ambulatory monitor was worn. They concluded that the level of physical activity during ambulatory monitoring had obscured the laboratory–ambulatory relationship and re-analysed their results after adjusting for this. The net effect was a slight improvement in the correlations, but they were still not very good. In another recent study, Fredrikson et al. [92] found high correlations between catecholamine and cortisol excretion during several laboratory stress tasks. However, the correlations between blood pressure reactivity measured in the laboratory and in the field (obtained by hourly readings while at work and at home using a semi-automatic but not ambulatory recorder) were uniformly low, with only three out of 12 correlations reaching statistical significance for systolic pressure, and one out of 12 for diastolic pressure. It should be noted that the laboratory measures were taken 4 months after the ambulatory pressures. In another recent study, which examined the relationship between reactivity measures obtained during laboratory testing and ambulatory measures, Langewitz et al. [93] examined the correlations between change scores for two laboratory tasks (cold pressor and mental arithmetic) and ambulatory blood pressure variances, and found the correlation coefficients to be weak, in the range 0.30–0.40.

Fredrikson et al. [94] related blood pressure during mental arithmetic to ambulatory pressure, and found that systolic pressure during mental arithmetic was more closely related to ambulatory systolic pressure (particularly during work) than to the resting systolic pressure. The change scores during mental arithmetic were not associated with any measure of ambulatory pressure. A similar study by Ironson et al. [95] also found no correlations between the change scores during reactivity testing and ambulatory pressure. In their study the resting blood pressure in the laboratory was more closely related to the ambulatory pressure than the pressure during the reactivity tasks.

Similar conclusions were obtained from a different viewpoint in a study of patients with paroxysmal elevations in

---

[2]The Stroop test is performed by showing subjects a series of names of colours printed in another colour, and asking them to read out the latter colour.

blood pressure and phaeochromocytoma-like symptoms [96]. These patients had a greater blood pressure variability during the day (but not during the night) than a comparative group of essential hypertensive individuals, but their response to mental arithmetic, bicycle exercise and a cold pressor test was the same.

Viewed as a whole, these studies suggest that if there is an association between reactivity measured in the laboratory and blood pressure variability or reactivity of daily life, it is either rather weak or obscured by the problems of measurement. Furthermore, it appears to be non-specific, as it can be demonstrated equally well (or badly) with laboratory challenges both with and without a strong behavioural component. The simplest explanation of findings such as those of Floras *et al.* is that there are significant inter-individual differences in blood pressure variability that may be detected both by laboratory testing and by ambulatory monitoring. As they stand, the results of these studies provide little evidence that the type of reactivity testing commonly used in the laboratory is an ecologically valid representation of the stresses of everyday life. Yet, the assumption of such validity is the basis for much of the work being done in this field. It seems clear that a great deal of research in this area is required before conclusions can be drawn.

It could be argued, however, that it is unreasonable to expect a laboratory task to predict overall blood pressure variability, and that it would be more appropriate to look for correlations with blood pressure changes during specific activities of daily life which more closely resemble the laboratory tasks. Such an approach was used by Matthews *et al.* [97], who found a significant correlation between blood pressure changes during a laboratory speaking task and a similar task in the classroom. However, the response to directly comparable tasks may be difficult to replicate outside the laboratory. Palatini *et al.* [98] compared the blood pressure response to exercise in the laboratory (bicycle ergometry) and in real life (running, bicycling and weight lifting). Blood pressure was measured directly from the brachial artery. They concluded

> '...blood pressure changes recorded during athletics are not well reproduced by the laboratory tests which...appear to underestimate the blood pressure elevations occurring in actual race situations.'

Another study [99] that compared heart rate responses to a flight simulator and real flight in airmen also found that the laboratory situation underestimated the changes occurring in real life. The question how restricted such correlations should be is important for those interested in the role of psychosocial factors in the development of hypertension. If it is possible to demonstrate correlations only between very similar activities in the laboratory and real life, the findings will be of comparatively limited interest. At the other extreme, if significant correlations can be demonstrated between all measures of reactivity in the laboratory and 24-hour variability, as suggested by Floras' results, it is unlikely that psychosocial factors play a major role in determining these associations because much of the diurnal blood pressure variability results from changes in physical activity that have little to do with psychosocial factors.

The reactivity hypothesis would receive its strongest support if the degree of generalization of changes measured in the laboratory to real life fell somewhere between these two extremes. It would be necessary to demonstrate that the response to a number of behavioural challenges in the laboratory predicts the response to psychologically stressful tasks measured by ambulatory monitoring situations during daily life. So far this has not been achieved. It will be very difficult to demonstrate in practice, because at any one moment the blood pressure will represent the summation of the effects of a number of different physical and mental activities, which cannot readily be disentangled.

Reactivity and left ventricular hypertrophy

Schmieder *et al.* [100] related two measures of reactivity — mental arithmetic and bicycle exercise — with LVH, and found that neither the change in pressure nor the absolute level correlated significantly. Furthermore, the subjects showing the greatest reactivity did not have any greater left ventricular mass than the others. Since left ventricular mass is generally thought to be determined by some aspect of the prevailing pressure, whether it be the average level or the variability, this finding also fails to support the idea that reactivity is representative of blood pressure variability.

Reactivity and prognosis

Reactivity and prognosis are discussed in Chapter 13.

Effect of antihypertensive treatment on blood pressure reactivity

In Chapter 10 we saw that antihypertensive treatment, while lowering the average level of pressure, has little or no effect on short-term variability or the diurnal profile of blood pressure. Many of the studies on which this conclusion was based also examined the effects of standardized reactivity tasks, using both physical and mental challenges.

Dynamic exercise has been one of the most widely studied challenges. In this situation systolic pressure increases markedly, as a result of an increased cardiac output, without much change in diastolic pressure. Most antihypertensive agents, including diuretics [101], calcium antagonists [102–104] and angiotensin converting enzyme inhibitors [105], have little effect on the rise in blood pressure during exercise. Beta blockers, by virtue of their negative inotropic effects, reduce the increase in systolic pressure during maximum exercise [105], although they may have little effect at lower levels [103].

During isometric exercise diastolic pressure increases to the same extent as systolic pressure. This change is not affected by calcium antagonists [103,104], angiotensin converting enzyme inhibitors [105] or beta blockers [103,105]. The latter merely change the haemodynamic pattern during isometric exercise from an increased cardiac output to an increased peripheral resistance, without affecting the pressor response [106], as was shown in Fig. 4.9. Even combined alpha/beta blockade has little effect [107]. Clonidine has been reported to attenuate the increase in systolic pressure but not diastolic pressure [107]. According to one report [108], acute alpha-adrenergic blockade with phentolamine does inhibit the response.

The pressor response to the cold pressor test is also not affected by antihypertensive treatment, whether it be with diuretics [109,110], reserpine [109] or beta blockers [110].

Mental stress has been less extensively studied in this context, but diuretics [110], calcium antagonists [111] and clonidine [111] have no effect. Beta blockers have been reported to have no effect in some studies [110,111] and to diminish the increase according to others [112].

Few animal studies have been carried out in this area. LeDoux et al. [113] evaluated the effect of methyldopa on the tonic level of pressure and on the increase occurring during conditioned emotional responses. They concluded that although both were suppressed by the drug, the drug effects were independent of each other.

These studies all support the concept, first discussed in Chapter 4, that the central nervous system acts to maintain the acute increases in blood pressure which occur during mental or physical activity even in the presence of agents which block the pathways which normally mediate this response (i.e. vasoconstriction or an increased cardiac output). This does not, of course, mean that the acute responses, which are thought to be mediated by the sympathetic nervous system, cannot be prevented, for example with combined and complete alpha and beta blockade [109]. However, it does support the view that there is a dissociation between the effects of antihypertensive agents on the tonic and phasic components of blood pressure, and that the two are regulated separately. The same conclusion can be reached from the effects on blood pressure variability reviewed in Chapter 10.

Summary and conclusions

The evaluation of blood pressure reactivity to standardized mental and physical tasks under controlled laboratory conditions has become a popular technique for evaluating the influence of behavioural factors in hypertension. Although this approach can yield valuable insights into the physiological mechanisms of such transient blood pressure changes, its relevance to the development of sustained hypertension is dubious. According to the fashionable, but unsubstantiated, reactivity hypothesis, individuals who show an increased blood pressure reactivity to stressful stimuli are at increased risk of becoming hypertensive, as a result of the cumulative effect of multiple pressor episodes eventually leading to a sustained rise in pressure. As it applies to human hypertension, there are several problems with this schema. Thus, the reliability of reactivity measures is not very good (in part because of measurement error) and individual differences in reactivity may be specific to the type of challenge used. Hypertensive subjects tend to show a greater reactivity than normotensive subjects, particularly to behavioural rather than physical challenges, but whether this precedes or follows the hypertension is unclear. Studies of normotensive individuals with a positive family history of hypertension have yielded conflicting results. Individual differences in reactivity could, in theory, be attributable to a variety of physiological variables, including the perception of the stimulus, central sympathetic outflow, adrenergic receptor density, baroreflex sensitivity and vascular hypertrophy. If reactivity does play a role in mediating the effects of environmental stress on the development of hypertension, it is important to know whether the individual differences can be localized to the central nervous system. Attempts to answer this question by measuring venous plasma noradrenaline responses to challenging stimuli have mostly yielded inconsequential results. More sophisticated techniques, however, indicate that hypertensive subjects may show a greater increment of sympathetic outflow during behavioural challenges than normotensive subjects.

Another requirement of the reactivity hypothesis is that the response to laboratory testing should reflect the response to the stressors of daily life. Several studies have attempted to relate laboratory reactivity measures to ambulatory blood pressure variability, with mostly negative results.

Antihypertensive treatment generally has little effect on blood pressure reactivity, and provides another example of the dissociation of the regulation of the steady-state level of blood pressure and its phasic variations.

References

1.   MANUCK SB, KRANTZ DW: Psychophysiologic reactivity in coronary heart disease and essential hypertension. In *Handbook of Stress, Reactivity, and Cardiovascular Disease* edited by Matthews KA, Weiss SM, Detre T, et al. New York: Wiley, 1986, pp 11–34.

2.   FOLKOW B: Cardiovascular structural adaptation: its role in the initiation and maintenance of primary hypertension. *Clin Sci Mol Med* 1978, 55 (suppl IV):IV3–IV22.

3.   JULIUS S, LI Y, BRANT D, KRAUSE L, BUDA AJ: Neurogenic pressor episodes fail to cause hypertension, but do induce cardiac hypertrophy. *Hypertension* 1989, 13:422–429.

4.   PICKERING TG, GERIN W: Reactivity and the role of behavioral factors in hypertension: a critical review. *Ann Behav Med* 1990, 12:3–16.

5.   LEDOUX JE, SAKAGUCHI A, REIS DJ: Behaviorally selective cardiovascular hyperreactivity in spontaneously hypertensive

rats: evidence for hyperemotionality and enhanced appetitive motivation. *Hypertension* 1982, 4:853–863.

6.   HALLBÄCK M: Consequences of social isolation on blood pressure, cardiovascular reactivity in spontaneously hypertensive rats. *Acta Physiol Scand* 1975, 93:455–465.

7.   FOLKOW B, HALLBÄCK M, WEISS L: Cardiovascular response to acute mental stress in spontaneously hypertensive rats. *Clin Sci Mol Med* 1973, 45:1315–1335.

8.   BEVEGARD BS, SHEPHERD JT: Regulation of the circulation during exercise in man. *Physiol Rev* 1967, 47:178–213.

9.   MANUCK SB, SCHAEFER DC: Stability of individual differences in cardiovascular reactivity. *Physiol Behav* 1978, 21:675–678.

10. MANUCK SB, GARLAND FN: Stability of individual differences in cardiovascular reactivity: a thirteen month follow-up. *Physiol Behav* 1980, 24:621–624.

11. MCKINNEY ME, MINER MH, RUDDELL H, ET AL: The standardized mental stress test protocol: test-retest reliability and comparison with ambulatory blood pressure monitoring. *Psychophysiology* 1985, 22:453–463.

12. PARATI G, POMIDOSSI G, RAMIREZ A, ET AL: Reproducibility of laboratory tests evaluating neural cardiovascular regulation in man. *J Hypertens* 1983, 1 (suppl 2):S88–S90.

13. MYRTEK M: Adaptation effects and the stability of physiological responses to repeated testing. In *Clinical and Methodological Issues in Cardiovascular Psychophysiology* edited by Steptoe A, Rüddel H, Neus H. New York: Springer-Verlag, 1985, pp 93–106.

14. EICH RH, JACOBSEN EC: Vascular reactivity in medical students followed for 10 years. *J Chron Dis* 1967, 20:583–592.

15. LANGEWITZ W, RÜDDEL H, NOACK H, WACHTARZ K: The reliability of psychophysiological examinations under field conditions: results of repetitive stress testing in middle-aged men. *Eur Heart J* 1989, 10:657–665.

16. GERIN W, PIEPER K, MARCHESE L, PICKERING TG: Measurement reliability of cardiovascular reactivity change scores: a comparison of intermittent and continuous methods of assessment. *Psychophysiology* (in press).

17. VAN EGEREN LF, SPARROW AW: Laboratory stress testing to assess real-life cardiovascular reactivity. *Psychosom Med* 1989, 51:1–9.

18. PARATI G, POMIDOSSI G, CASADEI R, ET AL: Limitations of laboratory stress testing in the assessment of subjects' cardiovascular reactivity to stress. *J Hypertens* 1986, 4 (suppl 6):S51–S53.

19. FREDRIKSON M, DIMBERG U, FRISK-HOLMBERG M, STROM G: Arterial blood pressure and general sympathetic activation in essential hypertension during stimulation. *Acta Med Scand* 1985, 217:309–317.

20. ALAM M, SMIRK FH: Blood pressure raising reflexes in health, essential hypertension, and renal hypertension. *Clin Sci* 1938, 3:259–266.

21. AMBROSIONI E, COSTA FV, MONTEBUGNOLI C, BORGHI JC, MAGNANI JB. Intralymphocytic sodium concentration as an index of response to stress and exercise in young subjects with borderline hypertension. *Clin Sci* 1981, 61:25s–27s.

22. BAHLMAN J, BROD J, CACHOVAN M: Stress-induced changes of the venous circulation. *Contrib Nephrol* 1982, 30:43–48.

23. BOHLIN G, ELIASSON K, HJEMDAHL P, ET AL: Personal control over work pace – circulatory, neuroendocrine and subjective responses in borderline hypertension. *J Hypertens* 1986, 4:295–305.

24. BOYER JT, FRASER JRE, DOYLE AE: The haemodynamic effects of cold immersion. *Clin Sci* 1960, 19:539–550.

25. BROD J, FENCL V, HEJL Z, JIRKA J: Circulatory changes underlying blood pressure elevation during acute emotional stress (mental arithmetic) in normotensive and hypertensive subjects. *Clin Sci* 1959, 18:269–279.

26. BROD J, CACHOVAN M, BAHLMANN J, ET AL: Haemodynamic changes during acute emotional stress in man with special reference to the capacitance vessels. *Klin Wochenschr* 1979, 57:555–565.

27. DRUMMOND PD: Cardiovascular reactivity in borderline hypertensives during behavioural and orthostatic stress. *Psychophysiology* 1985, 22:621–628.

28. ELIASSON K, HJEMDAHL P, KAHAN T: Circulatory and sympathoadrenal responses to stress in borderline and established hypertension. *J Hypertens* 1983, 1:131–139.

29. ESLER MO, NESTEL PJ: Renin and sympathetic nervous system responsiveness to adrenergic stimuli in essential hypertension. *Am J Cardiol* 1973, 32:643–649.

30. FREDRIKSON M, DIMBERG U, FRISK-HOLMBERG M, STROM G: Haemodynamic and electrodermal correlates of psychogenic stimuli in hypertensive and normotensive subjects. *Biol Psychol* 1982, 15:63–73.

31. FRISK-HOLMBERG M, ESSEN B, FREDRIKSON M, STROM G, WIBELL L: Muscle fibre composition in relation to blood pressure response to isometric exercise in normotensive and hypertensive subjects. *Acta Med Scand* 1983, 213:21–26.

32. GREENE NA, BOLTAX AJ, LUSTIG GA, ROGOW E: Circulatory dynamics during the cold pressor test. *Am J Cardiol* 1965, 16:54–60.

33. GROEN JJ, HANSEN B, HERRMANN JM, ET AL: Effects of experimental emotional stress and physical exercise on the circulation in hypertensive patients and control subjects. *J Psychosom Res* 1982, 26:141–154.

34. HINES EA, BROWN GE: The cold pressor test for measuring the reactibility of the blood pressure: data concerning 571 normal and hypertensive subjects. *Am Heart J* 1936, 11:1–9.

35. HODAPP V, WEYER G, BECKER J: Situational stereotypy in essential hypertension patients. *J Psychosom Res* 1975, 19:113–121.

36. KALIS BL, HARRIS RE, SOKOLOW M, CARPENTER LG: Response to psychological stress in patients with essential hypertension. *Am Heart J* 1957, 53:572–578.

37. KEANE TM, MARTIN JE, BERLER ES, ET AL: Are hypertensives less assertive? A controlled evaluation. *J Consult Clin Psychol* 1982, 50:499–508.

38. LAMID S, WOLFF FW: Drug failure in reducing pressor effect of isometric handgrip stress test in hypertension. *Am Heart J* 1973, 86:211–215.

39. LINDEN W, FEURSTEIN M: Essential hypertension and social coping behavior: experimental findings. *J Hum Stress* 1983, 9:22–31.

40. LORIMER AR, MACFARLANE PW, PROVAN G, DUFFY T, LAWRIE TDV: Blood pressure and catecholamine responses to 'stress' in normotensive and hypertensive subjects. *Cardiovasc Res* 1971, 5:169–173.

41. MILLER JH, BRUGGER M: The cold pressor reaction in normal subjects and in patients with primary (essential) and secondary (renal) hypertension. *Am Heart J* 1939, 18:329–333.

42. MURAKAMI E, HIWADA K, KOKUBU T: Pathophysiological characteristics of labile hypertensive patients determined by the cold pressor test. *Jpn Circ J* 1980, 44:438–442.

43. MUSUMECI V, BARONI S, CARDILLO C, ET AL. Cardiovascular reactivity, plasma markers of endothelial and platelet activity and plasma renin activity after mental stress in normals and hypertensives. *J Hypertens* 1987, 5 (suppl 5):S1–S4.

44. NESTEL PJ: Blood pressure and catecholamine excretion after mental stress in labile hypertension. *Lancet* 1969, i:692–695.

45. PERKINS KA, BUBBERT PM, MARTIN JE, FAULSTICH ME, HARRIS JK: Cardiovascular reactivity to psychological stress in aerobically trained versus untrained mild hypertensives and normotensives. *Health Psychol* 1986, 5:407–421.

46. SAFAR ME, WEISS YA, LEVENSON JA, LONDON GM, MILLIEZ PL: Hemodynamic study of 85 patients with borderline hypertension. *Am J Cardiol* 1973, 31:315–319.

47. SANNERSTEDT R, JULIUS S: Systematic haemodynamics in borderline arterial hypertension: responses to static exercise before and under the influence of propranolol. *Cardiovasc Res* 1972, 6:398–403.

48. SCHACHTER J: Pain, fear, and anger in hypertensives and normotensives. *Psychosom Med* 1957, 19:17–29.

49. SHAPIRO AP, MOUTSOS SE, KRIFCHER E: Patterns of pressor response to noxious stimuli in normal, hypertensive and diabetic subjects. *J Clin Invest* 1963, 42:1890–1898.

50. SICONOLFI SF, LASSATER TM, ELDER JP, GERBER CE, CARLETON RA: Normal blood pressure reactivity to mental stress in

patients with borderline hypertension. *J Cardiopul Rehab* 1986, 6:383–398.

51. STEPTOE A, MELVILLE DR, ROSS A: Behavioural response demands, cardiovascular reactivity, and essential hypertension. *Psychosom Med* 1983, 45:33–48.

52. SULLIVAN P, SCHOEUTGEN S, DEQUATTRO V, *ET AL*: Anxiety, anger, and neurogenic tone at rest and in stress in patients with primary hypertension. *Hypertension* 1981, 3 (suppl II):II119–II123.

53. SVENSSON JCH, THEORELL T: Cardiovascular effects of anxiety induced by interviewing young hypertensive male subjects. *J Psychosom Res* 1982, 26:359–370.

54. VOUDOUKIS IJ: Cold pressor test and hypertension. *Angiology* 1978, 29:429–439.

55. WESTHEIM A, OS L, KJELDSEN SE, *ET AL*: Increased circulatory and sympathetic response to tilting in essential hypertension. *J Hypertens* 1987, 5 (suppl 5):S341–S343.

56. WOLF S, CARDON PV, SHEPARD EM, WOLFF HG: *Life Stress and Essential Hypertension.* Baltimore: Williams and Wilkins, 1955.

57. LUND-JOHANSEN P: Hemodynamics in early essential hypertension. *Acta Med Scand* 1967, (suppl 428):1–101.

58. FREDRIKSON M, MATTHEWS KA: Cardiovascular responses to behavioural stress and hypertension: a meta-analytic review. *Ann Behav Med* 1990, 12:30–39.

59. RAVOGLI A, TRAZZI S, VILLANI A, *ET AL*: Early 24 hour blood pressure elevation in normotensive subjects with parental hypertension. *Hypertension* (in press).

60. MCCRORY WW, KLEIN AA, ROSENTHAL RA: Blood pressure, heart rate, and plasma catecholamines in normal and hypertensive children and their siblings at rest and after standing. *Hypertension* 1982, 4:507–513.

61. HAMADA M, KAZATAIM Y, SHIGEMATSU Y, *ET AL*: Enhanced blood pressure response to isometric handgrip exercise in patients with essential hypertension: effects of propranolol and prazosin. *J Hypertens* 1987, 5:305–309.

62. GRAAFSMA SJ, VAN TITS LJ, VAN HEIJST P, *ET AL*: Adrenoceptors on blood cells in patients with essential hypertension before and after mental stress. *J Hypertens* 1989, 7:519–524.

63. LENDERS JWM, WILLEMSEN JJ, DE BOO T, LEMMENS WAJ, THIEN T: Disparate effects of mental stress on plasma noradrenaline in young normotensive and hypertensive subjects. *J Hypertens* 1989, 7:317–323.

64. PALERMO A, BERTALERO P, BORCHINI M, *ET AL*: Sympathetic response to mental stress in borderline hypertensive patients. *J Cardiovasc Pharmacol* 1987, 10 (suppl 4):S156–S158.

65. GOLDSTEIN DS: Plasma norepinephrine during stress in essential hypertension. *Hypertension* 1981, 3:551–556.

66. NIELSEN JR, GRAM LF, PEDERSEN PK: Plasma noradrenaline response to a multistage exercise test in young men at increased risk of developing essential hypertension. *J Hypertens* 1989, 7:377–382.

67. CHODAKOWSKA J, NAZAR K, WOCIAL B, JARECKI M, STORKA B: Plasma catecholamines and renin activity in response to exercise in patients with essential hypertension. *Clin Sci Mol Med* 1975, 49:511–514.

68. GOLDSTEIN DE, EISENHOFER G, GARTY M, *ET AL*: Implications of plasma levels of catechols in the evaluation of sympathoadrenomedullary function. *Am J Hypertens* 1989, 2:133S–139S.

69. ESLER M, JENNINGS G, LAMBERT G: Noradrenaline release and the pathophysiology of primary human hypertension. *Am J Hypertens* 1989, 2:140S–146S.

70. MIYAJIMA E, YAMADA Y, MATSUKAWA T, *ET AL*: Neurogenic abnormalities in young borderline hypertensives. *Clin Exp Hypertens [A]* 1988, 10 (suppl 1):209–223.

71. MCALLISTER RG, LOVE DW, GUTHRIE GP, DOMINIC JA, KOTCHEN TA: Peripheral beta-receptor responsiveness in patients with essential hypertension. *Arch Intern Med* 1979, 139:879–881.

72. BERTEL OM, BÜHLER FR, KIOSSKI W, LÜTOLD B: Decreased beta-adrenoceptor responsiveness as related to age, blood pressure and plasma catecholamines in patients with essential hypertension. *Hypertension* 1980, 2:130–138.

73. TRIMARCO B, VOLPE M, RICCIARDELLI B, *ET AL*: Studies of the mechanisms underlying impairment of beta-adrenoceptor

mediated effects in human hypertension. *Hypertension* 1983, 5:584–590.

74. FELDMAN RD, LIMBIRD LE, NADEAU J, ROBERTSON D, WOOD AJJ: Leukocyte beta-receptor alterations in hypertensive subjects. *J Clin Invest* 1984, 73:648–653.

75. EISENHOFER G, LAMBIE DG, JOHNSON RH: Beta-adrenoceptor responsiveness and plasma catecholamines as determinants of cardiovascular reactivity to mental stress. *Clin Sci* 1985, 69:483–492.

76. JONES CR, ELLIOTT HL, DEIGHTON N, HOWIE CA, REID JL: Alpha-adrenoceptor number and function in platelets from treated and untreated patients with essential hypertension and age- and sex-matched controls. *J Hypertens* 1985, 3 (suppl 3):S153–S155.

77. BRODDE OE, DAUL A, O'HARA N, BOCK KD: Increased density and responsiveness of alpha and beta-adrenoceptors in circulating blood cells of essential hypertensive patients. *J Hypertens* 1984, 2 (suppl 3):S111–S114.

78. CONTINSOUZA-BLANC D, ELGHOZI J-L, DAUSSE J-P: Alteration of platelet alpha$_2$-adrenoceptors in human hypertension. *J Hypertens* 1984, 2 (suppl 3):S155–S157.

79. JIE K, VAN BRUMMELEN P, VERMEY P, TIMMERMANS PMBWM, VAN ZWIETEN PA: Alpha$_1$- and alpha$_2$-adrenoceptor mediated vasoconstriction in the forearm: differences between normotensive and hypertensive subjects. *J Hypertens* 1985, 3 (suppl 3):S89–S91.

80. AMMANN FW, BOLLI P, KIOWSKI W, BÜHLER FR: Enhanced alpha-adrenoceptor-mediated vasoconstriction in essential hypertension. *Hypertension* 1981, 3 (suppl I):I119–I123.

81. EGAN B, PARIS R, HINDERLITER A, SCHORK N, JULIUS S: Mechanism of increased alpha adrenergic vasoconstriction in human essential hypertension. *J Clin Invest* 1987, 80:812–817.

82. SIVERTSSON R: *The Hemodynamic Importance of Structural Vascular Changes in Essential Hypertension.* Acta Physiol Scand 1970, suppl 343.

83. SLEIGHT P, FOX P, LOPEZ R, BROOKS DE: The effect of mental arithmetic on blood pressure variability and baroreflex sensitivity in man. *Clin Sci* 1978, 55:381s–282s.

84. CUNNINGHAM DJC, STRANGE PETERSEN E, PETO R, PICKERING TG, SLEIGHT P: Comparison of the effects of different types of exercise on the baroreflex regulation of heart rate. *Acta Physiol Scand* 1972, 86:444–455.

85. HARBIN TJ: The relationship between the type A behavior pattern and physiological responsivity: a quantitative review. *Psychophysiology* 1989, 26:110–119.

86. WEIDNER G, FRIEND R, FICAROTTO TJ, MENDELL NR: Hostility and cardiovascular reactivity to stress in women and men. *Psychosom Med* 1989, 51:36–45.

87. SMITH TW, ALLRED KD, MORRISON CA, CARLSON SD: Cardiovascular reactivity and interpersonal influence: active coping in a social context. *J Pers Soc Psychol* 1989, 56:209–218.

88. MELVILLE DI, RAFTERY EB: Blood pressure changes during acute mental stress in hypertensive subjects using the Oxford intra-arterial system. *J Psychosom Med* 1981, 24:487–497.

89. FLORAS JS, HASSAN MO, JONES JV, SLEIGHT P: Pressor responses to laboratory stresses and daytime blood pressure variability. *J Hypertens* 1987, 5:715–719.

90. WATSON RD, STALLARD TJ, FLINN RM, LITTLER WA: Factors determining direct arterial pressure and its variability in hypertensive man. *Hypertension* 1980, 2:333–341.

91. HARSHFIELD GA, JAMES GD, SCHLUSSEL Y, *ET AL*: Do laboratory tests of blood pressure reactivity predict blood pressure variability in real life? *Am J Hypertens* 1988, 1:168–174.

92. FREDRIKSON M, TUOMISTO M, LUNDBERG U, MELIN B: Blood pressure in healthy men and women under laboratory and naturalistic conditions. *J Psychosom Res* (in press).

93. LANGEWITZ W, RÜDDEL H, SCHÄCHINGER H, SCHMIEDER R: Standardized stress testing in the cardiovascular laboratory: has it any bearing on ambulatory blood pressure values? *J Hypertens* 1989, 7 (suppl 3):S41-S48.

94. FREDRIKSON M, BLUMENTHAL JA, EVANS DD, SHERWOOD A, LIGHT KC: Cardiovascular responses in the laboratory and in the natural environment: is blood pressure reactivity to laboratory-induced mental stress related to ambulatory

blood pressure during everyday life? *J Psychosom Res* 1989, 33:753–762.

95. IRONSON GH, GELLMAN MD, SPITZER SB, *ET AL*: Predicting home and work blood pressure measurements from resting baselines and laboratory reactivity in black and white Americans. *Psychophysiology* 1989, 26:174–184.

96. TAKABATAKE T, YAMAMOTO Y, OHTA H, *ET AL*: Blood pressure variability and hemodynamic response to stress in patients with paroxysmal elevation of blood pressure. *Clin Exp Hypertens [A]* 1985, 7:235–242.

97. MATTHEWS KA, MANUCK SB, SAAB PG: Cardiovascular responses of adolescents during a naturally occurring stressor and their behavioral and psychophysiological predictors. *Psychophysiology* 1986, 23:198–209.

98. PALATINI P, MOS L, DI MARCO A, *ET AL*: Intra-arterial blood pressure recording during sports activities. *J Hypertens* 1987, 5 (suppl 5):S479–S481.

99. WILSON G, PURVIS B, SKELLY J: Physiological data used to measure pilot workload in actual flight and simulator conditions. In *Proceedings of the 31st Annual Meeting of the Human Factors Society*, 1987.

100. SCHMIEDER RE, GRUBE E, RÜDDEL H, SCHÄCHINGER H, SCHULTE W: Relation of hemodynamic reaction during stress to left ventricular hypertrophy in essential hypertension. *Am J Hypertens* 1990, 3:281–287.

101. RAFTERY EB, MELVILLE DJ, GOULD BA, MANN S, WHITTINGTON JR: A study of antihypertensive action of xipamide using ambulatory intra-arterial monitoring. *Br J Clin Pharmacol* 1981, 12:381–385.

102. HORNUNG RS, GOULD BA, JONES RI, SONECHA T, RAFTERY EB: Nifedipine tablets for hypertension: a study using continuous ambulatory intra-arterial monitoring. *Postgrad Med J* 1983, 59 (suppl 2):95–97.

103. HORNUNG RS, JONES RI, GOULD BA, SONECHA T, RAFTERY EB: Twice-daily verapamil for hypertension: a comparison with propranolol. *Am J Cardiol* 1986, 57:93D–98D.

104. CARDILLO C, MUSUMECI V, MORES N, FOLLI G: Effects of sustained-release verapamil on 24-hour ambulatory blood pressure and on pressor response to isometric exertion in hypertensive patients. *J Cardiovasc Pharmacol* 1989, 13 (suppl 4):S31–S33.

105. ENSTROM I, THULIN T, LINDHOLM L: A plea for more comprehensive blood pressure measurements when evaluating drug treatment of hypertension. *J Hypertens* 1988, 6:959–964.

106. GARAVAGLIA GE, MESSERLI FH, SCHMIEDER RE, NUNEZ DB: Antihypertensive therapy and cardiovascular reactivity during isometric stress. *J Hum Hypertens* 1988, 2:247–241.

107. WATT SJ, THOMAS RD, BELFIELD PW, GOLDSTRAW PW, TAYLOR SH: Influence of sympatholytic drugs on the cardiovascular response to isometric exercise. *Clin Sci* 1981, 60:139–143.

108. MCALLISTER RG: Effect of adrenergic receptor blockade on the responses to isometric handgrip: studies in normal and hypertensive subjects. *J Cardiovasc Pharmacol* 1979, 1:253–263.

109. SHAPIRO AP: Pressor responses to noxious stimuli in hypertensive patients. Effects of reserpine and chlorothiazide. *Circulation* 1962, 26:242–250.

110. ELIASSON K, KAHAN T, HYLANDER B, HJEMDAHL P: Reactivity to mental stress and cold provocation during long-term treatment with metoprolol, propranolol, or hydrochlorothiazide. *J Hypertens* 1986, 4 (suppl 6):S263–S265.

111. RÜDDEL H, SCHNEIDER R, LANGEWITZ W, SCHULTE W: Impact of antihypertensive therapy on blood pressure reactivity during mental stress. *J Hum Hypertens* 1988, 1:259–265.

112. GUAZZI M, FIORENTINI C, POLESE A, OLIVAN MT, MAGRINI F: Antihypertensive action of propranolol in man: lack of evidence for a neural depressive effects. *Clin Pharmacol Ther*, 1976, 20:304–309.

113. LEDOUX JE, SAKAGUCHI A, REIS DJ: Alpha-methyldopa dissociates hypertension, cardiovascular reactivity and emotional behavior in spontaneously hypertensive rats. *Brain Res* 1983, 259:69–76.

13 Which measures of blood pressure give the best prediction of target organ damage and prognosis?

The relationship between blood pressure and cardiovascular morbidity has been appreciated for many years. It is based on both actuarial studies [1] and population surveys [2]. It is, however, derived from a relatively small number of blood pressure readings taken from each individual in an office or clinic setting. As we have seen in earlier chapters, blood pressure varies considerably within individuals, and clinic pressure may not be representative of the pressure at other times. It is therefore relevant to ask whether other measures of pressure, including ambulatory pressure, will provide a better prediction of risk than clinic pressure. It is generally assumed that the damage due to hypertension is related to the average level of pressure over time (the true blood pressure). However, this assumption should not go unchallenged, because it is probable that the peaks of pressure and the shape of the arterial pressure waveform also contribute [3]. Recent findings from the Framingham survey indicate that the average pressure measured over 30 years gives a closer correlation than measurements made on a single occasion with ECG-LVH [4], which is the most reliable measure of target organ damage available at present [5].

The need for improved prediction of individual risk

The Veterans Administration trial [6] of the treatment of hypertension demonstrated that the treatment of patients with severe hypertension resulted in a significant reduction in cardiovascular morbidity. A number of other clinical trials have since examined the benefits of treating patients with mild hypertension [7–10]. Although the results have generally been positive, they have also been disappointing, because when studied from the point of view of the individual patient rather than the population, the probability of benefit from treatment is very low. Therefore, as we have seen in Chapter 1, treatment can be said to benefit the population, but not the individual patient.

As an individual's level of blood pressure is not a fixed entity, a good case can be made for supposing that a more representative estimate of the 'true' or average level of pressure than can be obtained with a small number of clinic measurements will improve the prediction of risk and hence the need for treatment. On theoretical grounds, it can be argued that the relationship between blood pressure and risk will be closer for the true (or ambulatory) pressure than for casual or screening pres-

sures. Most of the information about this relationship has come from screened populations in whom a small number of measurements were taken, which are subject to regression to the mean. Thus, those individuals found to have the highest screening pressure are likely to have a somewhat lower true pressure; at the other extreme those with the lowest screening pressure will have a higher true pressure (Fig. 13.1): hence the steeper relationship between true blood pressure and risk. The association between blood pressure and risk has recently been re-analysed by McMahon et al. [11], who used data from nine major prospective observational studies comprising 420 000 individuals. Using data from the Framingham study, they adjusted the blood pressure values for the 'regression dilution effect' and concluded that there was a steep log-linear relationship between the 'usual' (or true) diastolic pressure and the incidence of disease.

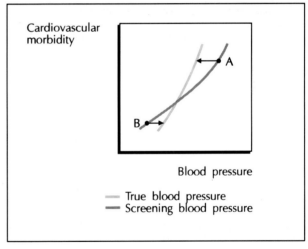

Fig. 13.1. Hypothetical relationship between screening blood pressure, true blood pressure, and risk of cardiovascular morbidity. In most individuals (e.g. A in the figure), the screening blood pressure overestimates the true blood pressure; in some (e.g. B) it underestimates it.

The question which measure of blood pressure will give the best prediction of risk can, in principle, be answered in two ways: either by relating different measures of blood pressure to target organ damage on a cross-sectional basis (the quick and easy way), or by relating them directly to prognosis with longitudinal or prospective studies. The latter is both more desirable and more difficult. The main limitation of cross-sectional studies is the difficulty of drawing causal inferences from them. To give one example, it has been found that patients with increased blood pressure variability have more extensive target organ damage [12] than patients with more stable pressures. It was therefore claimed that the variability is itself pathogenic. However, the opposite explanation is equally plausible: vascular damage may impair baroreflex sensitivity, which would result in an increased blood pressure variability. Longitudinal studies also present problems: for example, most people with hypertension are now treated, so that it is almost impossible to carry out a true natural history study.

The relationships between blood pressure, target organ damage and cardiovascular morbidity

The relationships between blood pressure and other risk factors affecting cardiovascular morbidity are illustrated schematically in Fig. 13.2, with target organ damage viewed as an intermediate risk factor resulting from the interactions of blood pressure and other primary risk factors, which contributes directly to cardiovascular morbidity. At present, echocardiography gives the most sensitive measurement of target organ damage. The best established echocardiographic index is LVH [13], but diastolic dysfunction may be an even more sensitive marker of the effects of hypertension on the heart [14]. Although the major brunt of the effects of hypertension is borne by the arteries, there is unfortunately no generally accepted clinical method for the evaluation of the structural changes in the arteries.

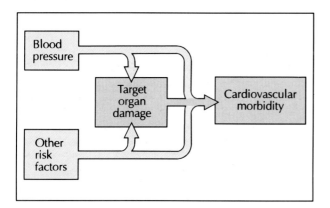

Fig. 13.2. Hypothetical relationships between blood pressure, other risk factors, target organ damage and cardiovascular morbidity.

I shall review here the utility of different ways of measuring blood pressure in predicting future disease states. At least six measures of blood pressure can be considered: clinic (or casual), basal, home, ambulatory and exercise pressures, and also blood pressure reactivity. The first five are usually expressed as absolute numbers and the last as a change score. The three outcome measures to be considered are future levels of blood pressure, target organ damage and morbidity.

The relationships between blood pressure and morbidity can be examined in three ways: by relating blood pressure directly to morbidity, by relating it to target organ damage, and by relating target organ damage to morbidity (Fig. 13.2). Studies relating blood pressure and target organ damage have been mainly cross-sectional, while studies relating these variables to morbidity are, of necessity, longitudinal. The remainder of this chapter is divided into five sections, each of which reviews one aspect of these relationships.

Cross-sectional studies relating blood pressure and target organ damage

Several studies have compared the correlation between different measures of blood pressure and target organ damage. The six measures of blood pressure and the four measures of target organ damage to be considered are shown in Fig. 13.3. Most studies have compared clinic pressure (usually averaged over several visits) with daytime or 24-hour ambulatory pressure, and have used LVH as the dependent measure. These studies are reviewed in detail below.

Ambulatory blood pressure and target organ damage
Aggregate measures of target organ damage
The first study relating clinic and ambulatory pressure to target organ damage was reported in the classic paper by Sokolow *et al.* [15], in which three measures were used: LVH evaluated from the ECG, heart size from the chest radiograph, and fundal changes. This aggregate measure of target organ damage was more closely related to ambulatory daytime blood pressure (r = 0.63 for systolic pressure and r = 0.65 for diastolic pressure) than to clinic pressure.

A similar composite index of target organ damage was used in a more recent study by Parati *et al.* [12], who also found a closer correlation between target organ damage and ambulatory pressure (in this case 24-hour pressure) than clinic blood pressure.

Left ventricular hypertrophy
LVH has traditionally been evaluated by the ECG, although echocardiography has the advantage of being both more sensitive and more specific. Thus, the prevalence of LVH by ECG criteria may be as low as 5% in patients with mild hypertension, whereas by echocardiographic criteria it may be between 20 and 50% [4]. The importance of LVH as a predictor of morbidity is discussed later.

The results of studies relating clinic and ambulatory pressure to LVH are summarized in Fig. 13.4. Most have used echocardiographically determined LVH (expressed as left ventricular mass). All the studies shown in the figure found a closer correlation for ambulatory than clinic blood pressure with left ventricular mass, with one ex-

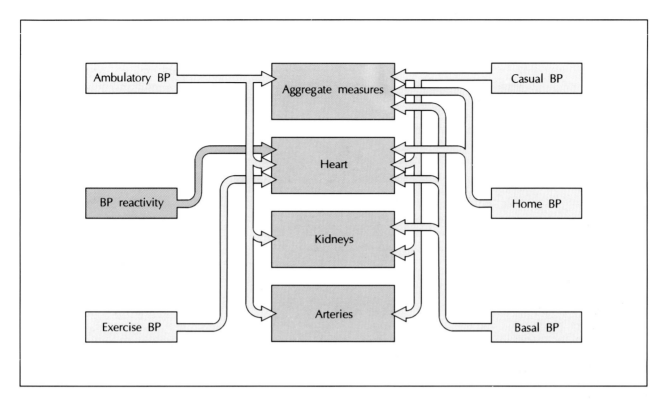

Fig. 13.3. Cross-sectional studies relating blood pressure (BP) and target organ damage. The blue arrows show associations that have been reported in at least one study; the grey arrow shows an association that has been evaluated with negative results.

ception [26], but even here measures of inter-ventricular septal and posterior wall thickness were more closely related to ambulatory than to clinic pressure. Verdecchia et al. [31] analysed their data in a different manner, by first computing the regression line relating clinic pressures to ambulatory pressures. Patients whose ambulatory pressure was high relative to their clinic pressure were much more likely to have LVH than those whose ambulatory pressure was low. This study provided further evidence that white coat hypertension is associated with an absence of target organ damage.

One study used ECG criteria for assessing LVH, but instead of the more frequently used 12-lead recording, the orthogonal vector cardiogram system was used, on the grounds that this gives a more reliable estimate of LVH [16]. In 180 patients with mild to moderate hypertension, no significant correlation was found with clinic pressure, whereas highly significant correlations were found with daytime ambulatory pressure.

We also found [19] that the correlation between ambulatory pressure and LVH was closer when the pressure was measured on a work than on a non-work day (Fig. 13.5). This, by analogy with the effects of physical conditioning on LVH, suggests that intermittent elevations in pressure, such as occur during working hours, may be important in the development of LVH.

Although most studies have found slightly higher correlations for daytime than for night-time blood pressures

with LVH (Fig. 13.4), a recent report by Verdecchia et al. [23] stated that patients whose blood pressure remains elevated during the night have more LVH than those whose pressure shows the normal decrease at night (Fig. 13.6).

These apparently conflicting results may be resolved as follows. In most people blood pressure falls at night by approximately the same degree, so that most of the inter-individual variation in 24-hour blood pressure will be determined by differences in daily activity, and hence better correlations will be obtained between daytime pressure and LVH (on the assumption that it is the average or 24-hour level of pressure which determines LVH). If, however, the population studied contains a significant portion of individuals whose pressure remains high at night (non-dippers), the correlation may be closer for night-time pressure.

The better correlation with ambulatory pressure than with clinic pressure could be due to a combination of two factors. First is the effect of the greater number of readings. This was elegantly demonstrated by Prisant and Carr [25], who showed not only that the correlations between clinic pressure and LVH were stronger if multiple clinic readings were used rather than a single reading, but also that they were weaker if a subset of ambulatory readings (e.g. from 8.00 a.m. to 12 noon) was used rather than the average for the full 24 h. The second factor is the more representative nature of the ambulatory readings, which was reviewed in Chapter 7.

Organ	Measured variable	Authors	n	Correlation coefficient		
				Clinic SBP	Ambulatory SBP (daytime)	Ambulatory SBP (night-time)
Heart	ECG-LVH	Vermeersch et al. [16]	180	0.19	0.36	–
	Echo-LVH	Rowlands et al. [17]	50	0.51	0.57	0.56
		Drayer et al. [18]	12	0.55	0.82	0.70
		Devereux et al. [19]	100	0.24	0.50	0.10
		Antivalle et al. [20]	84	0.26	0.45*	–
		Gosse et al. [21]	61	0.40	0.53	–
		White et al. [22]	47	0.55	0.61	0.58
		Verdecchia et al. [23]	237	0.38	0.40	0.47
		Palatini et al. [24]	42	0.52	0.62*	–
		Prisant and Carr [25]	55	0.32	0.59*	–
		Moulopoulos et al. [26]	40	0.39	NS	NS
		Baba et al. [27]	17 (HT)	−0.22	−0.07**	0.15
			21 (NT)	0.25	0.47**	0.15
Kidney	Albumin excretion	Opsahl et al. [28]	42	0.31	0.44*	–
		Dimmitt et al. [29]	25	0.60	0.52	–
	NAG excretion	Opsahl et al. [28]	42	0.14	0.32*	–
Arteries	Pulse wave velocity	Asmar et al. [30]	22	0.24	0.68	–
Combined	ECG, CXR, fundi	Sokolow et al. [15]	124	0.48	0.63	–

*Twenty-four-hour SBP used; **correlations with left ventricular wall thickness: work pressure used for daytime value.
NT, normotensive; HT, hypertensive; CXR, chest radiograph; NAG, N-acetyl-glucosaminidase.

Fig. 13.4. Correlations between different measures of blood pressure and target organ damage.

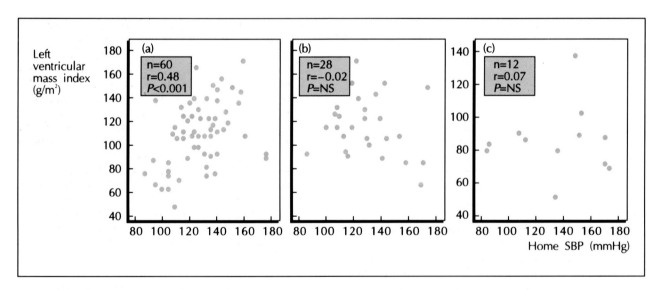

Fig. 13.5. Relationships between home systolic pressure measured by ambulatory monitoring and left ventricular mass index in groups separated by employment status. (a) Sixty employed subjects who wore the monitor on a work day; (b) 28 employed subjects who wore the monitor on a non-work day; (c) 12 unemployed subjects. Reproduced with permission [19].

Left ventricular filling

Abnormalities of left ventricular diastolic performance have recently become popular as possible early markers of the effects of hypertension on the heart. These can be investigated either by radionuclide ventriculography or by echocardiography [14,32,33]. Patients with LVH are more likely to show reduced diastolic filling rates than those without it [34]. An important point, however, is that fill-

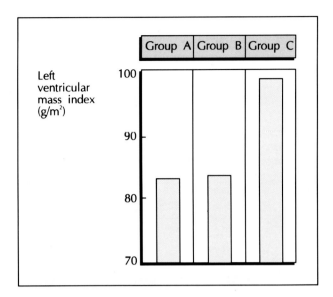

Fig. 13.6. Left ventricular mass index in three groups of subjects: A, normotensive; B, hypertensive dippers; C, hypertensive non-dippers. Reproduced with permission [23].

ing abnormalities are just as likely to be determined by functional as by structural changes, which may limit their usefulness as markers of target organ damage. Thus, they are likely to be less stable over time than LVH.

One study [22] related clinic and ambulatory blood pressures to diastolic filling abnormalities in normotensive and never-treated hypertensive subjects. The most potent determinant of filling rate was found to be age, followed by ambulatory blood pressure. Below the age of 55 years normotensive subjects had a higher filling rate than hypertensive subjects, but in older subjects it was uniformly depressed. Correlations between blood pressure and filling rate were less good for clinic pressure than for ambulatory pressure.

Microalbumin excretion
An increased rate of albumin excretion by the kidney may be one of the earliest detectable renal changes in hypertension. Three studies have related clinic and ambulatory pressures to albumin excretion; two [28,35] found a better correlation for ambulatory pressure, while the third [29] found the opposite. Dimmitt *et al.* commented that the variation in blood pressure resulting from changes in posture and exercise may account for the weaker correlations with ambulatory pressure. However, a more plausible explanation may be that they estimated albumin excretion from spot specimens of urine taken at the time of the clinic visit rather than by using 24-hour collections, as in the other two studies.

N-acetyl-glucosaminidase (NAG) excretion
NAG is an enzyme formed in renal tubules, and is detectable in the urine. It is found in increased quantities in hypertensive patients [36], although it may not be a

very specific marker for the effects of blood pressure on the kidney. Nevertheless, Opsahl *et al.* [28] reported a closer correlation between NAG excretion and ambulatory pressure than with clinic pressure.

Arterial stiffness
Increased arterial stiffness occurs in hypertension as a result of pressure-induced hypertrophy of the arterial wall, and it may also be a contributory factor in the development of systolic hypertension. One study has reported that pulse wave velocity (an indirect measure of arterial stiffness) correlated more closely with ambulatory pressure than with clinic pressure [30].

Home blood pressure and target organ damage
It has been known since the classic study of Ayman and Goldshine [37] that home blood pressure tends to be lower than clinic pressure. We subsequently demonstrated that home pressure readings taken by the patients agree more closely with the average 24-hour pressure than do clinic readings taken by the physician [38]. Despite the growing and widespread use of home blood pressure monitoring, there is relatively little information about its predictive value. In a study of the effects of antihypertensive treatment on blood pressure and LVH it was reported that regression of LVH evaluated by ECG correlated more closely with changes in home pressure than with clinic pressure [39]. Two studies have indicated [38,40] that the correlation between echocardiographically determined LVH and blood pressure is better for home readings than for clinic readings, as shown in Fig. 8.6.

Abe *et al.* [41] related clinic and home pressure to an aggregate measure of target organ damage (retinopathy, ECG-LVH, heart size on the chest radiograph and serum creatinine) in 100 hypertensive patients. Home pressure readings were, as might be expected, consistently lower than clinic readings, but gave generally similar correlations with target organ damage (for systolic pressure and diastolic pressure, respectively, these were r = 0.42 and 0.33 for home pressure, and 0.42 and 0.34 for clinic pressure). However, when a subset of 40 patients with clinic systolic pressures between 160 and 179 mmHg was divided into two groups, one with 'high' and the other with 'low' home pressure (i.e. white coat hypertension), target organ damage was more pronounced in the 'high' group, although the difference between the two groups was only significant for retinopathy.

Basal blood pressure and target organ damage
In a study of 471 hypertensive patients, Caldwell *et al.* [42] compared the correlations between blood pressure and target organ damage using both clinic and basal blood pressure. There was a considerable difference between the two measures, the average clinic pressure being 192/111 mmHg and the basal pressure being 146/89 mmHg. Four indices of target organ damage

were used: fundal changes ECG-LVH, chest radiograph changes and proteinuria, and each was correlated with clinic and basal pressure. The correlations were very similar for the two measures of pressure, leading the authors to conclude that the measurement of basal pressure had no practical value.

Schmieder *et al.* [43] measured blood pressure at a worksite screening and again during quiet rest in 73 hypertensive men. The latter readings were 13/0 mmHg lower than the former, but the correlations (for systolic pressure) with left ventricular mass were very similar (r = 0.28 for worksite pressure and r = 0.35 for resting pressure). Both these measures gave better correlations than the clinic readings (r = 0.16).

Exercise blood pressure and target organ damage

It is well recognized that individuals who exercise regularly are more likely to develop LVH, which may be concentric or eccentric depending on the type of exercise [44,45]. A number of studies have compared the correlation between blood pressure measured at rest (which may be considered to be intermediate between basal and clinic pressure) and during exercise with left ventricular mass or hypertrophy in hypertensive patients. The results are summarized in Fig. 13.7. In five out of eight studies the correlation with left ventricular mass was better for exercise systolic pressure. However, there is some disagreement about whether the correlation is closest with blood pressure measured during submaximal or maximal exercise. Most of the studies reported results for maximal exercise [21,46], but one [48] found a significant correlation with submaximal, but not maximal exercise.

The largest of these studies was conducted by Fagard *et al.* [51]. They measured blood pressure intra-arterially, at rest and during bicycle exercise, in 169 patients. Target organ damage was assessed by funduscopic examination and by ECG manifestations of LVH. Neither measure was more closely related to blood pressure measured during exercise than at rest. This negative result commands respect, both because it was the only study to use intra-arterial blood pressure recordings (and hence to avoid the errors of non-invasive blood pressure measurement during exercise), and because it had the largest sample size. The chief limitation of the study, however, was that it used ECG rather than echocardiography for measuring LVH.

It does not necessarily follow that the blood pressure achieved during regular exercise is influencing left ventricular mass. One of the studies [47] found that the correlation between exercise blood pressure and left ventricular mass was independent of the level of habitual physical activity. Furthermore, a hypertrophied ventricle may be capable of generating a higher systolic pressure during exercise. However, a study in children [52] found no correlation between left ventricular mass and peak systolic pressure during exercise. Another study of exercise performance in hypertensive adults found that patients

with LVH had a lower systolic pressure during maximal exercise [53].

Exercise	Authors	n	Correlation coefficient	
			Resting SBP	Exercise SBP
Treadmill	Ren *et al.* [46]	67	0.16	0.58
Treadmill	Nathwani *et al.* [47]	20	0.21	0.57
Treadmill	Papademetriou *et al.* [48]	–	0.35	0.48
Bicycle	Gosse *et al.* [21]	19	0.40	0.53
Bicycle	Schmieder *et al.* [43]	73	0.34	0.07
Treadmill	Gottdiener *et al.* [49]	39	0.40	0.65
Bicycle	Sau *et al.* [50]	103	0.34	0.26–0.34*
Bicycle	Fagard *et al.* [51]	169	0.24	0.19–0.29†

*Correlation coefficients included peak and submaximal exercise; †left ventricular hypertrophy assessed from ECG. SBP, systolic blood pressure.

Fig. 13.7. Correlations between blood pressure measured at rest and during exercise with left ventricular mass/hypertrophy.

Blood pressure reactivity and target organ damage

Despite the large literature on reactivity, this particular association has received little attention. One study [43] found no correlation between blood pressure measured during mental arithmetic and LVH (measured echocardiographically), despite the finding of a weak but significant correlation at rest.

Which measures of blood pressure give the best correlation with target organ damage?

So far, all the published studies addressing this question have shown that ambulatory pressure is superior to clinic pressure, and even that post-exercise and home pressure may give better correlations with target organ damage. There are several possible reasons for these findings. One is that ambulatory and home measurement provide a greater number of readings than clinic measurement, so that the average value is likely to be a closer approximation to the true level of pressure. Another may be that clinic pressure is less representative of the true level of blood pressure than the other measures, as discussed in Chapter 7. The white coat effect is variable from one patient to another, so that clinic pressure is, in general, a relatively poor predictor of pressures at other times.

Another point worthy of consideration is whether measurement of pressure at one particular time of day will give a better prediction than at another time. It is theoretically possible, for example, that there may be a threshold effect of blood pressure on LVH, such that pressures at the upper end of the range would give a better prediction of LVH than pressures at the lower end. Although it is not possible to draw definitive conclusions on this point at present, existing evidence is consistent with this view. This is exemplified by our finding [19] that work pressure provides the best correlation, and that most studies have found that pressures while awake are more closely related to LVH than sleeping pressures, which are, of course, lower. The observation of Verdecchia *et al.* [23] that night-time blood pressure is a better predictor of LVH than daytime pressure does not necessarily invalidate this idea. It could be that patients whose pressure remains high during the night exceed the threshold for longer periods of time than those whose pressure shows the normal decrease. The fact that clinic pressure tends to be higher than pressures at other times, and yet is a poor predictor of LVH, can also be reconciled because it correlates relatively weakly with blood pressure measured at other times, for example while at work [54]. All of these findings could equally well be explained by the assumption that it is the average level of pressure which influences target organ damage, and that there is no threshold level. On balance, this explanation seems more likely.

One important question that remains unanswered is whether the variability of blood pressure is also a determinant of target organ damage independently of the average level. Three studies, one using invasive monitoring [17] and two non-invasive monitoring [15,55], did not find any correlation between blood pressure variability and target organ damage. Two other studies did find a correlation, one of which used invasive monitoring [12] and the other non-invasive monitoring [56]. However, this finding of a positive relationship must be interpreted with caution, because in one of these studies [12] the patients had relatively advanced hypertension, and the increased blood pressure variability may have been the result, rather than the cause, of the target organ damage, as a consequence of impaired baroreceptor reflexes.

Prospective studies of blood pressure as a predictor of target organ damage

Surprisingly little information is available on this point. In a study of adolescents, Mahoney *et al.* [52] reported that resting systolic pressure did not predict left ventricular mass measured 3 years later, whereas exercise systolic pressure did.

Prospective studies of blood pressure as a predictor of hypertension

Essential hypertension is a creeping condition that develops over many years. It has sometimes been considered to be an acceleration of the normal increase in blood pressure associated with ageing, although this is not an inevitable process and may not occur in non-westernized societies. The prediction of future hypertension has been most extensively studied with casual blood pressure, measured either during screening surveys or during medical examinations. The problems associated with such measures have been discussed in Chapter 7. While they have provided an enormous amount of useful information, their limitations can be highlighted by two facts: only 20% of individuals with borderline hypertension are found to be hypertensive in later life [57]; and in the Australian trial of mild hypertension treatment [58], nearly 50% of patients in the placebo group became normotensive after 4 months.

Blood pressure is not the only factor that can be used to predict hypertension. A family history of hypertension is also of major importance. In Thomas and Duszyncki's prospective study of medical students [59] they found that subjects who had two hypertensive parents and a high initial clinic systolic pressure (above 125 mmHg) were 12.6 times more likely to become hypertensive over a 30-year follow-up period than subjects without these risk factors. Obesity and heart rate are also significant predictors of future blood pressure level [60]. The latter may reflect an increased sympathetic drive, which is characteristic in early hypertension. Echocardiographic left ventricular mass was also found to be a predictor in a recent study of 132 initially normotensive men and women followed for nearly 5 years [61]. This may be because it indicates the true blood pressure better than the clinic measurements with which it was compared in this study, but the result may also be interpreted as indicating that hypertension begins with changes in cardiac structure and function.

Not all of the blood pressure measures discussed in this chapter have been used in prospective studies (Fig. 13.8). In particular, no studies of ambulatory or home pressure have been reported. Apart from casual or clinic pressure, the greatest attention has been paid to reactivity and basal pressure, as discussed below.

Basal pressure
Several studies of the ability of the cold pressor test to predict hypertension also included measures of 'basal' blood pressure. In these instances the casual pressure was measured at the start of the experiment and the 'basal' pressure was taken as the last resting value before the stimulus. As the subjects were in some cases anticipating a noxious stimulus, these readings were probably not really basal. The Thousand Aviator Cohort study [62] found that the basal pressure was a better predictor (r = 0.32) of clinic blood pressure 18 years later than the initial clinic pressure (r = 0.18). Two other studies [59,63], however, found predictions with clinic pressures but not basal pressures.

Blood pressure reactivity
If the reactivity hypothesis is correct, an increased reactivity should predict future hypertension. Eight studies have used the cold pressor test for evaluating reactivity, in which from 73 to 1185 subjects were followed for periods ranging from 10 to 45 years [59,62–68]. The results of one study (the Precursors Study of medical students

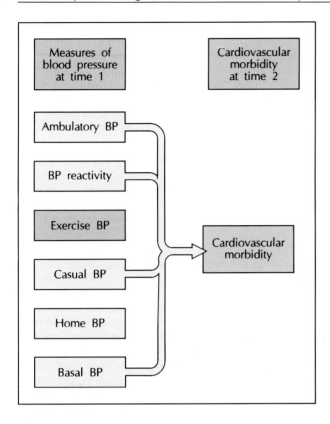

Fig. 13.8. Prospective studies relating blood pressure (BP) and development of cardiovascular morbidity.

Authors	n	Years of follow-up	Prediction of blood pressure status
Cold pressor test			
Barnett et al. [65]	207	27	Yes
Harlan et al. [62]	375	18	No
Eich and Jacobson et al. [66]	73	10	No
Thomas and Duszyncki [59]	1185	35	No
Menkes et al. [63]	910	20–36	Yes
Armstrong and Rafferty [64]	165	7	No
Wood et al. [67]	142	45	Yes
Gillum et al. [68]	106	32	No
Mental arithmetic			
Falkner et al. [69]	80	Up to 5	Yes
Borghi et al. [70]	44	5	Yes
Exercise test			
Wilson and Mayer [71]	3820	2.8	Yes
Franz [72]	173	3.8	Yes
Dlin et al. [73]	150	5.8	Yes
Jackson et al. [74]	114	3.0	Yes
Davidoff et al. [75]	721	5.8	Yes
Froom [76]	141	3.0	Yes
Gillum et al. [68]	106	32.0	Yes

Fig. 13.9. Reactivity tests and prediction of hypertension.

at Johns Hopkins University) were reported in two different analyses [59,63]. These studies are listed in Fig. 13.9. Five studies found no prediction of future hypertension or blood pressure level from the degree of reactivity [59,62,64,65,68]; one study claimed positive results, but only four out of 207 subjects became hypertensive, three of whom had a positive family history [65]. It therefore cannot be determined whether reactivity would predict hypertension independently of family history, which is the major predictive factor. Another study [67] also reported a significant role of reactivity in 142 individuals followed for 45 years, but the classification of hyper-reactivity was based on two cold pressor tests performed 27 years apart.

The most extensive study, and the one which deserves most attention, was the Johns Hopkins Precursors Study, which involved about 1000 male medical students who were followed for up to 35 years by Thomas. In the first report, published in 1982 [59], the cold pressor test failed to predict future hypertension. A subsequent analysis, published in 1989 [63] and using more sophisticated statistical techniques, found that after adjusting for age, obesity, baseline blood pressure and smoking, an exaggerated response to the cold pressor test did predict the development of hypertension after an interval of 20 years. However, without these adjustments there was still no association.

Two studies have reported that the reactivity to mental arithmetic, which has more of a psychological component than the cold pressor test, does predict future blood pressure. The first, by Falkner *et al.* [69], followed 80 adolescents with borderline hypertension for up to 5 years. The development of hypertension was predicted both by a positive family history and by an exaggerated blood pressure response to mental arithmetic. The relative importance of the two was not evaluated. The second study, by Ambrosioni's group [70], reported that subjects with a positive family history and borderline hypertension showed an increased reactivity to both behavioural and physical challenges, and that they were more likely to become hypertensive over a 5-year period.

Overall, the evidence that blood pressure reactivity is an independent predictor of future blood pressure status is unconvincing.

Exercise blood pressure

Although the blood pressure response to a standard dynamic exercise test can be considered a measure of reactivity, it will be dealt with separately because of its apparently much greater predictive value than other reactivity measures. No less than seven studies [68,71–76] have reported that the blood pressure measured during dynamic exercise predicts resting blood pressure measured 3 – 32 years later (see Fig. 13.9). Another study found that although the best single predictor of future hypertension was resting diastolic pressure, the prediction was significantly improved by including the pressure measured during either isometric or dynamic exercise [77].

An even simpler manoeuvre than exercise is change in posture, which in one study [78] was found to predict hypertension.

Prospective studies of blood pressure as a predictor of morbidity

The types of studies which have examined the relationships between different measures of blood pressure and cardiovascular morbidity are shown in Fig. 13.10 and reviewed below.

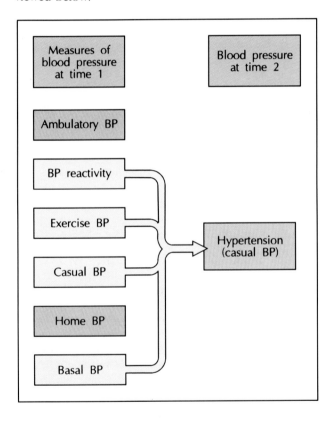

Fig. 13.10. Prospective studies relating blood pressure (BP) and cardiovascular morbidity.

Ambulatory pressure

From the point of view of both the clinician and the research scientist, the superior ability of ambulatory blood pressure compared with clinic pressure in predicting cardiovascular morbidity is crucial to the validity of the technique. Evidence for this rests largely on one prospective study, conducted by the pioneers of ambulatory monitoring, Perloff and Sokolow. It will be described in some detail, with references to the two papers that have so far been published from it. In the first, Perloff *et al.* [79]

analysed data from 1 076 patients followed for an average of 5 years. Ambulatory and clinic pressures were significantly correlated with each other, although ambulatory pressure was on average 16/9 mmHg lower. Patients were classified according to whether their ambulatory pressure was high or low relative to their clinic pressure. Those with higher ambulatory pressure had a higher mortality rate and incidence of cardiovascular morbidity than those with lower ambulatory pressure. Ambulatory pressure had the greatest predictive value in patients who were less than 50 years old, whose diastolic pressure at the time of entry to the study was less than 105 mmHg, and who had suffered no prior cardiovascular event. However, ambulatory pressure was not helpful in defining the prognosis of patients with more severe hypertension.

The second paper [80] was based on the same data but used a much more sophisticated analysis with the Cox proportional hazards linear regression model to control the influence of other predictor variables. The study criteria were met by 761 patients, with an average follow-up period of 66 months. Ambulatory blood pressure was expressed both as the 'predicted' and the 'residual' level. The former was derived from the regression equation relating clinic and ambulatory pressures for all the patients, and the latter was obtained by subtracting the predicted level from the observed level. Separate life table analyses were run for the 659 patients who had no previous cardiovascular event and for the 102 patients who had. The predictor variables included in the analysis were ambulatory and office pressures, age, sex, ECG-LVH, retinopathy, and use of antihypertensive therapy. For patients with no previous event the significant predictors were age, sex, ECG-LVH, and predicted and residual ambulatory pressures. For those with a previous event the predictors were age, sex, antihypertensive treatment and residual ambulatory pressures. As shown in Fig. 13.11, the morbidity rate was lower in patients whose ambulatory pressure was low in comparison to their clinic pressure.

Unlike the earlier analysis, therefore, which indicated that ambulatory pressure added to the prognostic ability of clinic pressure only in patients who had no previous cardiovascular event, the Cox model analysis showed that ambulatory pressure was also of value in patients with a previous event.

These findings support the hypothesis that patients with white coat hypertension are at lower risk than those with sustained hypertension, because they have a negative residual ambulatory pressure. Although Perloff *et al.* did not attempt to define a subgroup with white coat hypertension, from their published values of clinic and ambulatory pressures it appears likely that an appreciable number of patients in their low-risk group had normal ambulatory pressure. The authors also pointed out that their concept of the residual ambulatory pressure was different from Smirk's supplemental pressure [81], which he did not find predicted morbid events. This was defined as the difference between the clinic pressure and basal pressure (see Chapter 7), whereas the residual ambulatory pressure is derived from the difference between the clinic pressure and daytime pressure.

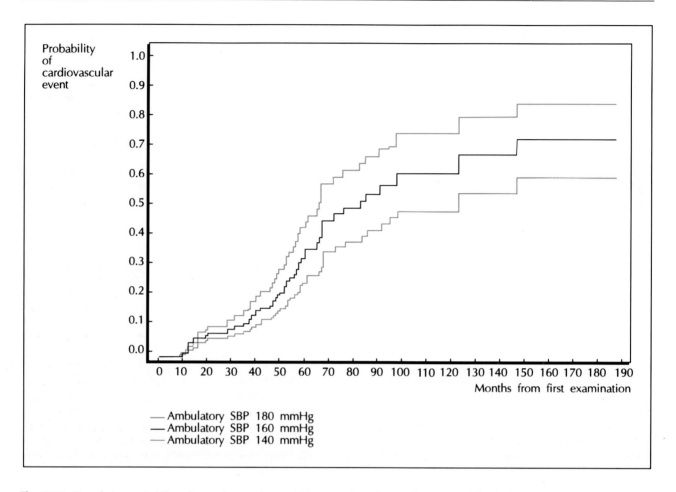

Fig. 13.11. Cumulative probability of a cardiovascular morbid event, plotted according to initial level of ambulatory systolic pressure. Data are from the prospective study of Perloff *et al.* [79,80].

A much smaller study was performed by Mann *et al.* [82]. They followed 137 patients for an average of 2 years, during which time 14 subjects experienced cardiovascular events. Combining the ambulatory and clinic pressures significantly improved the prediction of morbid events. In this study blood pressure variability did not appear to contribute to the prediction of morbid events. However, a more recent analysis of a larger series of 449 patients from the same group of investigators provided inconsequential results [83].

We have followed 729 patients with mild hypertension for an average follow-up of 5 years (unpublished results). We also used a Cox model analysis to evaluate the relative predictive power of a number of variables (including ambulatory blood pressure) measured at entry to the study, when none of the patients were on treatment. The analysis identified four predictors of risk: age, male sex, serum cholesterol, and diastolic blood pressure variability while awake, measured as the standard deviation of the ambulatory readings. Other measures of blood pressure did not achieve independent significance in the equation, but of the measures of the average level, ambulatory waking pressure was a better predictor than clinic pressure. If confirmed by other studies, this finding has several major implications. First, it appears to support the long-held

suspicion that blood pressure variability may be an independent predictor of risk. Second, it should be pointed out that of the 22 morbid events experienced by these patients, 18 were cardiac (myocardial infarction, coronary artery bypass surgery, or sudden cardiac death). In Chapter 6 the potential importance of acute surges in blood pressure as triggers of ischaemic myocardial events was discussed; these surges which may explain our findings. Whether or not blood pressure variability is also a prognostic factor for stroke cannot be determined from these data, and it cannot be assumed that it is. Third, numerous explanations have been proposed for the failure of antihypertensive treatment to prevent myocardial infarction, in contrast with the much greater success in preventing stroke [84–86]. As noted in Chapter 10, one of the paradoxical findings with antihypertensive medications is that they lower the tonic level of blood pressure while having little effect on blood pressure variability. If variability is indeed a major determinant of myocardial events, it may resolve this paradox.

Blood pressure reactivity

There are, in theory, several different ways in which blood pressure reactivity may be related to cardiovascular morbidity. First, it could be a marker for the development of hypertension, the evidence for which has been reviewed above. Second, it may affect the development of atherosclerotic lesions independently of any sustained effects on blood pressure. Third, it may be related to the triggering of acute thrombotic events and hence be a factor involved in the diurnal rhythm of cardiovascular morbidity, as discussed in Chapter 6. Some evidence relating to the second mechanism comes from studies in primates [87].

The only relevant study in man, which could be explained by either the second or the third mechanism, is the observation made many years ago by Keys *et al.* [88] that normotensive men who showed an exaggerated diastolic blood pressure response to the cold pressor test were at increased risk of suffering a myocardial infarction over the next 23 years.

Exercise blood pressure

Two studies have analysed the contribution of exercise blood pressure to the prediction of cardiovascular morbidity. Gosse *et al.* [89] claimed that blood pressure measured during exercise was a better prognostic indicator than clinic pressure. A limitation of their study was that half the patients were taking antihypertensive medication at the time of the baseline evaluation. The second study, by Fagard *et al.* [90], used invasive blood pressure measurement and compared the prediction based on resting and exercise blood pressure of morbidity in 143 men followed for more than 10 years. Using a Cox regression model, exercise blood pressure gave no additional information once resting presure had been entered into the equation.

This study illustrates one of the problems with this type of analysis. When different measures of blood pressure taken on the same occasion (e.g. at rest and during exercise) are related to a dependent variable, such as target organ damage or prognosis, there is such a high correlation between the measures (multi-collinearity) that it is very unlikely that one measure will give a significantly better prediction than another one.

Postural change in blood pressure

Postural change in blood pressure might be regarded as a form of blood pressure reactivity, in that it is a change in pressure occurring in response to a specific stimulus. However, in this case it appears to be an impairment of the normal responsiveness that is predictive of disease: in the Hypertension Detection and Follow-Up Program [91] it was found that a fall of more than 12 mmHg in systolic pressure on standing up was associated with an increased 5-year mortality. Patients who showed this were more likely to be overweight and diabetic.

Basal pressure

Two studies have examined the question of whether casual (clinic) or basal blood pressure gives a better prediction of morbidity. Smirk [81] followed 469 hypertensive patients for a minimum of 5 years. The basal pressure (obtained after 30 min of quiet rest while recumbent) gave a better prediction of mortality than the clinic pressure[1]. In the other study, by Simpson and Gilchrist [92], clinic pressure was compared with the blood pressure obtained after rest in hospital. As shown in Fig. 13.12, the resting pressure was clearly superior at predicting survival, particularly in those with less severe hypertension.

Does the diurnal pattern of blood pressure influence cardiovascular morbidity?

If it is accepted that the major determinant of cardiovascular morbidity is the integral of blood pressure over time, it would be expected that individuals whose blood pressure fails to fall during the night would be at greater risk than others with similar daytime pressures and a normal diurnal pattern. Although this prediction has not been adequately tested so far, the evidence that exists is generally consistent with it. As we saw in Chapter 6, sleep is associated with a relatively lower incidence of cardiovascular morbid events, as well as a lower blood pressure. In a study of 25 elderly patients, Kobrin *et al.* [93] observed that those whose pressure remained elevated during the night were more likely to show manifestations of atherosclerotic disease and LVH than those with a normal nocturnal fall. Gosse *et al.* [94] found that daytime ambulatory pressure correlated most closely with LVH in untreated patients, but night-time pressures gave a better correlation in patients on treatment. They argued (rather unconvincingly, in my opinion) that this implies that treatment which fails to lower nocturnal pressure also fails to reverse LVH.

Prospective studies of target organ damage as a predictor of morbidity

Although the presence of target organ damage is strongly associated with an increased risk of morbidity in hypertensive patients [95], this is of relatively little help in the evaluation of patients with mild hypertension, in most of whom elevation in blood pressure is the only abnormal finding. This discussion will, therefore, be restricted to a review of 'early markers' of target organ damage, which may be detectable before irreversible and clinically overt changes have occurred. Of these, the best established is echocardiographically determined LVH. Devereux *et al.* [96] found that the sensitivity of echocardiography for detecting LVH (85%) is much higher than for the ECG (43%). Therefore, many cases that would be otherwise

---

[1]Although this is an important paper, it is difficult to read. Its use of statistics is rudimentary, and it contains no less than 37 tables. Sir Horace Smirk was clearly fascinated by tables: some contained 396 compartments, and in the text he wrote with some relish that to do the job properly would require a table with 1000 compartments.

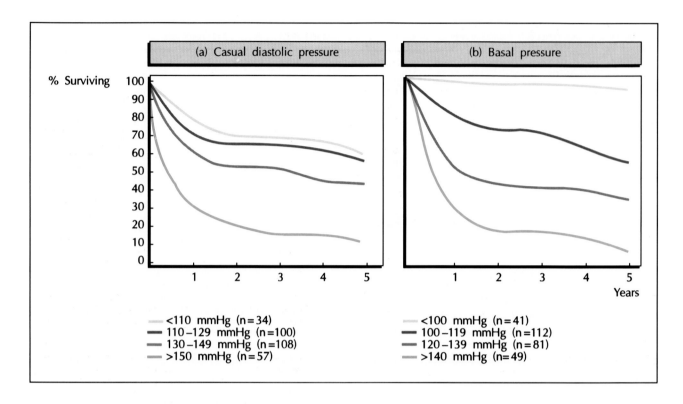

Fig. 13.12. Survival rates in subjects aged 40–60 years plotted according to casual diastolic pressure (a) or basal pressure (b). Data redrawn from Simpson and Gilchrist [92].

missed will be detected if an echocardiogram is included as part of the evaluation. The recognized associations between measures of target organ damage and morbidity are shown in Fig. 13.13.

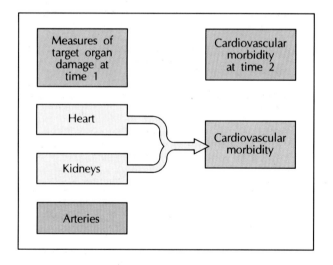

Fig. 13.13. Prospective studies relating target organ damage and cardiovascular morbidity.

Three published studies have related echocardiographically determined LVH to morbidity [97–99]. The first,

conducted by our group [97], was a prospective evaluation of 140 hypertensive men followed for 4.8 years. LVH was found to be a predictor of cardiovascular morbidity, which was independent of other risk factors such as clinic blood pressure, smoking and cholesterol. Men with an increased left ventricular mass were nearly four times as likely to suffer a morbid event as those without. Extension of this study to 10 years' follow-up of 250 men and women with initially uncomplicated hypertension revealed that only age and left ventricular mass were independent predictors of morbid events or death [100].

The second study was also a 4-year prospective study, which included 406 elderly men and 735 women who were participants in the Framingham Heart Study [98]. LVH was an independent predictor of CHD morbidity, even after adjusting for age, systolic pressure, smoking and cholesterol.

The third study was also from Framingham, and followed 3 220 subjects aged 40 years or more for 4 years [99]. Once again, left ventricular mass was a potent and independent predictor of risk of both non-fatal events and death.

There is also evidence that impairment of renal function, as manifested by an elevated blood urea [101] or albuminuria [102], is an independent risk factor in hypertensive patients.

Summary and conclusions

While clinic or casual pressure has provided almost all our knowledge relating blood pressure to target organ damage and prognosis, the acknowledgement that it may be a relatively poor index of the true blood pressure suggests that other measures less susceptible to regression to the mean, giving a better estimate of blood pressure variability, may prove prognostically superior. There is a need for improved predictors of risk, particularly in patients with mild hypertension. Five other measures of blood pressure have been reviewed (basal, home, ambulatory and exercise pressure, and also blood pressure reactivity) and compared with clinic pressure in their ability to predict target organ damage, future blood pressure status and cardiovascular morbidity.

Several cross-sectional studies have shown that ambulatory pressure correlates more closely with target organ damage (particularly LVH) than clinic pressure. There is some uncertainty whether the peaks (e.g. during work) or the troughs (e.g. during sleep) of blood pressure are more important. Limited data are available for home, basal and exercise blood pressure, but in each case the correlations with target organ damage tend to be closer than with clinic pressure. There is no evidence to suggest that blood pressure reactivity correlates more closely with target organ damage.

A much smaller number of prospective studies have compared clinic blood pressure with other measures for the prediction of hypertension. No data are available for home and ambulatory measurements in this regard, and data for basal pressure are equivocal. Several studies have examined the ability of reactivity (mainly using the cold pressor test) to predict future blood pressure status, the majority of which, with one or two notable exceptions, have yielded negative results. In marked contrast, blood pressure measured during exercise (which might be considered as reactivity to a purely physical stimulus) does appear to be a potent predictor of hypertension.

The prediction of cardiovascular morbidity is the most important determinant of utility of any clinical measure of blood pressure. According to one prospective study (and preliminary results from two others) ambulatory pressure does provide a better prediction than clinic pressure. There is also some evidence that basal pressure is better than clinic pressure, but data for the other potential measures (home and exercise pressure and blood pressure reactivity) are lacking.

One of the limitations of such studies is that the different measures of blood pressure compared for their ability to predict target organ damage (or prognosis) are often highly correlated with each other, which makes discrimination between them more difficult. This is particularly true for measures taken on the same occasion, such as rest and exercise blood pressure. Nevertheless, it appears that clinic pressure is not so good a predictor as other measures, with the possible exception of blood pressure reactivity. However, this may merely be another instance of the unrepresentative nature of clinic pressures, rather than any inherent superiority of any of the other measures.

References

1. PICKERING GW: *High Blood Pressure*. London: Churchill, 1968.
2. KANNEL WB: Role of blood pressure in cardiovascular morbidity and mortality. *Prog Cardiovasc Dis* 1974, 17:5–23.
3. O'ROURKE M: Basic concepts for the understanding of large arteries in hypertension. *J Cardiovasc Pharmacol* 1985, 7:S14–S21.
4. LEVY D, ANDERSON K, SAVAGE DD, KANNEL WB, CASTELLI WP: Influence of 30 year mean blood pressure levels on left ventricular mass: the Framingham Heart study. *J Am Coll Cardiol* 1987, 9 (suppl A):115A.
5. DEVEREUX RB, PICKERING TG, ALDERMAN MH, *ET AL*: Left ventricular hypertrophy in hypertension. Prevalence and relationship to pathophysiologic variables. *Hypertension* 1987, 9 (suppl II):II53–II60.
6. VETERANS ADMINISTRATION COOPERATIVE STUDY GROUP ON ANTIHYPERTENSIVE AGENTS: Effects of treatment on morbidity in hypertension: results in patients with diastolic blood pressure averaging 115 through 129 mmHg. *JAMA* 1967, 212:1028–1034.
7. AUSTRALIAN NATIONAL BLOOD PRESSURE STUDY MANAGEMENT COMMITTEE: The Australian Therapeutic Trial in Mild Hypertension. *Lancet* 1980, i:1261–1267.
8. MULTIPLE RISK FACTOR INTERVENTION TRIAL RESEARCH GROUP: Multiple Risk Factor Intervention Trial: Risk factor changes and mortality results. *JAMA* 1982, 248:1465–1476.
9. HYPERTENSION DETECTION AND FOLLOW-UP PROGRAM COOPERATIVE GROUP: Five-year findings of the Hypertension Detection and Follow-up Program. *JAMA* 1979, 242:2562–2571.
10. MEDICAL RESEARCH COUNCIL WORKING PARTY: MRC Trial of treatment of mild hypertension: principal results. *Br Med J* 1985, 291:97–104.
11. MCMAHON S, PETO R, CUTLER J, *ET AL*: Blood pressure, stroke, and coronary heart disease. Part 1. Prolonged differences in blood pressure: prospective observational studies corrected for the regression dilution bias. *Lancet* 1990, 335:765–774.
12. PARATI G, POMIDOSSI G, ALBINI F, MALASPINA D, MANCIA G: Relationship of 24-hour blood pressure mean and variability to severity of target-organ damage in hypertension. *J Hypertens* 1987, 5:93–98.
13. DEVEREUX RB: Importance of left ventricular mass as a predictor of cardiovacular morbidity in hypertension. *Am J Hypertens* 1989, 2:650–654.
14. JULIUS S, JAMESON K, MAJIA A, *ET AL*: The association of borderline hypertension with target organ changes and higher coronary risk. Tecumseh blood pressure study. *JAMA* 1990, 264:354–358.
15. SOKOLOW M, WERDEGAR D, KAIM HK, HINMAN AT: Relationship between level of blood pressure measured casually and by portable recorders and severity of complications in essential hypertension. *Circulation* 1966, 34:279–298.
16. VERMEERSCH P, DUPREZ D, PACKET L, CLEMENT DL: Left ventricular hypertrophy in mild hypertension: value of ambulatory recordings. *J Hypertens* 1987, 5 (suppl 5):S495–S496.
17. ROWLANDS DB, GLOVER DR, IRELAND MA, *ET AL*: Assessment of left ventricular mass and its response to antihypertensive treatment. *Lancet* 1982, i:467–470.
18. DRAYER JIM, WEBER MA, DE YOUNG JL: BP as a determinant of cardiac left ventricular muscle mass. *Arch Intern Med* 1983, 143:90–92.
19. DEVEREUX RB, PICKERING TG, HARSHFIELD GA, *ET AL*: Left ventricular hypertrophy in patients with hypertension: importance of blood pressure response to regularly recurring stress. *Circulation* 1983, 68:470–476.
20. ANTIVALLE M, LATTUADA S, PARAVIANI M, RINDI M, LIBRETTI A: Twenty-four hour noninvasive ambulatory blood pressure

monitoring in the assessment of early hypertension. *J Hypertens* 1986, 4 (suppl 5):S322–S324.

21. GOSSE P, CAMPELLO G, AOUIZERATE E, ET AL.: Left ventricular hypertrophy in hypertension: correlation with rest, exercise and ambulatory systolic blood pressure. *J Hypertens* 1986, 4 (suppl 5):S297–S299.

22. WHITE WB, SCHULMAN P, DEY JM, KATZ AM: Effects of age and 24-hour ambulatory blood pressure on rapid left ventricular filling. *Am J Cardiol* 1989, 63:1343–1347.

23. VERDECCHIA P, SCHILLACI G, GUERRIERI M, ET AL.: Circadian blood pressure changes and left ventricular hypertrophy in essential hypertension. *Circulation* 1990, 81:528–536.

24. PALATINI P, MORMINO P, DI MARCO A, ET AL.: Ambulatory blood pressure versus casual pressure for the evaluation of target organ damage in hypertension: complications of hypertension. *J Hypertens* 1985, 3 (suppl 3):S425–S427.

25. PRISANT LM, CARR AA: Ambulatory blood pressure monitoring and echocardiographic left ventricular wall thickness and mass. *Am J Hypertens* 1990, 3:81–89.

26. MOULOPOULOS SD, STAMATELOPOULOS SF, ZAKOPOULOS NA, ET AL.: Effect of 24-hour blood pressure and heart rate variations on left ventriuclar hypertrophy and dilatation in essential hypertension. *Am Heart J* 1990, 119:1147–1152.

27. BABA S, OZAWA H, NAKAMOTO Y, UESHIMA H, OMAE T: Enhanced blood pressure response to regular daily stress in urban hypertensive man. *J Hypertens* 1990, 8:647–655.

28. OPSAHL JA, ABRAHAM PA, HALSTENSON CE, KEANE WF: Correlation of office and ambulatory blood pressure measurements with urinary albumin and N-acetyl-beta-D-glucosaminidase excretion in essential hypertension. *Am J Hypertens* 1988, 1:1175–1205.

29. DIMMITT SB, WEST JNW, EAMES SM, ET AL.: Usefulness of ophthalmoscopy in mild to moderate hypertension. *Lancet* 1989, i:1103–1105.

30. ASMAR RG, BRUNEL PC, PANNIER BM, LACOLLEY PJ, SAFAR ME: Arterial distensibility and ambulatory blood pressure monitoring in essential hypertension. *Am J Cardiol* 1988, 61:1066–1070.

31. VERDECCHIA P, SCHILLACI G, BOLDRINI F, ET AL.: Risk stratification of left ventricular hypertrophy in systemic hypertension using invasive ambulatory blood pressure monitoring. *Am J Cardiol* 1990, 66:583–590.

32. FOUAD FM, TARAZI RC, GALLAGHER JH, McINTYRE RJ, COOK SA: Abnormal left ventricular relaxation in hypertensive patients. *Clin Sci* 1980, 59:411–414.

33. INOUYE I, MASSIE B, LOGE D, ET AL.: Abnormal left ventricular filling; an early finding in mild to moderate systemic hypertension. *Am J Cardiol* 1984, 53:120–126.

34. FOUAD FM, SLOMINSKI JM, TARAZI RC: Left ventricular diastolic function in hypertension: relation to left ventricular mass and systolic function. *JACC* 1984, 3:1500–1506.

35. GIACONI S, LEVANTI C, FOMMEI E, ET AL. Microalbuminuria and casual and ambulatory blood pressure monitoring in normotensives and in patients with borderline and mild essential hypertension. *Am J Hypertens* 1989, 2:259–261.

36. ALDERMAN MH, MELCHER L, DRAYER DE, REIDENBERG MM. Increased excretion of urinary N-acetyl-β-glucosaminidase in essential hypertension and its decline with antihypertensive therapy. *N Engl J Med* 1983, 309:1213–1217.

37. AYMAN D, GOLDSHINE AD: Blood pressure determinations by patients with essential hypertension. I. The difference between home and clinic readings before treatment. *Am J Med Sci* 1940, 200:465–474.

38. KLEINERT HD, HARSHFIELD GA, PICKERING TG, ET AL.: What is the value of home blood pressure measurement in patients with mild hypertension? *Hypertension* 1984, 6:547–578.

39. IBRAHIM MM, TARAZI RC, DUSTAN HP, GIFFORD RW: Electrocardiogram in evaluation of resistance to antihypertensive therapy. *Arch Intern Med* 1977, 137:1125–1129.

40. VERDECCHIA P, BENTIVOGLIA M, PROVIDENZA M, SAVINO K, COREA L: Reliability of home self-recorded arterial pressure in essential hypertension in relation to the stage of the disease. In *Blood Pressure Recording in the Clinical Management of Hypertension* edited by Germano G. Rome: Ediziono Pozzi, 1985, pp 40–42.

41. ABE H, YOKOUCHI M, SAITOH F, ET AL.: Hypertensive complications and home blood pressure: comparisons with blood pressure measured in the doctor's office. *J Clin Hypertens* 1987, 3:661–669.

42. CALDWELL JR, SCHORK MA, AIKEN RD: Is near basal blood pressure a more accurate predictor of cardiorenal manifestations of hypertension than casual blood pressure? *J Chron Dis* 1978, 31:507–512.

43. SCHMIEDER RE, GRUBE E, RÜDDEL H, SCHÄCHINGER H, SCHULTE W: Relation of hemodynamic reaction during stress to left ventricular hypertrophy in essential hypertension. *Am J Hypertens* 1990, 3:281–287.

44. IKAHEIMO MJ, PALATSI KJ, TAKKINEN JT: Noninvasive evaluation of the athletic heart: sprinters versus runners. *Am J Cardiol* 1979, 44:24–30.

45. PEARSON AC, SCHIFF M, MROSEK D, LABOVITZ AJ, WILLIAMS GA. Left ventricular function in weight lifters. *Am J Cardiol* 1986, 58:1254–1259.

46. REN JF, HAKKI AH, KOTTLER MN, ISKANDRIAM AS: Exercise systolic blood pressure: a powerful determinant of increased left ventricular mass in patients with hypertension. *J Am Coll Cardiol* 1985 5:1224–1231.

47. NATHWANI D, REEVES RA, MARQUEZ-JULIO A, LEENEN FHH: Left ventricular hypertrophy in mild hypertension: correlation with exercise blood pressure. *Am Heart J* 1985 104:386–387.

48. PAPADEMETRIOU V, NOTARGIACOMO A, SETHI E, ET AL.: Exercise blood pressure response and left ventricular hypertrophy. *Am J Hypertens* 1989, 2:114–116.

49. GOTTDIENER JS, BROWN J, ZOLTICK J, FLETCHER RD: Left ventricular hypertrophy in men with normal blood pressure: relation to exaggerated blood response to exercise. *Ann Intern Med* 1990, 112:161–166.

50. SAU F, SEGURO C, CHERCHI A: Relationship between exercise blood pressure and LV mass in hypertensive patients. *Eur Heart J* 1989, 10 (abstract suppl):127.

51. FAGARD R, STAESSEN J, AMERY A: Exercise blood pressure and target organ damage in essential hypertension. *J Hum Hypertens* (in press).

52. MAHONEY LT, SCHIEKEN RM, CLARKE WR, LAUER RM: Left ventricular mass and exercise responses predict future blood pressure. The Muscatine Study. *Hypertension* 1988, 12:206–213.

53. TUBAU JF, SZLACHCIC J, BRAUN S, MASSIE BM: Impaired left ventricular functional reserve in hypertensive patients with left ventricular hypertrophy. *Hypertension* 1989, 14:1–8.

54. PICKERING TG, HARSHFIELD GA, KLEINERT HD, BLANK S, LARAGH JH: Blood pressure during normal daily activities, sleep, and exercise. Comparison of values in normal and hypertensive subjects. *JAMA* 1982, 247:992–996.

55. GOSSE P, ROUDANT R, REYNAUD P, JULIEN E, DALLOCCHIO M: Relationship between left ventricular mass and noninvasive monitoring of blood pressure. *Am J Hypertens* 1989, 2:631–633.

56. PESSINA AC, PALATINI P, SPERTI G, ET AL.: Evaluation of hypertension and related target organ damage by average day-time blood pressure. *Clin Exp Hypertens [A]* 1985, 7:267–278.

57. JULIUS S, SCHORK MA: Borderline hypertension — a critical review. *J Chron Dis* 1971, 23:723–754.

58. A report by the Management Committee of the Australian Therapeutic Trial in Mild Hypertension: Untreated mild hypertension. *Lancet* 1982, i:185–191.

59. THOMAS CB, DUSZYNCKI KR: Blood pressure levels in young adulthood as predictors of hypertension and the fate of the cold pressor test. *Johns Hopkins Med J* 1982, 151:93–100.

60. JULIUS S, SCHORK MA: Predictors of hypertension. *Ann N Y Acad Sci* 1978, 304:38–42.

61. DE SIMONE G, DEVEREUX RB, ROMAN MJ, ET AL. Echocardiographic left ventricular mass and electrolyte intake predict subsequent hypertension in initially normotensive adults. *Ann Intern Med* (in press).

62. HARLAN WR, OSBORNE RK, GRAYBIEL A: Prognostic value of the cold pressor test and the basal blood pressure: based on an 18-year follow-up study. *Am J Cardiol* 1964, 13:683–687.

63. MENKES MS, MATTHEWS KA, KRANTZ DS *ET AL*: Cardiovascular reactivity to the cold pressor test as a predictor of hypertension. *Hypertension* 1989, 14:524–530.

64. ARMSTRONG HG, RAFFERTY JA: Cold pressor test. Follow-up study for seven years on 166 officers. *Am Heart J* 1960, 39:484–490.

65. BARNETT PH, HINES KA, SCHIRGER A, GAGE RP: Blood pressure and vascular reactivity to the cold pressor test. *JAMA* 1963, 183:845–848.

66. EICH RH, JACOBSON EC: Vascular reactivity in medical students followed for 10 years. *J Chron Dis* 1967, 20:583–592.

67. WOOD DL, SHEPS SG, ELVEBACK LR, SCHIRGER A: Cold pressor test as a predictor of hypertension. *Hypertension* 1984, 6:301–306.

68. GILLUM RF, TAYLOR HL, ANDERSON J, BLACKBURN H: Longitudinal study (32 years) of exercise tolerance, breathing response, blood pressure, and blood lipids in young men. *Arteriosclerosis* 1981, 1:455–462.

69. FALKNER B, ONESTI G, HAMSTRA B: Stress response characteristics of adolescents with high genetic risk for essential hypertension. A five-year follow-up. *Clin Exp Hypertens* 1981, 3:583–591.

70. BORGHI C, COSTA FV, BOSCHI S, MUSSI A, AMBROSIONI E: Predictors of stable hypertension in young borderline subjects: A five-year follow-up study. *J Cardiovasc Pharmacol* 1986, 8 (suppl 5):S138–S141.

71. WILSON NV, MAYER BM: Early prediction of hypertension using exericse blood pressure. *Prev Med* 1981, 10:62–68.

72. FRANZ IW: Assessment of blood pressure response during ergometric work in normotensive and hypertensive patients. *Acta Med Scand* 1982, (suppl 670):35–47.

73. DLIN RA, HANNE N, SILVERBERG DS, BAR-OR O: Follow-up of normotensive men with exaggerated blood pressure response to exercise. *Am Heart J* 1983, 106:316–320.

74. JACKSON AS, SQUIRES WG, GRIMES G, BEARD ER: Prediction of future resting hypertension from exercise blood pressure. *Cardiac Rehabil* 1983, 3:263–268.

75. DAVIDOFF R, SCHAMROTH CL, GOLDMAN AP, *ET AL*: Postexercise blood pressure as a predictor of hypertension. *Aviat Space Environ Med*, 1982, 53:591–594.

76. TANJI JL, CHAMPLIN JJ, WONG GY, *ET AL*: Blood pressure recovery curves after submaximal exercise. A predictor of hypertension at ten-year follow-up. *Am J Hypertens* 1989, 2:135–138.

77. CHANEY RH, EYMAN RK: Blood pressure at rest and during maximal dynamic and isometric exercise as predictors of systemic hypertension. *Am J Cardiol* 1988, 62:1058–1061.

78. SPARROW D, ROSNER B, VOKONAS PS, WEISS ST: Relation of blood pressure measured in several positions to the subsequent development of hypertension. The Normative Aging Study. *Am J Cardiol* 1986, 57:128–221.

79. PERLOFF D, SOKOLOW M, COWAN R: The prognostic value of ambulatory blood pressures. *JAMA* 1983, 249:2792–2798.

80. PERLOFF D, SOKOLOW M, COWAN RM, JUSTER RP: Prognostic value of ambulatory blood pressure measurements: further analyses. *J Hypertens* 1989, 7 (suppl 3):S3–S10.

81. SMIRK FH: Observations on the mortality of 270 treated and 199 untreated retinal grade I and II hypertensive patients followed in all instances for 5 years. *NZ Med J* 1964, 63:413–443.

82. MANN S, MILLAR-CRAIG MW, RAFTERY EB: Superiority of 24-hour measurements of blood pressure over clinic values in determining prognosis in hypertension. *Clin Exp Hypertens [A]* 1985, 7:279–281.

83. HEBER ME, WHITTINGTON JR, BROADHURST PA, BRIGDEN GS, RAFTERY EB: Prognostic value of 24 hour ambulatory blood pressure monitoring. *Eur Heart J* 1990, 11:274.

84. COOPE J: Hypertension: the cause of the J-curve. *J Hum Hypertens* 1990, 4:1–4.

85. WEINBERGER MH: Antihypertensive therapy and lipids. paradoxical influences on cardiovascular disease risk. *Am J Med* 1986, 80 (suppl 2A):64–69.

86. KJELDSEN SE, NEUBIG RR, WEDER AB, ZWEIFLER AJ: The hypertension-coronary heart disease dilemma: the catechol amine-blood platelet connection. *J Hypertens* 1989, 7: 876–860.

87. CLARKSON TB, MANUCK SB, KAPLAN JR: Potential role of cardiovascular reactivity in atherogenesis. In *Handbook of Stress, Reactivity, and Cardiovascular Disease* edited by Matthews KA, Weiss SM, Detre T, *et al.* New York: Wiley, 1986, pp 35–48.

88. KEYS A, TAYLOR HL, BLACKBURN H, *ET AL*. Mortality and coronary heart disease among men studied for 23 years. *Arch Intern Med* 1971, 128:201–214.

89. GOSSE P, DURANDET P, ROUDAUT R, BROUSTET JP, DALLOCCHIO M: Valeur prognostique de la tension artérielle d'effort chez l'hypertendu. *Arch Mal Coeur* 1989, 82:1339–1342.

90. FAGARD R, STAESSEN J, THIJS L, AMERY A: The prognostic significance of exercise versus rest blood pressure in hypertensive men. *Hypertension* (in press).

91. DAVIS BR, LANGFORD HG, BLAUFOX MD, *ET AL*: The association of postural changes in systolic blood pressure and mortality in persons with hypertension: the Hypertension Detection and Follow-up Program experience. *Circulation* 1987, 75:340–346.

92. SIMPSON FO, GILCHRIST AR: Prognosis in untreated hypertensive vascular disease. *Scot Med J* 1958, pp 31–39.

93. KOBRIN I, DUNN FG, OIGMAN W, *ET AL*: Essential hypertension in the elderly: circadian variation of arterial pressure. In *Ambulatory Blood Pressure Monitoring* edited by Weber MA, Drayer JIM. Darmstadt: Steinkopff, 1984, pp 181–185.

94. GOSSE P, CAMPELLO G, ROUDANT R, DALLACCHIO M: High night blood pressure in treated hypertensive patients: not harmless. *Am J Hypertens* 1988, 1 (suppl):195s–198s.

95. SOKOLOW M, PERLOFF DB: The prognosis of essential hypertension treated conservatively. *Circulation* 1961, 23:697–713.

96. DEVEREUX RB, CASALE PN, WALLERSON DC, *ET AL*: Cost-effectiveness of echocardiography and electrocardiography for detection of left ventricular hypertrophy in patients with systemic hypertension. *Hypertension* 1987, 9 (suppl II):II69–II76.

97. CASALE PN, DEVEREUX RB, MILNER M, *ET AL*: Value of echocardiographic measurement of left ventricular mass in predicting cardiovascular morbid events in hypertensive men. *Ann Intern Med* 1986, 105:173–178.

98. LEVY D, GARRISON RJ, SAVAGE DD, KANNEL WB, CASTELLI WP: Left ventricular mass and incidence of coronary heart disease in an elderly cohort. The Framingham Heart Study. *Ann Intern Med* 1989, 110:101–107.

99. LEVY D, GARRISON RJ, SAVAGE DD, KANNEL WB, CASTELLI WP: Prognostic implications of echocardiographically determined left ventricular mass in the Framingham Heart Study. *N Engl J Med* 1990, 322:1561–1566.

100. KOREN MJ, CASALE PN, SAVAGE DD, *ET AL*: Relation of left ventricular mass prognosis in essential hypertension. *Circulation* 1989, 80 (suppl II):II538.

101. BULPITT CJ, BEILIN LJ, CLIFTON P, *ET AL*: Risk factors for death in treated hypertensive patients. *Lancet* 1979, ii:1340–137.

102. SAMUELSSON O, WILHELMSEN L, ELMFELDT D, *ET AL*: Predictors of cardiovascular morbidity in treated hypertension: results from the Primary Prevention Trial in Göteborg, Sweden. *J Hypertens* 1985, 3:167–176.

14   Diaries

The use of diaries is an integral part of ambulatory monitoring studies. Diaries serve two purposes: first, they may be useful for patients in whom transient blood pressure changes may be the cause of intermittent symptoms such as dizziness. This procedure has been widely used in ambulatory ECG monitoring. The second and much more important use is to correlate what the subject is doing and feeling with what is happening to his or her blood pressure. This is important not only for studies focusing on the relationships between behaviour and blood pressure, but also, for example, for drug studies. This is because the effects of physical and mental activity on blood pressure are so powerful that very different levels of pressure will be recorded in different circumstances. Thus, if the effects of an antihypertensive drug are being studied by reported ambulatory monitoring of patients before and after they take the drug, a potential confounding factor would occur if the patient went to work on one of the study days and stayed at home on another. This can be recognized if adequate diaries are kept.

One of the advantages of the non-invasive recorders is that the intermittent inflation of the cuff warns the subject each time a reading is being taken, so that it is possible to record the activity at that precise moment. This is less easily achieved with continuous (e.g. intra-arterial or ECG) recorders, where two alternative strategies would be to make an entry either each time there is a significant change in activity or at intervals pre-set by a timer.

Diary design: variables that should be recorded

The number of variables that subjects are asked to record is always a compromise between what is desirable and what is feasible. It is generally agreed that an 'open-ended' diary in which subjects are merely asked to make comments about their activity is much less satisfactory than a structured format, where they are asked to enter a number of specific items. An example of an open-ended diary produced by the manufacturers of an ambulatory monitor is shown in Fig. 14.1. Clearly, only the crudest information can be obtained from such a diary.

Some commonly evaluated situational variables are listed in Fig. 14.2. One of the most important of these is position, which has a major influence on blood pressure [1]. At the time of each reading subjects should be asked to specify whether they are sitting, lying or standing. Another is location, the two most important items being whether the subject is at home or at work [2]. Commuting may be another major category, although it may also be a time when invalid blood pressure readings are obtained because of movement artefact. Activity should also

be recorded, although here there may be less standardization, and entries may need to be tailored to the particular group being studied. Furthermore, we have sometimes found it advantageous to separate activities conducted at work from those conducted at home by using different entry pages for the two locations. Examples of general activities include talking, eating, drinking and walking. Activities specific to the work situation may include typing or working at a video terminal, and home activities would include cooking and watching television.

Mood is also a determinant of blood pressure. We ask our subjects to record whether they are happy, angry or anxious [3]. For patients taking medications, it is important that the time of each dosage should be recorded in the diary. This is clearly important in drug studies, where the duration of effect is being evaluated, and also in studies of patients with intermittent symptoms which might be drug-induced. Symptoms should also be recorded.

A final consideration of the design of diaries is that they should be compact and easy to read.

Psychological issues in diary design

At least two psychological issues in diary design need to be discussed. The first concerns the compliance of the subjects in filling out the entries accurately, and the second concerns the potential effects that the self-monitoring process may have on individuals' behaviour. Both these issues have been reviewed previously by Chesney and Ironson [4].

The major determinant of compliance is undoubtedly the complexity of the diary. Diaries that have a high 'response cost' are likely to be completed less satisfactorily [5]. If, as is customary, blood pressure readings are taken every 15 min, the amount of time spent on each diary entry must be kept to a minimum. We have compromised on this point by having some entries completed every 15 min and others every 30 min. Another technique for improving compliance is a thorough briefing of the subjects before the recording is started, including asking subjects to fill out a sample record. Informing people that the accuracy of their entries will be checked has been shown to improve compliance [6]. Many people are naturally curious about how different activities and moods affect their blood pressure, and this may help improve their compliance.

The phenomenon of the effects of self-monitoring on behaviour been termed 'reactance' [7], and has been used in behavioural intervention studies [8]. An example of this phenomenon comes from a study of the smoking habits of college students, who were first monitored

Log Information

TIME RECORDING STARTED _____

TIME RECORDING COMPLETED _____

TIME INTERVAL 0001-0600 Hrs _____ Min.

0600-1200 Hrs _____ Min.

1200-1800 Hrs _____ Min.

1800-2400 Hrs _____ Min.

DISPLAY ON/OFF MONITOR # _____

ALARM ON/OFF RAM PAC # _____

Daytime NOON TO 6 PM

TIME	ACTIVITY/MEDICATION	COMMENTS/ SYMPTOMS

Daytime 6 AM TO NOON

TIME	ACTIVITY/MEDICATION	COMMENTS/ SYMPTOMS

Nighttime 6 PM TO MIDNIGHT

TIME	ACTIVITY/MEDICATION	COMMENTS/ SYMPTOMS

Fig. 14.1. A typical open-ended diary produced by one of the manufacturers of ambulatory monitors (Spacelabs).

unobtrusively during classes and then asked to monitor their own smoking frequency [8]. If the self-monitoring period was initiated by focusing on the positive aspects of smoking, the students smoked more, whereas if the negative aspects were emphasized, they smoked less. The direction of behaviour change may, to some extent, depend on the instructions that the subjects are given. Thus, if they are told to expect a high degree of variability of mood, they are likely to report this [9].

The reactance phenomenon is unlikely to be a major problem in most ambulatory monitoring studies, unless one aspect of the diary is emphasized in particular (as might, for example, occur in a study of the effects of smoking on blood pressure). Wearing a monitor is itself more likely to change a subject's behaviour pattern than having to fill out a diary.

Psychometric issues in diary design

Diaries should be as unambiguous as possible. An important question for each entry category is whether it should be unimodal or multidimensional. Some categories, such as location, clearly are of the former type: one cannot be in two places at once. Other categories, such as activity and mood, are not: one might be walking and talking at the same time, and it is possible to feel both anxious and depressed. A diary may be designed to allow for these possibilities or to permit only one entry for each category. In the case of mood, for example, the subject would have to choose whether anxiety or depression was the predominant emotion. In evaluating moods it is also helpful to include a scaling factor (e.g. very angry, moderately angry, a little angry, not at all angry), which should

Location	Posture
Work	Upright
Home	Sitting
Commuting	Lying
Miscellaneous	
Activity	
Walking	Reading
Talking	Writing
Eating/drinking	Watching television
Smoking	Sleeping
Interactions	**Mood**
Alone	Happy
Spouse	Sad
Children	Angry
Client	Anxious
Co-workers	Neutral
Medication	**Symptoms**
[Open-ended]	[Open-ended]

Fig. 14.2. Situational variables monitored in diaries.

include a neutral state. We have found that our subjects check the neutral categories more than either the positive or the negative ones. An example of a diary we are currently using for behavioural studies is shown in Fig. 14.3.

It may also be appropriate to attempt to evaluate more subtle influences on blood pressure, such as the social situation. Therefore, talking is known to raise blood pressure, but the effect varies according to the status of the person being spoken to (see Chapter 4). Consequently, it may be useful to include a note of the person whom the subject is with at the time of each blood pressure reading, and what sort of interaction is taking place. Examples would include family members, co-workers and friends.

Validity of diaries

In psychological studies it is customary to assess the validity of a measure, that is the extent to which the questionnaire or diary actually measures what it is supposed to measure. Although such an evaluation is usually undertaken before an instrument becomes widely used, it has not so far been reported for ambulatory monitoring diaries. They could be evaluated by asking an independent observer to note the subject's activities during the monitoring period. However, obtrusive monitoring by an observer may itself alter the subject's behaviour [11]. If a diary is too complex or too ambiguous, subjects may tend to make the same entries throughout. In addition, subjects may complete entries retrospectively, for example just before they return the diary to the investigator. This is likely to occur if the diary is too complex, and also if subjects are particularly busy or stressed at the time that the reading is being taken.

Another factor that is likely to affect the validity of diary entries is the personality of the subject. A compulsive individual is more likely to complete all the items than one who has a more casual approach to life. This could result in a systematic bias in behavioural studies.

Activity monitoring as a supplement to diaries

The correlation of activity and blood pressure would be greatly simplified if it were possible to monitor subjects' posture and movements automatically, rather than relying on diary entries. Such monitoring would also permit an assessment of the validity of the entries by correlating them with the objectively recorded physical activity. As described in Chapter 4, it is now possible to monitor physical activity continuously, using monitors which are about the size of a large wristwatch and which can be worn on the wrist or waist. It should be emphasized that such monitors record movement rather than position, so that they cannot replace the recording of posture in the diaries. In theory, they might also be expected to help

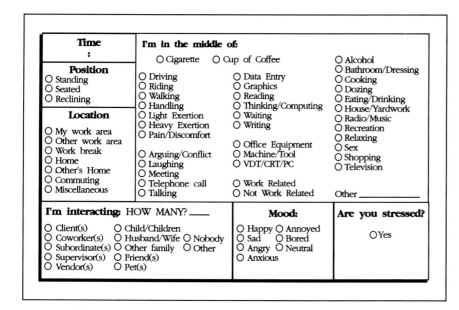

Fig. 14.3. A more elaborate diary than shown in Fig. 14.1, currently being used in behavioural studies.

separate the relative contributions of physical and mental activity to blood pressure changes, except that in practice the two are probably closely related: periods of acute mental stress are also likely to be periods of increased physical activity. At other times, increases in physical activity may be accompanied by mental relaxation.

Use of diaries for the evaluation of intermittent symptoms

A potential, but unsubstantiated, clinical application of ambulatory monitoring is the evaluation of patients with intermittent symptoms that might be related to a transient increase or decrease in blood pressure. In this instance the patient is asked to record the symptoms in a diary that can then be related to the ambulatory blood pressure readings.

Although this approach sounds reasonable, a much wider experience with the correlation of transient symptoms recorded in patient's diaries with arrhythmias occurring during ambulatory ECG recordings suggests that the results may be disappointing. Several studies have analysed data from patients referred for evaluation of intermittent symptoms, such as palpitations, light-headedness and syncope [11–13]. In one study [12], 371 patients kept a diary during the ECG recording. Typical symptoms occurred in 47% of patients, but the symptoms coincided with a significant arrhythmia in only 13%; symptoms unaccompanied by a significant arrhythmia occurred in 34%; and an arrhythmia without symptoms occurred in another 33%. In a similar study [13], only 2% of patients had symptoms coinciding with a major arrhythmia, while 42% had symptoms alone and 64% had asymptomatic major arrhythmias.

These studies show that the correlation between symptoms and arrhythmias is very weak, even in patients who have a high prevalence of both, and in many of whom

treatment of the arrhythmia results in an amelioration of the symptoms. It seems unduly optimistic to expect any better associations between blood pressure changes and symptoms, particularly if the symptoms are of short duration and blood pressure readings are taken intermittently.

Data entry and analysis

It has been our practice in research studies to enter at least four descriptors from the diary for each blood pressure reading: location, position, activity and mood. In principle, this allows blood pressure variability to be expressed in terms of each one of these descriptors. However, it should be realized that these are not truly independent measures: sleep is always associated with lying, and watching television is nearly always done while sitting. Consequently, these associations could be a source of confounding factors. When describing the effects of sleep on blood pressure, for example, one needs to distinguish the effects of lying down from the effects of sleep itself. The issue of multi-collinearity is discussed in Chapter 16.

Ideally, one would like to specify the effects of each activity on a subject's blood pressure. As described in Chapter 4, we found that 16 commonly occurring activities could account for a substantial portion of overall blood pressure variance [14]. We decided that at least five readings were needed to characterize the blood pressure for each activity or situation, a requirement that has subsequently been validated by Llabre *et al.* [15]. An example of the effects of specific activities on blood pressure based on such an analysis of diary entries by Van Egeren and Madarasini [16] is shown in Fig. 14.4. It should be pointed out that any such estimate is an over-simplification, because the blood pressure at any one moment will be the end result of a number of factors, both internal and external.

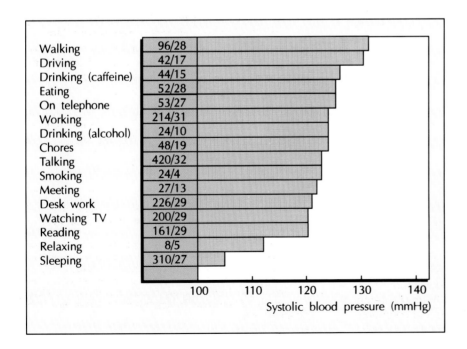

Fig. 14.4. Effect of specific activities on systolic blood pressure, based on data obtained with Van Egeren's computer-assisted diary. The numbers before each bar indicate the number of times the activity was reported and the number of subjects who reported it. Reproduced with permission [16].

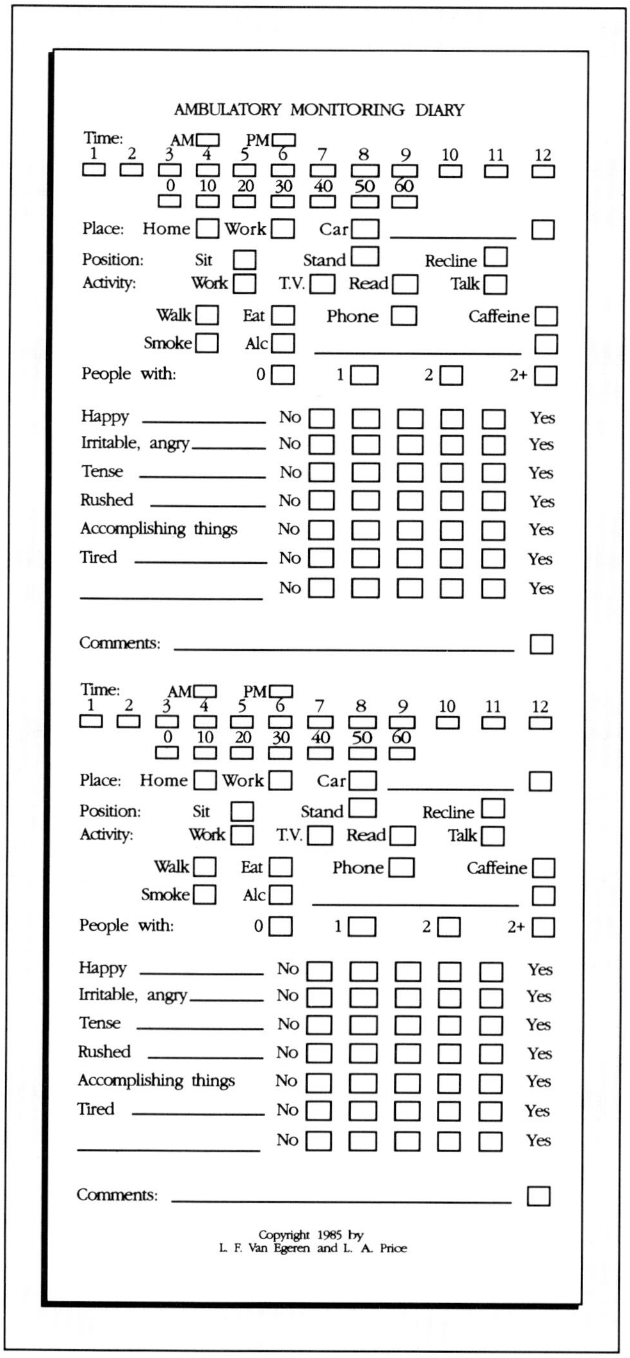

AMBULATORY MONITORING DIARY

Time: AM☐ PM☐
1 2 3 4 5 6 7 8 9 10 11 12
☐ ☐ ☐ ☐ ☐ ☐ ☐ ☐ ☐ ☐ ☐ ☐
0 10 20 30 40 50 60
☐ ☐ ☐ ☐ ☐ ☐ ☐

Place: Home ☐ Work ☐   Car ☐ _____ ☐

Position: Sit ☐   Stand ☐   Recline ☐
Activity: Work ☐   T.V. ☐   Read ☐   Talk ☐
            Walk ☐   Eat ☐   Phone ☐   Caffeine ☐
            Smoke ☐   Alc ☐ _____ ☐
People with: 0 ☐   1 ☐   2 ☐   2+ ☐

Happy _____ No ☐ ☐ ☐ ☐ ☐ Yes
Irritable, angry_____ No ☐ ☐ ☐ ☐ ☐ Yes
Tense _____ No ☐ ☐ ☐ ☐ ☐ Yes
Rushed _____ No ☐ ☐ ☐ ☐ ☐ Yes
Accomplishing things No ☐ ☐ ☐ ☐ ☐ Yes
Tired _____ No ☐ ☐ ☐ ☐ ☐ Yes
_____ No ☐ ☐ ☐ ☐ ☐ Yes

Comments: _____ ☐

Time: AM☐ PM☐
1 2 3 4 5 6 7 8 9 10 11 12
☐ ☐ ☐ ☐ ☐ ☐ ☐ ☐ ☐ ☐ ☐ ☐
0 10 20 30 40 50 60
☐ ☐ ☐ ☐ ☐ ☐ ☐

Place: Home ☐ Work ☐   Car ☐ _____ ☐

Position: Sit ☐   Stand ☐   Recline ☐
Activity: Work ☐   T.V. ☐   Read ☐   Talk ☐
            Walk ☐   Eat ☐   Phone ☐   Caffeine ☐
            Smoke ☐   Alc ☐ _____ ☐
People with: 0 ☐   1 ☐   2 ☐   2+ ☐

Happy _____ No ☐ ☐ ☐ ☐ ☐ Yes
Irritable, angry_____ No ☐ ☐ ☐ ☐ ☐ Yes
Tense _____ No ☐ ☐ ☐ ☐ ☐ Yes
Rushed _____ No ☐ ☐ ☐ ☐ ☐ Yes
Accomplishing things No ☐ ☐ ☐ ☐ ☐ Yes
Tired _____ No ☐ ☐ ☐ ☐ ☐ Yes
_____ No ☐ ☐ ☐ ☐ ☐ Yes

Comments: _____ ☐

Fig. 14.5. Computer-assisted diary developed by Van Egeren. Reproduced with permission [16].

Computer-assisted diaries

One of the problems with conventional diaries is that entry of the data recorded by the subjects into a computer is both very time-consuming and subject to error. This is particularly true of the more elaborate diaries used by behavioural scientists, which may require more than 1000 individual entries for a single 24-hour recording. Van Egeren has pioneered the development of computer-

assisted diaries using 'mark sense' cards [16], which the subject marks with a pencil at pre-set sites. These cards can then be read by a card reader connected to a personal computer. An example of such a card is shown in Fig. 14.5; each card accommodates two entries on each side, so that if blood pressure is taken every 15 min, the subject uses one card per hour, and it takes approximately 30–45 s to make each entry. The computer program not only collates the data but also checks it for missing or incompatible entries, and so on.

The advantages of this type of system include considerable savings in time, good acceptance from the subjects keeping the diary and improvements in accuracy and ease of data analysis.

Summary and conclusions

The effects of physical and mental activity on blood pressure are so pervasive that the proper interpretation of an ambulatory blood pressure recording requires at least some knowledge of the subject's activities during the recording. Subjects are, therefore, required keep a diary describing their activities. Several categories of situational variables may be recorded, the most important of which are location, position and activity. For patients in clinical studies, medication and symptoms should also be recorded, and for those in behavioural studies it may be helpful to include mood and social interactions.

No diary design is universally applicable, but diaries which require answers to specific questions are preferable to those with an 'open-ended' format. Diaries should be unambiguous, simple and compact. If they are too complex, subjects will either not fill them out at all or do so retrospectively. No information is available about the validity of diary entries, but it is likely that this could be improved by including automatic monitoring of physical activity, which is now possible with miniature ambulatory monitors.

A potential clinical application of ambulatory monitoring is the correlation of intermittent symptoms with transient changes in blood pressure. However, experience with attempts to relate similar symptoms to transient arrhythmias using ECG monitoring suggests that such correlations may be difficult to establish.

Most diaries require manual data entry by a technician, but a promising development is computer-assisted diaries that can be read by an optical card reader.

References

1. GELLMAN M, SPITZER S, IRONSON G, *ET AL*: Posture, place and mood effects on ambulatory blood pressure. *Psychophysiology* (in press).

2. HARSHFIELD GA, PICKERING TG, KLEINERT HD, BLANK S, LARAGH JH: Situational variations of blood pressure in ambulatory hypertensive patients. *Psychosom Med* 1982, 44:237–245.

3. JAMES GD, YEE LS, HARSHFIELD GA, BLANK S, PICKERING TG: The influence of happiness, anger, and anxiety on the blood pressure of borderline hypertensives. *Psychosom Med* 1986, 48:502–508.

4. CHESNEY MA, IRONSON GH: Diaries in ambulatory monitoring. In *Handbook of Research Methods in Cardiovascular Behavioral Medicine.* New York: Plenum, 1989, pp 317–332.

5. CONDIOTTE MM, LICHTENSTEIN E: Self-efficacy and relapse in smoking cessation programs. *J Consult Clin Psychol* 1981, 49:648–659.

6. EVANS RI, HANSEN WB, MITTLEMARK MB: Increasing the validity of self-reports of smoking behavior in children. *J Appl Psychol* 1977, 62:521–523.

7. KAZDIN AE: Reactive self-monitoring: the effects of response desirability, goal setting, and feedback. *J Consult Clin Psychol* 1974, 42:704–716.

8. McFALL RM: Effects of self-monitoring on normal smoking behavior. *J Consult Clin Psychol* 1970, 35:135–142.

9. CIMMINERO AR, NELSON RO, LIPINSKI DP: Self-monitoring procedures. In *Handbook of Behavioral Assessment: Self-Monitoring Procedures* edited by Cimminero AR, Calhoun KS, Adams HE. New York: Wiley, 1977, pp 195–232.

10. LONG J, LYNCH JJ, MACHIRAN NM, THOMAS SA, MALINOW KM: The effect of status on blood pressure during verbal communication. *J Behav Med* 1982, 5:165–172.

11. HINDMAN MC, LAST JH, ROSEN KM: Wolff-Parkinson-White syndrome observed by portable monitoring. *Ann Intern Med* 1973, 79:654–663.

12. ZELDIS SM, LEVINE BJ, MICHELSON EL, MORGANROTH J: Cardiovascular complaints: correlation with cardiac arrhythmias on 24-hour electrocardiographic monitoring. *Chest* 1980, 78:456–462.

13. CLARK PI, GLASSER SP, SPOTO E: Arrhythmias detected by ambulatory monitoring: lack of correlation with symptoms of dizziness and syncope. *Chest* 1980, 77:722–725.

14. CLARK L, DENBY L, PREGIBON D, *ET AL*: A quantitative analysis of the effects of activity and time of day on the diurnal variations of blood pressure. *J Chron Dis* 1987, 40:671–681.

15. LLABRE M, IRONSON GH, SPITZER SB, GELLMAN MD, WEIDLER DJ, SCHNEIDERMAN N: Blood pressure stability of normotensives and mild hypertensives in different settings. *Health Psychol* 1988 (suppl):127–137.

16. VAN EGEREN LF, MADARASINI S: A computer-assisted diary (CAD) for ambulatory blood pressure monitoring. *Am J Hypertens* 1988, 1 (suppl 1):179s–185s.

15 The potential contribution of ambulatory blood pressure monitoring to decision making in hypertension and its impact on the health-care system

The decision to start a patient with mild hypertension on a potentially life-long regimen of medication is not easy or simple. Like many other decisions in clinical medicine, it involves a number of 'trade-offs' between potential costs and benefits. Since all forms of pharmacological treatment currently in use have disadvantages, including side effects and financial costs, the success or failure of treatment will depend on whether the benefits outweigh the risks and costs. In this chapter we shall attempt to make some more rational recommendations than currently advocated, to discuss how the clinical role of ambulatory monitoring should be evaluated, and to predict its likely impact on the health-care system.

The present situation

In its latest report [1], the Joint National Committee (JNC) on the Detection, Evaluation, and Treatment of Hypertension recommended that treatment should generally be started if the diastolic pressure measured twice on each of two occasions is greater than 90 mmHg. The World Health Organization [2] recommends that patients with diastolic pressures between 90 and 104 mmHg on at least two occasions should be seen on two further occasions before treatment is started, and the British Hypertension Society [3] recommends pharmacological treatment only if the diastolic pressure exceeds 100 mmHg.

Typically, such recommendations define a cut-off point or dividing line, which is the same for all patients, above which treatment is recommended and below which it is withheld. This approach suffers from a number of deficiencies. First, the cut-off point is based solely on blood pressure, not on risk. Individual people with identical blood pressures may have quite different levels of cardiovascular risk. Furthermore, the rate at which risk changes with changing blood pressure is known to depend on the presence of other cardiovascular risk factors. This is illustrated in Fig. 15.1, which is based on data from the Framingham Heart Study. This shows how the relationship between blood pressure and morbidity is influenced by other risk factors. Reducing the blood pressure by the same amount in different individuals will therefore have different consequences. In the individual whose risk is low to begin with (line 1 in the figure), the absolute benefit is negligible, whereas in the high-risk individual it may be very large (line 3 in the figure). Therefore, the treatment threshold should ideally be individualized for each patient, reflecting other aspects of risk for cardiovascular disease.

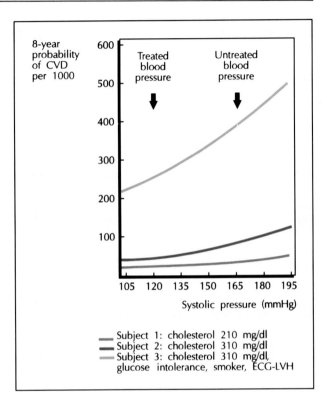

Fig. 15.1. Data from the Framingham Heart Study showing how the relationship between systolic pressure and cardiovascular risk varies according to the presence of other risk factors. Curves for three subjects are shown. Lowering systolic pressure from 165 (untreated) to 120 (treated) mmHg should produce greater benefit (reduction of risk) in subject 3 than in subject 1.

A second deficiency of the JNC recommendations is that although the call for multiple readings is intended to compensate for variability of blood pressure in an individual patient, the guidelines are not based on any quantitative assessment of the known variability of blood pressure. Using an analysis of the spontaneous variability of blood pressure over multiple clinic visits, Schechter and Adler [4] estimated that the JNC procedure (two readings on each of two visits) would yield a positive predictive value of only 60%: that is, only 60% of patients diagnosed as having diastolic pressures above 90 mmHg would have a true blood pressure above this level.

A third deficiency of the recommendations is that they take no account of the white coat effect. As we have seen in Chapter 7, this may also lead to a significant misclassification of hypertension.

Cost–benefit and cost-effectiveness analysis

The two principal ways of assessing the utility and economic impact of a diagnostic test or intervention are cost–benefit and cost-effectiveness analysis [5]. In both, the financial costs of the procedure form one side of the equation. With cost–benefit analysis the other side is the calculated financial savings (or losses), and with cost-effectiveness analysis the benefit is expressed in non-monetary terms. In analyses of hypertension treatment it has typically been expressed as QALYs (quality-adjusted life years of survival resulting from the intervention) but might also be expressed in other terms such as the amount of blood pressure reduction.

The limitation of both types of analysis is that although many of the factors entered into the equations are relatively easy to quantify in comparable units of measurement (such as the cost of performing an ambulatory recording or the cost of antihypertensive medications), others are not (such as the experience of side effects from medications). Cost–benefit analysis requires that some monetary value be placed on these factors; this may be extremely difficult in practice because they are often highly subjective. One approach used is 'willingness to pay'; in the case of drug-induced side effects, this would be the amount one would be willing to pay to be freed of the side effects. This method has not been found to be very reliable, limiting the application of cost–benefit analysis [5].

How cost-effective is the treatment of mild hypertension?

Treatment of hypertension is expensive: in the United States nearly $10 billion is spent on it annually [6]. Furthermore, with the current trend towards increasing use of newer and more expensive agents such as angiotensin converting enzyme inhibitors and calcium antagonists, the costs of treatment are increasing dramatically. According to Louis [7], in Australia the average cost per month for blood pressure treatment was A$5 in 1977 and A$10 in 1987, but rose to A$36 in 1988, when angiotensin converting enzyme inhibitors were introduced. This was probably just the tip of the iceberg, because in 1988 these agents accounted for only 5% of prescriptions for hypertension and heart failure, and their use is growing rapidly.

One of the factors that should determine the approach to the treatment of hypertension is its cost-effectiveness. This was the subject of an extensive analysis by Weinstein and Stason [8]. It took into account the risks resulting from a particular level of blood pressure (based on the data from the Framingham Study), the costs of treatment and the costs associated with a stroke or myocardial infarct. Cost-effectiveness was expressed as the dollar cost per year of QALY. A number of findings are relevant to the present discussion. First, the medical costs saved by the prevention of cardiovascular morbidity do not come close to paying for the costs of treatment. Even in patients with diastolic pressure above

105 mmHg, only 22% of the costs of treatment can be saved. Second, the treatment of patients with mild hypertension is much less cost-effective than of those with more severe hypertension. If treatment is restricted to those with diastolic pressures above 105 mmHg the cost-effectiveness ratio would be $4850 per QALY (in 1976 dollars), whereas for treatment of pressures between 95 and 105 mmHg the cost would be $9880. Third, it is more cost-effective to treat younger men and older women. The explanation for this somewhat surprising result is that younger men have a greater prospect of increased life expectancy as a result of treatment than older men; in young women, however, the risk attributable to hypertension is so small that the cost-effectiveness is low. As a result of such considerations Weinstein and Stason suggested that one of the best ways to reduce costs without compromising the quality of care would be to limit treatment to patients with well documented, sustained hypertension.

A more recent analysis by Littenberg et al. [9] found higher (i.e. less optimal) cost-effectiveness ratios than those of Weinstein and Stason, partly because the clinical trials of treating hypertension have shown smaller benefits than the projections made by Weinstein and Stason in 1976. Littenberg et al. also concluded that the cost-effectiveness was very dependent on the costs of antihypertensive treatment.

Alternative strategies: the sequential threshold decision-making approach

A useful approach to making more rational therapeutic medical decisions that has not yet been applied in hypertension is decision analysis. This technique, imported from engineering, business and operations research, is particularly suitable as a decision aid when quantifiable gains and losses are at stake, the consequences of actions taken are known only probabilistically, and the decision must be individualized. Decision analysis has also been recommended as a substitute for clinical trials in situations where they are not practical.

In the clinical situation there are commonly three therapeutic options: treatment if the diagnosis is virtually certain, withholding treatment if the probability of disease is very low, and performing further diagnostic tests if it is somewhere in between. Pauker and Kassirer [10] have analysed this paradigm and shown how the threshold probabilities defining 'sufficiently certain' and 'very low' probabilities of disease can be calculated in terms of the costs, risks and benefits of treatment. In the case of hypertension the patient's blood pressure may be substituted for probability of disease. As shown in Figure 15.2, the three zones corresponding to these three options are separated by two thresholds. The first is the treatment threshold, which is the level of pressure above which the benefits of treatment are judged to outweigh the risks. The second is the testing threshold: if the blood pressure is below this level, treatment can be withheld without any further testing. Between these two thresholds uncertainty prevails: further testing is indicated and treatment is given only to those with positive test results.

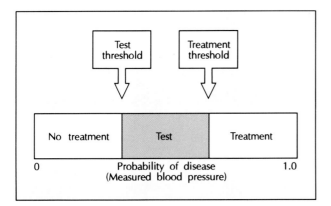

Fig. 15.2. The 'threshold decision' model of Pauker and Kassirer [10], adapted for the diagnosis of hypertension. Treatment, no treatment or further testing is recommended on the basis of the estimated probability of disease, which in this case is the measured blood pressure.

Schechter [11,12] has adapted this model for making the decision to treat hypertension, but in its initial form the model uses only clinic pressure. It allows for the fact that the disease state is a continuum rather than a present–absent dichotomy. The diagnostic procedure (measurement of blood pressure) also produces a quantitative result rather than a confirmation or refutation of a diagnosis. The model takes into account the spontaneous variability of blood pressure between clinic visits and assumes that the benefits of treatment are linearly related to the true pretreatment blood pressure. The hypothetical relationship between blood pressure and the benefits of treatment (measured as the gain in QALYs) is shown in Fig. 15.3 for two patients, one aged 20 years and the other 50, based on the data of Weinstein and Stason [8]. The costs and benefits of treatment are defined by four parameters: the slope and intercept of the line relating net treatment benefits to true blood pressure (Fig. 15.3), the cost of having the patient return for further evaluation, and a term attenuating the benefits when institution of treatment is delayed to obtain further measurements (this last item is relatively unimportant). The values assigned to these parameters are necessarily subjective, though methods for relating them to the established relationship of blood pressure to cardiovascular morbidity and reaching reasonable values are described. The model assumes that treatment also has some negative effects (such as the costs and side effects of medication). Thus, the cut-off point above which treatment is preferred to no treatment can be defined mathematically.

A strength of the model is that both the intercept and the slope of the line relating treatment benefit to blood pressure, which defines this cut-off point, can be tailored to the individual.

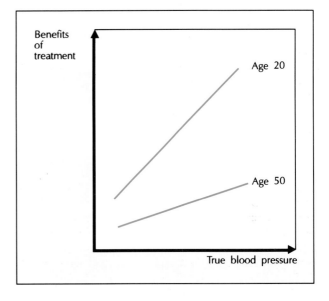

Fig. 15.3. Hypothetical relationship between blood pressure and the benefits of treatment (measured as the gain in QALYs) for two individuals, one aged 20 and one 50. Based on data from Weinstein and Stason [8].

One of the advantages of this model is that it permits an estimation of the treatment and testing thresholds. It is thus possible to decide what course of action should be taken after a blood pressure reading is taken. If the diastolic pressure is above the treatment threshold, treatment is started. If it is sufficiently low (e.g. below 85 mmHg, which is below the testing threshold), treatment is withheld. If it is between the two thresholds, further measurements are indicated. As shown in Fig. 15.4, as more readings are taken the two thresholds gradually converge, so that it is eventually possible to decide whether treatment should be started or not.

With this approach, the number of measurements needed to make the decision is not the same for every patient; it is greatest for those whose pressures are closest to the dividing line. It is of some interest to note that Monte Carlo simulation[1] studies of this approach applied to a medical clinic population reveal that the average number of blood pressure measurements required to make a decision is only slightly greater than that recommended by the JNC, but the effort is selectively applied to the most borderline patients. The most clear-cut hypertensives and normotensives, constituting about 80%

---

[1]Monte Carlo simulation is a computer modelling technique for estimating the outcome of a complex chain of events of varying probability. In the present instance, the consequences of choosing to treat people whose blood pressures meet certain criteria are estimated by generating a hypothetical patient population whose blood pressure distribution corresponds to a real population and applying these criteria to them. An advantage of this technique is that the impact of many different criteria can be studied quickly and easily, which could otherwise only be done through costly clinical trials.

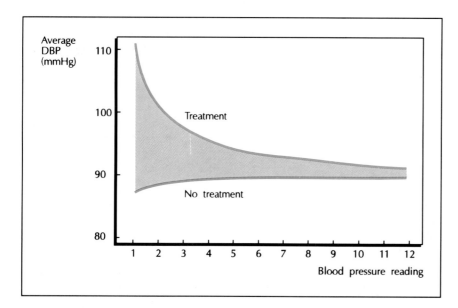

Fig. 15.4. Application of Schechter's threshold decision model [12] to the diagnosis of hypertension (defined as a measured diastolic pressure of 90 mmHg or higher), showing the effects of repeated clinic readings.

of the population, are identified at the first or second measurement, whereas the most marginal cases undergo a long series of measurements. By the fifth reading, a decision will have been reached in 95% of patients, and less than 1% of the population ultimately require 10 or more measurements to reach a decision.

Because the borderline cases are more carefully evaluated, many are spared unnecessary treatment. The same simulation reveals that whereas approximately 19% of the population is assigned to treatment using JNC recommendations, the sequential approach leads to treatment of approximately 14% of patients. These findings are consistent with the earlier observation that the positive predictive value of the JNC procedure is near 60%.

This model is not something that can be readily used by practising clinicians in its present form, but it provides the basis for the development of a more rational and individualized approach to the problem. It could also be adapted for home blood pressure measurement and for ambulatory monitoring, as described below.

Evaluating the impact of new diagnostic technology

When a new diagnostic test is first introduced it is generally hoped that it will improve the standards of medical care and in some cases also reduce costs. Despite the enormous number of tests adopted by clinicians over the past 30 years, few have been subjected to any rigorous analysis of their effectiveness. The primary purpose of any diagnostic test is to direct patient care, but in fact this outcome is the exception rather than the rule. In an analysis of two widely used and powerful advances in cardiac diagnostic technology, echocardiography and thallium scanning, Goldman et al. [13,14] concluded that in

the former case 8% of tests contributed to an important change of patient management and in the latter 12%. In both cases, however, it was concluded that the majority of tests were ordered appropriately.

In a review of the impact of advances in medical technology, Knaus [15] concluded that most new diagnostic tests increase the costs of medical care and argued that there may be a vicious cycle, because the new test may provide more diagnostic and therapeutic options that make it more rather than less difficult to take definitive action. It should also be recognized that any technological advance has an enormous potential for abuse: patients complaining of headache are routinely investigated with computed tomography scans, even though the yield of useful new information is pitifully small [16]. It is not hard to imagine that if ambulatory blood pressure monitoring were approved for general reimbursement, it too could be grossly over-utilized.

Guyatt et al. [17] have proposed a useful framework for the evaluation of new diagnostic technology in a series of six steps summarized in Fig. 15.5. The first is to establish the technological capability of the test: in the case of ambulatory monitoring, most experts are agreed that the current generation of monitors are sufficiently reliable and accurate to pass this test, although there are some dissenting opinions [18], and the accuracy is certainly not ideal.

Step two is the establishment of the range of possible uses of the test. With ambulatory monitoring the overriding issue is its use in patients with borderline hypertension.

Step three is the evaluation of the test's diagnostic accuracy by comparison with a 'gold standard'. In the present case the question is not whether the devices can measure blood pressure accurately, but whether they can give a more accurate estimate of the true blood pressure and

1. Technological capability
2. Range of possible uses
3. Diagnostic accuracy
4. Impact on health-care providers
5. Therapeutic impact
6. Patient outcome

Fig. 15.5. Framework for the evaluation of new diagnostic procedures (after Guyatt et al. [17])

of cardiovascular risk. The problem here is that there is no gold standard. The only existing candidate is clinic blood pressure, but the entire rationale of ambulatory blood pressure is that it is more reliable and valid than clinic pressure. Guyatt et al. suggest that when there is no gold standard, one must rely on construct validity. In this instance, this would involve the assessment of which measure of blood pressure gives a better prediction of target organ damage and prognosis, as was discussed in Chapter 13.

Step four is an evaluation of the impact on health-care providers. This is basically a question of whether the test is regarded by the medical community as providing useful information. Acceptability by patients might be an additional criterion.

Step five is an evaluation of the therapeutic impact of the test. Guyatt et al. suggested that the best way to do this is with a randomized controlled trial, in which patients would be randomized to be evaluated with the new test or not, and the effects on their outcome would be assessed. In the case of ambulatory monitoring this would be difficult to carry out. It might be relatively easy to demonstrate that patients' antihypertensive therapy was altered by ambulatory monitoring, but would these changes be appropriate? One way of answering this question would be to assess the effects on target organ damage, for example by comparing the regression of LVH in two groups of patients, in one of which the dose of antihypertensive medications was regulated according to clinic pressures and in the other according to ambulatory pressures.

The sixth and final step concerns the effects on patient outcome. Ideally, one would like to show that patients evaluated with ambulatory monitoring have fewer morbid events and fewer drug-related side effects than those evaluated only with clinic pressures. While the former outcome could be properly assessed only in an expensive long-term study of a very large population, the latter could feasibly be addressed in a clinical trial.

It should be pointed out that these six steps are a counsel of perfection. Although a few diagnostic procedures have been evaluated in this way [19,20], the results have often been inconclusive. It is universally accepted that computed tomography scanning is of diagnostic value in patients with acute strokes, and yet the only study to assess its impact on patient outcome (which used historical controls rather than randomized groups) failed to demonstrate any [21].

The role of ambulatory monitoring in evaluating the need for treatment

The decision-making strategy of Schechter described above was based on clinic readings and optimizing the number of readings that can be obtained in an individual patient. It can thus reduce the error associated with the spontaneous variability of blood pressure between clinic visits and hence improve the estimate of the true pressure. It cannot, however, correct for the error associated with the white coat effect. As we have noted, approximately 20% of patients with mild hypertension may be misclassified even on the basis of multiple clinic readings.

If it is accepted that such patients, once identified, do not need to take antihypertensive medication, the question arises whether the extra cost incurred by performing the additional monitoring can offset the savings from treatment. So far, little attempt has been made to answer this question. Krakoff et al. [22] performed a simplified cost–benefit analysis using the blood pressure data of 60 patients, all of whom were advised to take medication on the basis of their clinic readings. Thirty-eight per cent of these patients had average ambulatory systolic and diastolic pressures below 130/85 mmHg and were hence considered not to need treatment. It was estimated that if the cost of the ambulatory monitoring was equal to the yearly cost of treatment, monitoring every patient would increase the first year's cost by 60%. By 3 years, however, the total cost with this strategy would be less than with the traditional approach because of the accumulated savings in the costs of treatment. In our own institution, a single clinic visit costs $60, and an ambulatory recording $175. Advocates of ambulatory monitoring would argue that in many cases a single recording would provide more useful information than three additional clinic visits.

Fahs et al. ('The cost-effectiveness of ambulatory blood pressure.' Unpublished working paper) have carried out a preliminary analysis comparing the traditional JNC strategy with a strategy incorporating ambulatory monitoring and echocardiography. The two strategies are illustrated in Fig.15.6.

With the ambulatory monitoring strategy, patients whose clinic diastolic pressure falls between 90 and 104 mmHg on three occasions have an ambulatory blood pressure evaluation. For those with ambulatory diastolic blood pressures under 85 mmHg, treatment is withheld. Treatment is given to those whose average ambulatory blood pressure exceeds 90 mmHg. When the average ambulatory blood pressure is between 85 and 90 mmHg (approximately 18% of those who are monitored), the next diagnostic step is an echocardiogram. If this reveals early LVH or diastolic dysfunction (estimated to occur in 40% of those studied), treatment is prescribed.

The model has been applied to a hypothetical general population of 40- to 50-year-old men, of whom about 22% are assumed to have a clinic diastolic pressure above 90 mmHg. Under the JNC guidelines, these men are all prescribed treatment. With the ambulatory monitoring strategy the 10.5% of this population who have clinic di-

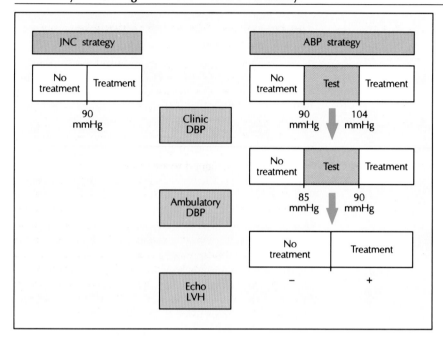

Fig. 15.6. Two strategies for the evaluation of patients with mild hypertension, compared in the model of Fahs *et al.* (unpublished working paper). (a) The 'traditional' JNC strategy, where treatment is decided solely on the basis of clinic diastolic blood pressure (DBP). (b) The ambulatory blood pressure (ABP) strategy, where patients with borderline clinic DBP are evaluated with ambulatory monitoring and, if still borderline, by echocardiography.

astolic pressures between 90 and 104 mmHg are monitored. Two per cent have echocardiograms.

Morbidity and mortality rates are derived from Vital Statistics of the United States [23], which are combined with the data of Perloff *et al.*'s prospective study [24] to give differential values for clinic and ambulatory pressures. The model assumes that treatment reduces morbidity and mortality by 50% in both hypertensives and normotensives. In this respect, it is heavily biased in favour of treatment, as the benefits of treating myocardial infarction (the major risk for this hypothetical population) have been found to be closer to 10% in clinical trials [25]. The model predicts that whereas 22% of the population would be treated according to the JNC guidelines, only 7% would be treated by the ambulatory monitoring strategy. The life expectancy would be the same with both treatment strategies, but the rate of non-fatal myocardial infarcts over the first 10 years is slightly higher under the ambulatory monitoring strategy (9.6 versus 8.5%). With no treatment at all, the estimated rate is 10.3%.

The difference in the projected rates of myocardial infarction with the two strategies may be attributable to the assumption that treating normotensive individuals confers some benefit, which remains unproven. However, because of the lack of better prospective data, the conclusions based on this model can only be considered tentative. Even though formal cost-effectiveness analysis has not yet been applied to it, it nevertheless suggests that appropriately constrained use of ambulatory monitoring could result in substantial cost savings in the long run.

Recognition of ambulatory blood pressure monitoring by government agencies and insurance companies

The evidence that ambulatory monitoring can give a more reliable estimate than clinic pressures of the damage caused by hypertension and of its prognosis is becoming increasingly hard to ignore. Nevertheless, regulatory agencies have been reluctant to approve it for routine clinical use and most still regard it as an experimental procedure[2]. The same view has been expressed by influential bodies such as the American College of Physicians [26]. In the United States, the procedure is listed in the *Physicians' Current Procedural Terminology*, the standard manual used for filing insurance claims. While many of the smaller private insurance companies do reimburse for it, the main determinant of reimbursement is recognition by Medicare (the federal scheme for patients older than 65), which does not. The biggest private insurance company, Blue Cross/Blue Shield, tends to follow Medicare policies, and provides reimbursement in only a few states.

In other countries the situation is generally similar. Although its use is approved in government-owned hospitals in some countries (e.g. Germany, Japan, Australia and Switzerland), most do not reimburse its costs. Two exceptions are Germany and Singapore, and it is expected that Japan will provide some reimbursement starting in 1991.

[2]We are indebted to Mr Bill Neiger and Mr Harvey Hauschildt of Spacelabs for providing much of this information.

Should ambulatory monitoring be approved for routine clinical use?

The findings presented above show that, although ambulatory monitoring does add to the cost of investigating patients with mild hypertension, it has the potential of saving overall costs. This, of course, rests on the assumption that it would identify a certain percentage of patients for whom treatment would not be prescribed, but who would have been treated on the basis of their clinic pressures.

At present, it must be admitted that the evidence supporting this assumption is inconclusive, although it generally points in that direction. Whether or not ambulatory monitoring would actually save costs and improve the quality of life for those excused treatment is another story altogether. It has to be admitted that practising physicians do not follow an idealized algorithm for making decisions. This is well illustrated by a study of how internists and family physicians use the stress test, the diagnostic value of which has been the subject of hundreds of scientific articles. When asked how they would evaluate a patient presenting with a history of chronic stable angina, 81% of physicians said they would order a stress test [28]. Fifty-three per cent said that the results of the test would not alter their decision to refer the patient to a cardiologist, and 82% said they would still prescribe antianginal medication even if the test was negative. This finding illustrates the way in which a diagnostic test is ordered routinely, without much consideration of how the results will be used. It is not hard to imagine ambulatory blood pressure monitoring being used in a similar way. Another consideration must be addressed: like any other professionals, doctors like to make money, and in the United States they do this by performing tests and procedures rather than by talking or listening to patients. Most specialists have at least one test which serves as a 'cash cow'[3]; for cardiologists this might be stress testing, and for gastroenterologists endoscopy. Hypertension specialists have so far lacked such a test, and ambulatory blood pressure monitoring would certainly make an ideal candidate.

If there were some way of restricting the use of ambulatory monitoring and ensuring that it would not be over-utilized, we would recommend that it be approved for clinical use. Unfortunately, this is not like to happen; in practice, a test is either approved or it is not.

Summary and conclusions

The decision to treat a patient with mild hypertension with antihypertensive medication involves a delicate balance between potential harms and benefits. The current recommendations, based on a small number of clinic readings, are deficient for a number of reasons: first, they take little account of the influence of other risk factors on the relationship between risk and blood pressure; second, they ignore the spontaneous variability of blood pressure between visits; and third, they take no account of the white coat effect.

The cost-effectiveness of treatment based solely on a few clinic readings is low, and can be greatly increased by better stratification of patients according to their level of risk. One way in which this can be done is by using a decision analysis approach, whereby patients whose blood pressures fall into the 'grey zone' of uncertainty are subjected to further evaluation. This approach can reduce the number of patients assigned to treatment, even when it uses only clinic pressures in the decision analysis. By incorporating ambulatory monitoring and echocardiography a further reduction in the number of treated patients ensues, which may offset the additional cost of testing. However, the ultimate determinant of the cost-effectiveness of ambulatory monitoring is whether or not physicians are prepared to withhold pharmacological treatment in patients with white coat hypertension, who can only be reliably identified by ambulatory monitoring. At present, opinions are sharply divided on this question.

Although a case can be made that the clinical use of ambulatory monitoring could be cost-effective if used appropriately, experience with other new diagnostic tests shows that they often increase rather than decrease costs, and that they are often ordered without any assurance that the results which they provide will significantly alter patient management. In most countries, ambulatory monitoring has not been approved for general use by governmental agencies on the grounds that it is still an experimental procedure. Given the huge number of individuals who occasionally show marginally elevated blood pressures, there can be no doubt that the indiscriminate and widespread use of the procedure could add significantly to the cost of health care.

References

1. The 1988 Report of the Joint National Committee on the Detection, Evaluation, and Treatment of High Blood Pressure. *Arch Intern Med* 1988, 148:1023–1050.
2. 1989 Guidelines for the management of mild hypertension: Memorandum from a WHO/ISH meeting. *J Hypertens* 1989, 7:689–693.
3. Report of the British Hypertension Society working party. Treating mild hypertension. *Br Med J* 1989, 298:694–698.
4. SCHECHTER CB, ADLER RS: Bayesian analysis of diastolic blood pressure measurement. *Med Decision Making* 1988, 8:182–190.
5. O'BRIEN R, RUSHBY J: Outcome assessment in cardiovascular cost-benefit studies. *Am Heart J* 1990, 199:740–748.
6. STASON WB: Opportunities for improving the cost-effectiveness of antihypertensive treatment. *Am J Med* 1986, 81 (suppl 6C):45–49.
7. LOUIS WJ: Regulatory demands for cost-benefit studies. *Am Heart J* 1990, 119:771–775.
8. WEINSTEIN MC, STASON WB: *Hypertension: A Policy Perspective.* Cambridge: Harvard University Press, 1976.
9. LITTENBERG B, GARBER AM, SOX HC: Screening for hypertension. *Ann Intern Med* 1990, 112:192–202.
10. PAUKER SG, KASSIRER JP: The threshold approach to clinical decision making. *N Engl J Med* 1980, 302:1109.

[3]This is not a pejorative term, but is widely used in business circles to denote a regular source of income.

11.   SCHECHTER CB: Sequential decision making with continuous disease states and measurements. I. Theory. *Med Decision Making* 1990, 10:242–255.

12.   SCHECHTER CB: Sequential decision making with continuous disease states and measurements. II. Application to diastolic pressure. *Med Decision Making* 1990, 10:256–265.

13.   GOLDMAN L, COHN PF, MUDGE GH, ET AL.: Clinical utility and management impact of M-mode echocardiography. *Am J Med* 1983, 75:49–56.

14.   GOLDMAN L, FEINSTEIN AR, BATSFORD WP, COHEN LS, GOTTSCHALK A, ZARET BL: Ordering patterns and clinical impact of cardiovascular nuclear medicine procedures. *Circulation* 1980, 62:680–687.

15.   KNAUS WA: Medical care and medical technology: the need for new understanding. In *The U.S. Health Care System. A look to the 1990s* edited by Ginzberg E. Totowa: Rowman and Allanheld, 1985, pp 70–88.

16.   LARSON EB, OMENN GS. LEWIS H: Diagnostic evaluation of headache. Impact of computerized tomography and cost-effectiveness. *JAMA* 1980, 243:359–362.

17.   GUYATT GH, TUGWELL PX, FEENY DH, HAYNES RB, DRUMMOND M: A framework for clinical evaluation of diagnostic technologies. *Can Med Assoc J* 1986, 134:587–594.

18.   BROADHURST P, HUGHES LO, RAFTERY EB: Non-invasive ambulatory blood pressure monitors: a cautionary note. *J Hypertens* 1990, 8:595–597.

19.   DIXON AK, FRY IK, KINGHAM JG, ET AL.: Computed tomography in patients with an abdominal mass: effective and efficient? A controlled trial. *Lancet* 1981, i:1199–1205.

20.   DRONFIELD MW, LANGMAN MJS, ATKINSON M, ET AL.: Outcome of endoscopy and barium radiography for acute upper gastrointestinal bleeding: controlled trial in 1037 patients. *Br Med J* 1982, 284:545–548.

21.   CHRISTIE D: Before and after comparisons: a cautionary tale. *Br Med J* 1979, 2:1629–1630.

22.   KRAKOFF LR, EISON H, PHILLIPS RH, LEIMAN SH, LEV S: Effects of ambulatory pressure monitoring on the diagnosis and cost of treatment for mild hypertension. *Am Heart J* 1988, 116:1152–1154.

23.   NATIONAL CENTER FOR HEALTH STATISTICS: *Vital Statistics of the United States, 1980.* US Department of Health and Human Services publication (PHS) 85–1102. Public Health Service, 1985.

24.   PERLOFF D, SOKOLOW M, COWAN R: Prognostic value of ambulatory blood pressures: further analyses. *J Hypertens* 1989, 7 (suppl 3):S3–S10.

25.   MCMAHON SW, CUTLER JA, FURFBERG CD, PAYNE GH: The effects of drug treatment for hypertension on mortality and morbidity for cardiovascular disease: a review of randomized controlled trials. *Prog Cardiovasc Dis* 1986, 19 (suppl 1):99–118.

26.   HEALTH AND POLICY COMMITTEE, AMERICAN COLLEGE OF PHYSICIANS: Automated ambulatory blood pressure monitoring. *Ann Intern Med* 1986, 104:275–278.

27.   HARTZ A, HOUTS P, BARTHOLOMEW M, GOLDMAN S, KANTER T, DEBER R: How physicians use the stress test for the management of angina. *Med Decision Making* 1989, 9:157–161.

16 Methods of analysis of ambulatory blood pressure data

A single ambulatory blood pressure recording session may produce up to 100 readings per subject. This chapter discusses how the readings should be used and analysed, and may therefore be of more interest to the researcher than the clinician.

It was argued in earlier chapters that ambulatory recordings have several advantages over clinic measurements. First, because so many readings are taken, ambulatory monitoring should give a more precise estimate of a subject's true level of blood pressure and its variability. Second, readings can be taken in a wide variety of settings. Third, the readings are less likely to be confounded by factors such as observer error and the white coat effect. However, the situations in which ambulatory blood pressure readings are made are much less controlled than in the clinic; this creates both a problem and an opportunity. The problem is the difficulty of comparing the data obtained from one recording with those from another, because the circumstances in which the recordings were made are unlikely to be identical for each individual and the total number of readings is also likely to vary. These factors need to be taken into consideration when the data are analysed and interpreted. The opportunity is that ambulatory monitoring allows quantitative study of the influences of these factors on blood pressure. This chapter will focus on measures of centrality (e.g. means and medians) and of variability, including a discussion of how diurnal changes in blood pressure can be quantified. As the initial step in any data analysis usually concerns data editing and a consideration of missing values, we shall address these questions first.

Although issues that may be important are discussed and suggestions for analyses are proposed, it must be stressed that no single method is appropriate to answer all research questions. Furthermore, we would expect all reasonable approaches to arrive at similar conclusions. Finally, the analytical problems for ambulatory blood pressure data are so complex that it is most unlikely that any single analytical approach will answer all the potential questions.

Data editing and outlier detection

All ambulatory recordings include readings that are considerably above or below the average reading. These readings could be either outliers or artefacts caused by faulty equipment or movement. Artefacts may have a disproportionate effect on measures of blood pressure variability as well as on measures of centrality, especially if the number of artefacts is large relative to the number of true readings.

A typical, but not ideal, example of a 24-hour diastolic pressure recording is shown in Fig. 16.1. Most of the readings lie between 80 and 90 mmHg, but one clearly high reading was recorded while the subject was at work, and one low reading was recorded during sleep. It is clearly difficult to decide retrospectively which readings are artefacts, but a number of techniques have been used. The most common is perhaps subjective assessment, whereby the technician or investigator scans the series of readings and picks out those which look suspicious. This can be done using a number of criteria, such as an abnormally narrow pulse pressure, disparity with previous readings, or incongruence with the time of day or activity. This method is theoretically unsatisfactory because it is inconsistent and subject to the biases of individual researchers, but is nonetheless widely used.

The alternative technique is based on a rigorous set of rules that can be built into a computer algorithm, the simplest of which eliminates readings that are physiologically improbable. An example is a program currently incorporated into the Spacelabs software system that identifies readings as artefactual if any of the following criteria are met:

1. Systolic pressure is below 70 or above 260 mmHg;
2. Diastolic pressure is below 40 or above 150 mmHg;
3. Pulse pressure (systolic minus diastolic) is greater than 150 or less than 20 mmHg.

It is certainly possible for physiological levels to exceed these criteria; however, most of the readings excluded by this algorithm are probably artefacts. On the other hand, in some normotensive people (e.g. young women), blood pressure during sleep may at times be lower than 70/40 mmHg, and it may therefore be appropriate to reinstate readings identified as errors by the computer.

In our early studies [1] we used a similar algorithm, based on an empirically observed relationship between systolic and diastolic pressure. It was designed to exclude readings where the pulse pressure was too narrow, for example 140/120 mmHg. The algorithm was as follows: for diastolic pressure between 60 and 125 mmHg, readings were excluded if the pulse pressure was less than $(0.41 \times \text{diastolic pressure}) - 17$.

Another approach, which may be used in conjunction with the algorithms described above, is to identify those readings which are out of line with the bulk of the data. The criteria here are thus relative rather than absolute. Two ways of defining such outliers have been employed. The first method [2] identifies readings that are extreme

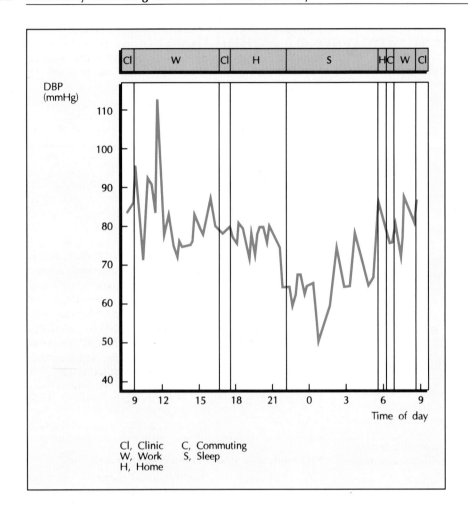

Cl, Clinic   C, Commuting
W, Work   S, Sleep
H, Home

Fig. 16.1. A 24-hour recording showing diastolic pressure values in one subject. Note the outliers at noon and 1.00 a.m.

relative to the other readings in the series. This method is based on the relationship between systolic and diastolic pressure. Figure 16.2 shows a scatterplot of 917 readings from 15 subjects, analysed by two versions of this procedure. The readings form an ellipse-shaped cluster; the lower right-hand part of the plot is empty because diastolic pressure cannot exceed systolic pressure. It is possible to construct an ellipse which will include a desired percentage of readings, for example 95%, so that the remaining 5% of readings outside the boundary of the ellipse can be identified as outliers.

The second method is to label readings as outliers if they have a disproportionately large influence on the estimation of the effect of interest (e.g. the average level of pressure in a particular situation). For example, elimination of a single reading could have a major effect on the estimate of mean blood pressure. Marler *et al.* [3] used an algorithm called the DFFITS statistic [4] to identify particularly influential readings and excluded them from some sets of analyses. Numerous other algorithms have been described to identify outliers and disproportionately influential readings; these have been reviewed by Cook and Weisberg [4]. These algorithms usually give similar results, although exceptions may occur.

How much should the data be edited?

We can never be absolutely sure whether an individual reading is an artefact or not. Elimination of artefacts and outliers has both benefits and costs. The extent to which editing should be applied may vary from one study to another, depending on issues such as the nature of the population being studied, the statistical procedures which will be used to analyse the data, the estimates or parameters to be derived and other considerations.

Most investigators agree that algorithms which detect physiologically improbable readings in most commercially available software packages are on the whole appropriate. It is highly likely that these readings are artefacts, which can bias the summary statistics.

Readings that are not automatically eliminated but are labelled as suspicious by one of the outlier detection methods described above are less likely to be extreme, less likely to be artefactual and less likely to bias the summary statistics. By eliminating such outliers a set of readings which are more similar to each other, that is with a lower variance, is created. Although this similarity will tend to give a more precise estimate of the effect of interest, this apparent precision may give a false sense of security if non-artefactual readings are eliminated. Further-

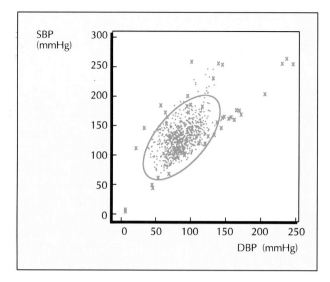

Fig. 16.2. Scatter diagram of systolic pressure and diastolic pressure enhanced with an ellipsoid region for detecting likely artefacts. Points outside the region are readings identified by one analytical model, and those labelled with an x by another model. Reproduced with permission [2].

more, these outliers, if they are genuine readings, are potentially the most interesting data points.

Very little work has been done to evaluate the consequences of editing data. Staessen *et al.* [5] used editing criteria similar to those described in the previous section, and concluded that whether the data points identified by these criteria were excluded or included made very little difference to the estimates of mean blood pressure. Further work of this type should be encouraged.

Test theory, reliability and generalizability

'Reliability' is an important concept in the analysis of ambulatory blood pressure data. It is defined as the proportion of variance in a measure that is attributable to true variability as opposed to measurement error. Such errors may be random or non-random; the latter are discussed in the next section. Estimates of reliability can be obtained using formulae derived from classic test theory [6,7], originally developed to assess the validity of psychometric tests measuring constructs such as intelligence. The procedures are also useful in blood pressure research, where many independent replications of measurement are made and many sources of variation need to be considered: between-person, within-person, within-situation and so forth. The procedures allow estimation of the precision of individual readings, of the average value for an individual subject and also of the number of readings needed to obtain a particular degree of reliability. We [8] have also used classic test theory measurement models to criticize and refine the methodology of laboratory reactivity testing, discussed in Chapter 12.

Reliability theory predicts that when the reliability of a particular measure is low, the relationships between that measure and any other are also likely to be low. We have provided evidence [8] suggesting that a major reason for the inconclusive findings relating cardiovascular reactivity to blood pressure variability may be the low reliability of the measures of reactivity. Under assumptions of constancy of effect and variance, one solution to the reliability problem is to obtain more measurements. This, of course, can be done with ambulatory monitors. Although any single reading taken by a monitor is likely to be less reliable than a single casual measurement, the greater number of readings that can be obtained means that monitoring should provide a more reliable summary measure than casual measurement.

Cronbach *et al.* [7] have extended the reliability model to incorporate estimates of reliability for measurements taken under different conditions. This generalizability or G-theory model enables one to derive estimates of reliability across a range of measurement conditions or occasions. The statistical procedure involves the allocation of variation according to its various determinants — individual, location, occasion and so on — using analysis of variance. This model was used by Llabre *et al.* [9] to estimate the number of blood pressure readings needed to achieve a given precision in laboratory, clinic and ambulatory settings.

Non-random sources of measurement error

Each blood pressure measurement is subject to a certain degree of error, some of which is non-random. An example of this was provided by a validation study of the Spacelabs 90207 ambulatory recorder [10], in which we found that the combination of being young and female was associated with a tendency for the recorder to overestimate blood pressure; overestimation was not apparent in subjects who were older and male [10]. Another example is exercise: in a study of the Oxford Medilog recorder [11] good agreement was observed between the recorder and observer at rest, but as the level of exercise (walking) increased there was a progressively greater overestimation of blood pressure by the recorder.

Clearly, these types of error may introduce a significant bias in estimates of the effects of situational variables on blood pressure and in the comparisons of blood pressure between groups.

Measures of centrality

Since ambulatory monitoring was first introduced, estimation of the average or mean level of blood pressure has been the most widely used method of describing the data. Estimates can be made over varying time periods, for example over 4 h, during the waking hours or over 24 h, or according to situational variables (e.g. work and home). These estimates permit comparisons of levels in previously defined groups (e.g. normotensives and hypertensives, blacks and whites).

Mean or median?

Ambulatory blood pressure data can be characterized in three distinct ways: as interval, ordinal or nominal measurements. For each of these, different statistical procedures are used. With interval measurements it is assumed that the absolute difference between measurements has meaning: for example, the difference between 90 and 100 mmHg is the same as between 50 and 60 mmHg. With ordinal measurements only their ranking has meaning: 100 mmHg is higher than 90 mmHg. Nominal measurements are simply categorized in groups, for example normotensives and hypertensives.

In most cases, blood pressure data are assumed to be interval measurements (and also to be normally distributed). Parametric procedures are used for interval measurements, and means and standard deviations are derived. If the measurements are assumed to be ordinal, non-parametric procedures are used, and medians and interquartile ranges calculated. Finally, if the measurements are assumed to be nominal, categorical procedures are appropriate, and statistics such as odds and rates are calculated.

Although most reports of ambulatory blood pressure data have used the arithmetical mean to describe the level of pressure for any given situation, a case could be made for using the median value instead. Unlike the mean, the median is a non-parametric statistic and has the advantage of being influenced less by outliers at one or other extreme of the range of values. If the data are highly skewed, the median will be closer to the centre or peak of the distribution curve than the mean. However, blood pressure data are usually only slightly skewed (towards the higher readings), so that the mean and median are likely to be very close, as demonstrated in Fig. 16.3, which shows the data from Fig. 16.1 replotted as histograms, with and without adjustment for location.

We recommend the use of the mean rather than the median, for several reasons. First, most of the available data is expressed as mean values; second, more statistical procedures are based on the use of means; and third, statistical theory has shown that the estimate of a measure of centrality is more efficient using the mean (i.e. it is more precise and has a lower variance), provided the data are normally distributed[1]. This assumption of normality implies that a larger than expected number of extreme values or artefacts is not present.

Area under the curve

The AUC has gained some adherents, both for expressing the average level of ambulatory pressure and for defining the effects of antihypertensive medication. In a plot of

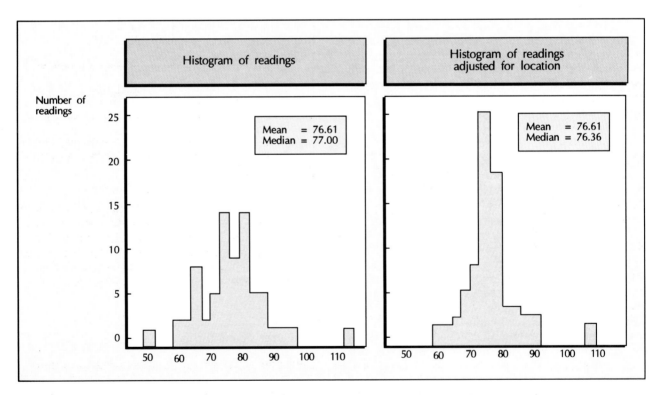

Fig. 16.3. Data from Fig. 16.1 replotted as histograms: (a) unadjusted data; (b) data adjusted for location. Note that in each case the distribution is approximately normal, and that the mean and median values are very similar.

---

[1]The 'normal distribution' of blood pressure has two aspects to it, which should not be confused with each other. The first is the distribution of true blood pressure within a population; whether this distribution curve was unimodal or bimodal provided the basis of the celebrated Pickering–Platt debate [12]. The second aspect is the variation of individual subjects' blood pressure around the true pressure. As it happens, both these distribution curves are approximately normal, with some skewness towards the higher end of the curves.

blood pressure against time, the AUC is the area enclosed by lines joining successive data points at the beginning and end of the measurement period and the lines joining the first and last points to the x axis (zero blood pressure). This approach is conceptually appealing as a measure of the overall burden or load of blood pressure. As a general rule, it will give values that are very close to the average level, but the correspondence will not be exact. Two individuals with the same average blood pressure but different variability will have different AUCs, with the more labile individual probably showing a smaller AUC.

A potential advantage of the AUC is that when the interval between readings increases (e.g. because of missing data), these readings are weighted more than readings separated by shorter intervals. In contrast, the simple average does not incorporate any such time weighting.

The AUC suffers from many of the same problems as the mean. If there are periods during the recording where the error rate is high (e.g. because of movement artefact), the remaining readings will have a disproportionately large influence on the AUC, and if they too are erroneous, they may introduce a significant bias. We do not favour the use of the AUC because it is influenced both by the mean level and by the variability of blood pressure, and we prefer to analyse these two components separately.

Blood pressure load
Several investigators have used this measure, particularly for correlating ambulatory blood pressure with target organ damage [13,14], as reviewed in Chapter 9. The basic concept is simple, but in our opinion is of limited validity. The blood pressure load is expressed as the percentage of readings above a fixed threshold level, typically 140/90 mmHg, as proposed by Zachariah *et al.* [13], or 140/90 mmHg during the day and 120/80 mmHg at night, as proposed by White *et al.* [14]. The estimate of load will be greatly influenced by the policy adopted for editing extreme values. If the number of readings is relatively small, the variance of the estimate of the percentage of readings above the threshold level will be much greater than for the estimate of the mean level. In other words, load is likely to be a less reliable measure than the mean. Although it has been claimed that the load correlates more closely with measures of target organ damage than the average pressure [14], it is likely that this will be true only over a relatively narrow range of blood pressure, for reasons given below.

The conceptual problem is illustrated in Fig. 16.4, which shows the relationship between blood pressure load and the average (true) blood pressure. The fact that the relationship is sigmoid means that above a certain level of average blood pressure the load plateaus at 100%. It seems most unlikely that the relationships between blood pressure and its consequences are of this type, and indeed all the evidence points to the opposite view, namely that the relationship becomes steeper rather than flatter at the

highest levels of pressure [15,16], as shown in Fig. 16.4. Furthermore, the relationship between load and average pressure depends on the threshold value used to define the load, the choice of which is arbitrary. Thus, there is no convincing evidence that any sudden increase in risk occurs above a blood pressure of 140/90 mmHg (see, for example, Fig. 1.2). Another argument against the use of blood pressure load may be used by its advocates in its support: it is influenced both by the average level and by the variability of blood pressure. If one is interested in deciding which of these two components is more important it is essential to analyse them separately.

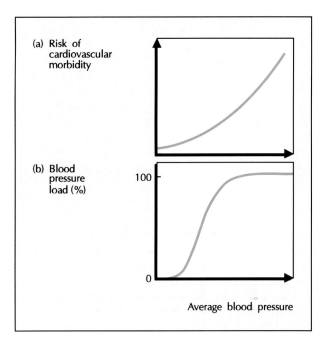

Fig. 16.4. Hypothetical relationship (a) between blood pressure and its consequences, and (b) between average blood pressure and blood pressure load.

White [17], one of the original advocates of the concept of blood pressure load, has suggested a refinement which incorporates two measures (AUC and load) and overcomes some of the limitations described above. This estimates the AUC above the threshold level used to define the blood pressure load, as shown in Fig. 16.5.

Estimates of mean levels according to activity

An alternative method of analysis is based on activity or location, rather than on a fixed period of time. This type of analysis obviously depends on accurate diaries being kept by the subjects. We routinely analyse our data according to whether the subject is at work, at home or asleep, and have argued elsewhere (Chapters 4 and 5) that activity is a more important determinant of blood pressure than the time of day [18]. The effects of a wide range of physical and mental activities on blood pressure are discussed in detail in Chapter 4. Here, we will confine ourselves to the analytical issues.

Ambulatory monitoring is normally performed in free-ranging subjects, whose activities will almost certainly show significant between-subject differences. If these differences are very large, they will introduce a significant bias in the overall mean level of blood pressure. A prime example of this would be the comparison of data from one subject studied on a work day and another subject studied on a non-work day. This confounding factor is equally important for within-subject comparisons. An example of this would be a study assessing the effects of an antihypertensive medication, in which the same subjects are monitored on and off medication. Activity should, as far as possible, be held constant from one occasion to another in order to minimize the potential confounding of the effects of the medication from changes in activity between occasions.

When examining the effects of situational variables on blood pressure in a group of subjects it is important to adjust for individual differences in baseline blood pressure, as pointed out by Van Egeren and Madarasmi [19]. If, for example, the effects of smoking and watching television are being compared, this adjustment will distinguish between the transient effects of smoking on blood pressure and a generally higher mean blood pressure in smokers than in non-smokers. An important consideration is which pressure should be taken as the baseline. One frequently used measure is the calibration readings taken at the start of the ambulatory recording. Although this measure has the advantage of being taken under highly standardized conditions, it may not be very representative of the individual's true blood pressure. An alternative is to use the average waking pressure, which avoids

this problem, but is itself influenced by the effects of the situational variables of interest.

Another question that should be addressed here is whether the readings that define the blood pressure for any specific activity are consecutive. If, for example, the pressure at work is being estimated, this is nearly always the case. However, if the pressure during telephoning is of interest, there may be several periods during the day when such readings are available, but they are likely to be interspersed with other activities. The same applies to home readings, which may include two distinct periods, the early morning and the evening, that are likely to be characterized by different activities and blood pressures.

It is customary to take readings every 15 min during the day and every 30 min at night. If the interval between readings varies in this way, the level of blood pressure at night will be under-represented if the simple 24-hour average is computed. Therefore, a time-weighted average level would be more appropriate.

The level of blood pressure for any location or activity is likely to be confounded by other co-factors. For example, we are more likely to be standing while at work than at home, and most of the readings taken lying down will be during sleep. Therefore, the apparent difference between work and home blood pressure could be due to the effects of changes in posture rather than the effects of work itself. Several strategies have been used to address this problem. One common technique is to study the effects of each location for each level of the confounding variables. For example, Llabre *et al.* [9] and Gellman *et al.* [20] calculated the average blood pressure level for each location (at work and at home) separately for two positions (seated and standing). They concluded that the effects of posture accounted for more of the overall vari-

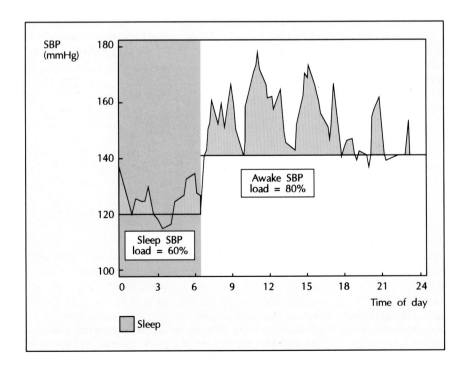

Fig. 16.5. Two methods of analysing the overall level of blood pressure over 24 h, as proposed by White [17]: (a) as blood pressure load (the percentage readings above 140 mmHg during the day and above 120 mmHg during sleep), and (b) as the area under the curve above the threshold level (blue shaded areas).

ance of blood pressure than the effects of location. The obvious problem with this strategy is that the number of possible confounders must be small, otherwise the number of combinations of activities, postures and locations could easily become too unwieldy.

An alternative strategy is to derive estimates of the effects of activities and other variables by statistically controlling for the effects of potential confounders. Clark *et al.* [18], Pieper [21], Pieper *et al.* (submitted for publication) and Marler *et al.* [3] all used regression techniques to estimate the effects of location while controlling for differences in posture, whereas James *et al.* [22] used analysis of covariance to estimate the effects of emotion while controlling for posture, location and time of day.

Potential problems with the use of mean values

The calculation of a summary measure such as the mean is a standard procedure and is usually the measure of choice: it is not, however, without its problems. In particular, it may lead to biased results in some conditions and may not necessarily be the most efficient measure. Some of the more important problems are considered below.

Co-factors and multicollinearity

Many of the variables of interest are likely to be highly correlated with each other. This correlation needs to be taken into account when performing the analyses. In the present context this factor applies both to the independent variables (the situational factors) and to the dependent variables (the different measures of blood pressure). Thus, sleeping and reclining are obviously closely related with each other. In statistical terms, when multiple regression analysis is performed with correlated variables, the regression coefficients will have unduly large standard errors.

If the research question involves the calculation of a summary measure for one of the sources of variation, it is essential to control for the confounding effect of the other sources by statistical or experimental means. This point can also be illustrated by the example of the higher blood pressure recorded at work than at home, which has often been attributed to the higher level of stress at work. An alternative explanation is that people are standing for a greater proportion of time at work than at home, and that the higher pressure is merely a consequence of this. Thus, in one of our early studies, we reported a blood pressure difference of 5/4 mmHg between work and home [1]. A later analysis (admittedly on a different set of data), which controlled for the effects of posture, estimated this difference to be only 2/2 mmHg [21]. Gellman *et al.* [20] used a method that estimated the effects

of location separately for each position. In their study, the average work–home difference for diastolic pressure was 4 mmHg. When only the readings taken in the two locations while seated were included, the difference was exactly the same. However, there was no difference between the pressures measured while standing at work and standing at home. This suggests that the effects of standing on blood pressure override the effects of location. One could take this co-factor argument further and claim that it is not the effects of standing itself but the other activities associated with standing that are responsible for the higher pressures. This can, of course, be investigated experimentally as well as statistically. In Chapter 4 it was pointed out that postural change *per se*, in controlled laboratory conditions, has a negligible effect on systolic pressure, although diastolic pressure changes markedly. In a statistical analysis of data from 211 men studied with ambulatory monitoring, Pieper [21] found that standing raised blood pressure by 5/3 mmHg relative to sitting, while reclining (but not sleeping) lowered blood pressure by 4/6 mmHg, after controlling for location.

Differential precision and heteroscedasticity

In any field study using ambulatory monitoring, it is likely that the numbers of readings for any activity will vary considerably from one individual to another, and different individuals may have quite different activities. As noted above, failure to allow for these differences may affect the estimate of the average 24-hour blood pressures. Furthermore, the variability of blood pressure for any activity is unlikely to be the same for all subjects, although the assumption of equal variability (homoscedasticity)[2] is an important component of many statistical procedures. The problems of comparing ambulatory blood pressure recordings made in different subjects, and even in the same subject on different occasions, are emphasized by Fig. 16.6. This figure shows the timing of readings made in 27 subjects (13 hypertensives and 14 normotensives), studied on two separate days according to the same protocol, with readings taken every 15 min during the day and every 30 min at night [23]. Both factors (the number and the variability of readings) will affect the precision with which mean levels of blood pressure can be estimated. If the purpose of the research is to estimate the population value for a group of subjects, the precision of the estimate can be improved by incorporating these two factors into the summary estimation procedure. Each subject's mean would be weighted by some function of each of these two factors, using techniques such as those described by Hedges and Olkin [24].

Autocorrelation

Ambulatory blood pressure readings are typically made at regular intervals, often every 15 min. Many statisti-

---

[2]Homoscedasticity exists if the variance of a function is the same for all individuals and situations. Because, as described in Chapter 4, the variability of blood pressure usually increases at higher levels of pressure and some people's pressure is more labile than others', independent of the average level, heteroscedasticity between individuals may exist. Within-person heteroscedasticity may also occur if different activities are associated with different blood pressure variability, independent of level. Both types can have effects on the precision of the estimates, and if heteroscedasticity is extreme remedial statistical procedures may be necessary.

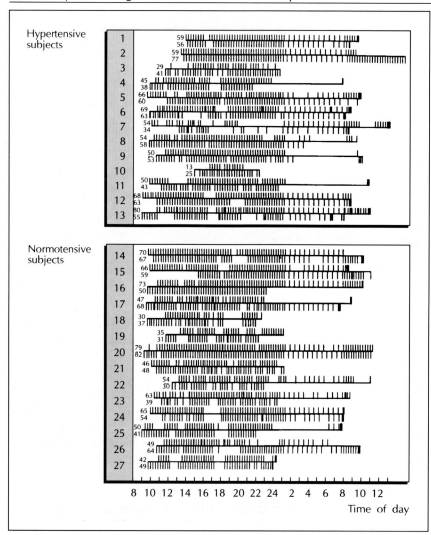

Hypertensive subjects

Normotensive subjects

8 10 12 14 16 18 20 22 24 2 4 6 8 10 12

Time of day

Fig. 16.6. The timing of ambulatory blood pressure readings in 27 subjects (13 hypertensive and 14 normotensive), each of whom was monitored on 2 days. The readings for day 1 are plotted as vertical bars above the horizontal line, and those for day 2 below. The number of readings for each of the days is shown at the beginning of the line. Reproduced with permission [23].

cal procedures operate on the assumption that individual measurements are independent of each other, but when serial measurements of a variable such as blood pressure are made over short time intervals (referred to as a time series), this assumption is not necessarily valid [25]. It is reasonable to suppose that measurements made at shorter time intervals from each other will show a higher degree of autocorrelation (i.e. correlation with each other) than ones made over longer intervals. This type of correlation is generally expressed in terms of the residuals, that is the deviation of each reading from the average level rather than the readings themselves, after first controlling for the influence of factors which are thought to influence blood pressure. Autocorrelation expressed in this way could, in principle, occur for two reasons: first, as a result of a prolonged response time to a perturbation or stimulus, and second, as a result of a prolonged stimulus. For readings made every 15 min or so, the former possibility is less likely to apply, since blood pressure can change from very high to very low levels over much shorter periods than 15 min. An example of the latter would be the combination of drinking coffee and smoking a cigarette, which can increase blood pres-

sure for more than 2 h, as shown in Fig. 4.9. The degree of autocorrelation is of particular relevance in the analysis of the effects of situational variables such as posture, activity and mood on blood pressure. The analytical procedures described above all assume that individual readings are independent of each other, and that the corresponding diary entries can be related to each reading.

For data obtained with ambulatory blood pressure monitoring at intervals ranging from every 5 min to every hour, it has been suggested that there may be some autocorrelation between consecutive readings [26]. However, it is likely to be relatively small in most experimental settings: in an analysis of the autocorrelation between residuals of readings measured very 15 min, controlling for position and location, Pieper [21] found first-order autocorrelation coefficients of 0.10 for systolic pressure and 0.15 for diastolic pressure. Similar results were obtained by Van Egeren and Madarasmi [19], who found coefficients of 0.18 for systolic and 0.17 for diastolic pressure. Thus, fewer than 4% of the variability of blood pressure readings can be explained by the value of the immediately preceding readings. Using a statistical measure that is affected by autocorrelation, the root of the mean squared successive differences (RMSSD), Schachinger *et al.* [27] found that, for an individual subject, the standard deviation of the blood pressure was often greater than the RMSSD, indicating that a positive autocorrelation may have been present. These findings of a generally low level of autocorrelation indicate that it is valid to relate individual blood pressure readings to the corresponding situational variables.

It is important to note that even if autocorrelation is present, it does not affect the estimate of the mean level of pressure. However, under the conditions generally found in ambulatory blood pressure recordings, it will result in an underestimate of the variability (e.g. the standard error of the mean). For an autocorrelation coefficient of 0.15, failure to incorporate the autocorrelation will result in a confidence interval for the estimate of the mean value which is as much as 30% too small.

Multiple tests and type I error

A type I error is the chance finding of a statistically significant relationship when in fact none exists. Type I errors are likely to occur if multiple comparisons are made. In most analyses of ambulatory blood pressure data, the mean values corresponding to several different periods of time or activity are reported. These calculations are commonly followed by tests of whether the mean values are significantly different from each other, for example between locations, activities or groups of subjects. While such multiple comparisons may reveal differences that truly exist, they also increase the likelihood of a type I error. Clearly, the more comparisons that are made, the greater is the likelihood of this occurring. Type I errors can be reduced by employing correction factors for multiple testing [28].

Furthermore, if the tests indicate that two groups differ significantly for one comparison (e.g. work blood pressure), but not for another (e.g. home blood pressure), it cannot be concluded that the difference between the two variables is significantly different between the groups. One method to overcome this problem is to use multivariate or repeated measure designs in the analyses [29]. This permits the simultaneous comparison of several different means, and also controls for type I errors. Another technique would be to use hierarchical linear models, as proposed by Marler *et al.* [3]. A problem with the standard repeated measures designs is that complete data are required for every subject. The greater the number of measures being compared, the greater is the chance that for an individual subject data will be missing from one of the measures; the subject will therefore be eliminated from the entire analysis. This problem is well illustrated by a study reported by Gellman *et al.* [20], who compared the mean pressure levels for four situational variables (supine, sitting, standing and walking) in 131 subjects. Data for all four measures were obtained from only 53 subjects. The exclusion of so many subjects from the analysis may lead to biased results and conclusions, unless the subjects are a random subset of the total sample, which is unlikely.

Measures of variability

The important but neglected issue of blood pressure variability was discussed in Chapter 4, where it was argued that, as conventionally used, the term encompasses a number of sources of variability with different physiological mechanisms and time courses. The short-term variability that is associated with respiration and Mayer waves can only be evaluated by beat-to-beat measurement of blood pressure and, with intermittent blood pressure sampling, merely serves as a source of random error. With sampling every 15 min, the main source of variability is likely to be changes in physical and mental activity. The overall level of variability will be determined by two factors: the frequency and intensity of different activities on the one hand, and blood pressure reactivity to these different stimuli on the other. For research purposes it may be important to separate the relative contributions of these two factors. In principle, this could be done statistically or experimentally. Using a statistical method, variability would be standardized for changes in the levels of situational variables (for example posture, location and activity); an experiment could involve putting subjects through a standardized protocol; such a protocol is used for reactivity testing in the laboratory, but has so far rarely been used in ambulatory monitoring.

Absolute or relative measures of variability

An important question concerns whether variability should be expressed in absolute terms (e.g. as the standard deviation) or in relative terms (e.g. as the coefficient of variation). As pointed out in Chapter 4, within-subject short-term variability (measured over half-hour intervals with intra-arterial monitoring) increases as the average level of blood pressure increases, regardless of whether it is expressed in absolute or in relative terms [30]. On the other hand, comparison of variability between subjects (normotensive versus hypertensive subjects) shows that it is higher in absolute terms at higher levels of pressure but not in relative terms.

From the above considerations, it is clear that, in statistical terms, blood pressure variability is heteroscedastic. When variability is positively correlated with the mean level, as may be the case with blood pressure, it may be appropriate to use a simple power transformation to equalize the variance across levels [31]. However, there is no guarantee that this procedure, which may stabilize within-subject variability, will also stabilize between-subject variability.

In our research, we generally prefer to use absolute measures of variability, because they keep the variability and the level of blood pressure distinct from each other. If, for example, we want to determine whether blood pressure level or variability is a more potent predictor of cardiovascular morbidity, we might obtain a very similar estimate of risk using level and relative variability of pressure, because the latter measure incorporates level. Given the fact that variability is not independent of the average level, we really want to know whether variability adds anything to the prediction of outcome over and above the mean level (i.e. controlling for mean level). This can be done best by using an absolute measure of variability.

Thus, for any investigation comparing the variability and level of pressure, it is first appropriate to analyse the relationship between the two and then to relate variability to the outcome measure after controlling for level. This would apply not only when blood pressure is the independent variable (as in the example quoted above), but also when it is the dependent variable, for example in an analysis of the effects of antihypertensive treatment on the level and variability of blood pressure.

Which measure of variability should be used?

Several possible measures can be used to express blood pressure variability. The standard deviation has been most widely used, and is a valid measure if the data are normally distributed, as is usually true for blood pressure. The standard deviation has the additional advantage of being expressed in the same units as the mean (mmHg) whereas the variance (another possible measure) is expressed as squared units (mmHg^2).

It is important to stress that outliers in the data will have a much greater effect on the variance or standard deviation than on the mean, because the first two measures are derived from the square of the differences of individual readings from the mean. Furthermore, extreme positive and negative outliers will balance each other out for the estimate of the mean level, but will increase the estimate of variability disproportionately. If such outliers are artefactual readings, they should be eliminated from the data. However, we cannot know which values are artefacts and which are true, but extreme, readings. This was discussed above but it should be stressed here that any editing can have a major influence on the estimates of blood pressure variability.

A way out of this dilemma is to use non-parametric measures of variability, such as the interquartile range, which are less susceptible to the influence of outliers. This type of measure has been used relatively infrequently [32], but is valid and particularly useful where there are outliers and artefacts.

Another measure, the use of which has been advocated by Schachinger et al. [27], is the RMSSD. The important difference of this from other measures of variability is that it takes into consideration the time sequence of the readings. Figure 16.7 shows three examples of hypothetical data which have the same mean and standard deviation but different variabilities: this would be revealed by the RMSSD. The RMSSD is, therefore, useful in situations where short-term blood pressure variability needs to be

distinguished from a trend or step-change in blood pressure. Schachinger et al. suggested that it might be useful for expressing 24-hour variability, although it would not distinguish between dippers and non-dippers. When variability is expressed over shorter periods, or for a situational variable (e.g. at work), the RMSSD would not have any advantage over the standard deviation.

Conditional measures of variability

In most ambulatory studies the variability of blood pressure is determined by two factors: behavioural (variations of activity during the recording) and non-behavioural (the individual's intrinsic blood pressure lability). As with the mean level of blood pressure, it may be appropriate to relate measures of variability to situational variables such as activity. Comparing variability in individuals whose level of physical activity is very different may give spurious results if one is interested in endogenous differences in blood pressure variability. In such instances it may be appropriate to control statistically for the relevant situational variables. This would be particularly relevant in studies relating blood pressure reactivity measured in the laboratory to ambulatory blood pressure variability. An ingenious method for separating the behavioural and non-behavioural components of blood pressure variability has been used by Van Egeren and Sparrow [33], who assumed that the latter could be represented by the variability during sleep. Daytime variability was adjusted for variability during sleep to evaluate the behavioural component.

Analysis of diurnal rhythms

The existence of a diurnal rhythm of blood pressure was recognized long before the introduction of ambulatory monitoring. The phenomenon has been reviewed extensively in Chapter 5. It provides an alternative method for analysing blood pressure changes, based on the time of day rather than on situational variables such as activity and location. Its chief advantage is that the analysis is much simpler, as there is only one independent variable, time, which proceeds monotonically and predictably. It is not essential to have a diary, because all the non-invasive recorders automatically record the time of each reading. However, all statistical methods for analysing time series work best if the data are collected at equal time intervals. The common use of less frequent readings during the night presents a problem, therefore, which may be further exacerbated if many readings are missing.

There has been considerable controversy about whether time of day is a primary determinant of blood pressure, or whether it is merely a proxy measure of the activities that occur at regular intervals throughout the day and night. In Chapter 5 we argued that the bulk of evidence favours the view that activity is the prime determinant. Below we discuss three methods for analysing diurnal rhythms for which the major determining factor is as-

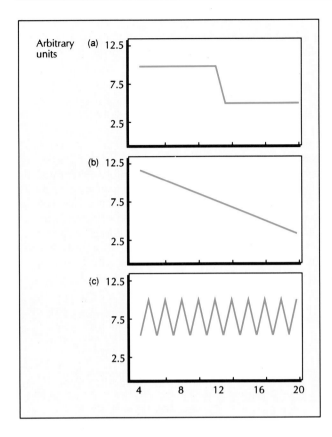

Fig. 16.7. Three hypothetical series of data points, which have the same mean and standard deviation (2.5 arbitrary units). The RMSSD shows the difference in the pattern of variations, and is 1.15 in (a), 0.43 in (b), and 5 in (c). Reproduced with permission [27].

sumed to be time of day, and also methods for which it is assumed to be activity.

Whatever the final verdict on this controversy, there is a definite need for methods of analysis which can quantify the diurnal profile of blood pressure. There is extensive evidence (again reviewed in Chapter 5) that individual subjects may show substantial deviations from the usual diurnal rhythm by showing little or no decrease in blood pressure during the night (the 'non-dippers'). So far as is known, these deviations are not dependent on differences in physical activity or arousal.

Cosinor analysis

Cosinor analysis has been widely used for analysing biological parameters that show a true circadian rhythm (of which blood pressure may or may not be an example). The basic principle is to fit the data to a cosine wave with a periodicity of 24 h [34,35]. The basis for this type of analysis is a three parameter equation of the form:

$$f(t) = a_o + A\cos(2\pi t + \phi)$$

where $f(t)$ is the blood pressure at time t, a_o is the average 24 hour blood pressure, A is the amplitude of the diurnal wave, and ϕ is the phase angle (equivalent to the

timing of the peak and trough of the wave). The data points are fitted to the cosine curve by a least squares method which permits the estimation of A and ϕ. We argued in Chapter 5 that this procedure makes the assumption that the peak and trough of the blood pressure are exactly 12 h apart, and equidistant from the mean level (or, more precisely, the mesor). Unfortunately, this is rarely the case, and so a more empirical, if mathematically less pure, approach is needed. An example of the relatively poor fit with the data points provided by this type of analysis is shown in Fig. 16.8. In one of the most thoughtful papers on the topic, Streitberg *et al.* [26] pointed out other deficiencies of this model. These are as follows.

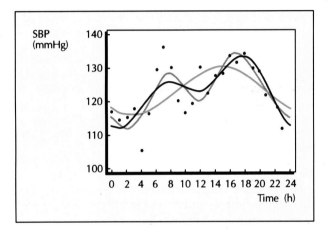

Fig. 16.8. Twenty-four-hour blood pressure readings from a normotensive subject analysed according to the cosinor method (blue line), and with addition of a second (black line) and third (grey line) harmonic with periods of 12 and 8 h, respectively. Reproduced with permission [5].

(1) If there is a high degree of autocorrelation between successive blood pressure readings, the gradual changes after any change of activity (e.g. the sleep–waking cycle) may be misinterpreted as a sine wave.

(2) The model is very sensitive to the effects of missing readings, or readings taken at irregular intervals.

(3) The model assumes that the residuals (i.e. the deviations of individual values from the ideal curve) are independent, homoscedastic and normally distributed.

(4) The diurnal pattern of blood pressure is assumed to be biphasic, whereas in practice it is often multiphasic (for example, in Italians who take a siesta).

(5) The model predicts that a histogram of blood pressure values would be bimodal, as most of the readings should occur at the two extremes of blood pressure. In practice, the predicted distributions of blood pressure are not observed, and, as shown in Fig. 16.3, are unimodal and slightly skewed to the right.

The limitations of cosinor analysis are described in greater mathematical detail by Van Cauter and Huyberechts [36].

Fourier analysis

Given that a single cosine function may not adequately describe the diurnal rhythm of blood pressure, a more elaborate analysis can be undertaken using a Fourier analysis, which involves adding a series of harmonics with periods such as 12, 8, 6, 4, 3, 2 and 1 h to the analysis. This process has been applied by Van Cauter to the analysis of the diurnal variations of blood hormone levels, and is referred to as 'periodogram' analysis [36,37]. A number of steps are recommended. First, the means and standard deviations for 24 h, day and night, are calculated. This will give an estimate of whether there are significant day–night differences. Second, the presence of rhythmical changes can be tested for in two ways: one examines whether consecutive readings are autocorrelated, and the second tests whether the oscillations about the mean correspond to 'white noise', in which case the integrated spectrum is a linear function of the frequency. Fourier analysis is then applied to the data. This is likely to provide a better fit to the data than the simpler cosine analysis, as shown in Fig. 16.8.

Spline models[3]

The use of spline models has been advocated by Streitberg [26], and has the advantage of being empirical and non-parametric. It also provides a smoothed curve of the data points, but makes no *a priori* assumptions about its shape. The data series is divided into a series of 'knot sequences', in which each knot is a point where the data points suddenly change direction. Knots can be chosen either idiometrically (i.e. fitted individually for each subject or data series) or as a fixed sequence. For both practical and statistical reasons, Streitberg advocates using a fixed sequence of eight knots, with times corresponding to 0200, 0530, 0800, 1000, 1200, 1600, 2030 and 2200 hours. The data points are fitted for each interval between successive knots, and the end result is a smoothed curve of the diurnal profile of blood pressure. It could be argued that this type of analysis is more activity-dependent than time-dependent, since the knots clearly correspond to times at which activities are likely to change. This type of analysis is not available in standard statistical packages and has not so far been used in published studies.

Analysis based on activity

The alternative approach to the analysis of diurnal rhythms is to assume that activity and arousal are the primary determining factors, and to base the analysis on the subjects' diary entries or (less satisfactorily) on some arbitrary time when most subjects are usually asleep (e.g. 10.00 p.m. to 6.00 a.m.). We have argued elsewhere (Chapter 5) that there is a 'step change' in blood pressure both on falling asleep and on waking up, and that this is of greater magnitude than the changes occurring during the hours of sleep.

In general, two strategies have been employed to assess the effects of activities on blood pressure. According to the first, all data from all subjects are pooled and analyses are then performed on the entire set of readings. This strategy has been used by a number of investigators, including our own group [2,19,22], and has the advantage that it is possible to control for confounders and cofactors. Furthermore, individual differences in overall blood pressure level can be allowed for by adjusting for baseline and standardizing the readings before analysis. However, this method is open to criticism because of the variable number of readings per subject and because it assumes independence of measurements both within and between subjects.

According to the second strategy, the means for each activity are calculated separately for each subject. The means are then averaged to arrive at a summary estimate of the effects of the activities in the population. We have also used this method to estimate the effects of situational variables such as work, home and sleep [1]. Although this method is probably more sound statistically, because it does not rest so much on an assumption of independence of observation, it does not control for cofactors and confounders. Furthermore, the differential precision of the estimates for each subject do not allow for the different numbers of readings per subject.

A more sophisticated approach is based on a recently described set of statistical procedures called hierarchical linear models [38], such as that used by Marler *et al.* [3] and Pieper [21]. These models show promise as a method for addressing many of the statistical and analytical concerns outlined in this chapter. The general approach involves two stages: first, estimating the effects of the situational variables separately for each subject; second, summarizing the estimates across subjects to arrive at estimates for the population, and then testing for differences between groups of subjects. The model can be adapted to address statistical concerns such as confounding factors and cofactors, precision, autocorrelation and heteroscedasticity. However, this area is still actively evolving in the statistical literature and is not yet available in commercial software.

Evaluation of treatment effects

As we have seen in Chapter 10, ambulatory monitoring is becoming a routine part of the evaluation of new antihypertensive medications. The standard procedure is to compare at least two recordings for each patient, one made while untreated and one during treatment. Ambulatory monitoring permits the analysis of two factors which cannot be evaluated by conventional measurements: the duration of action of a medication, and its effects on the diurnal rhythm of blood pressure. How these should be analysed is discussed below.

---

[3]A spline is a flexible strip used by draughtsmen for drawing curves.

Duration of action

It is generally assumed that effective antihypertensive treatment requires a sustained reduction in blood pressure throughout the day and night (although this assumption has never been empirically tested). Traditionally, to test this with ambulatory blood pressure data, consecutive hourly averages with and without treatment are compared, for example by using multiple t-tests [39–41]. However, such multiple testing greatly increases the probability of a type I error, as discussed above. In a typical study, 24 hourly comparisons would be made. If a significance value (α) of 0.05 is chosen, a correction factor such as the Bonferroni criterion could be applied, according to which each individual t test would require an α of 0.05/24 (0.002) or less to be considered significant. Although this procedure is statistically correct, it clearly reduces the chances of finding significant differences.

A better strategy would be to examine the effects of treatment over longer periods of time, for example 4 h, or by situation (work, home, sleep). The latter would be more powerful statistically, although at some sacrifice of temporal discrimination.

Repeated measures procedures have also traditionally been used to analyse this type of problem. They are included in most standard statistical software packages. However, this approach is severely limited by the fact that all data points must be present; this is rarely the case with ambulatory blood pressure data.

Effects on diurnal rhythm of blood pressure

The possibility that different types of treatment may have different effects on the diurnal rhythm of blood pressure is of considerable interest. An extension of the method proposed by Marler et al. [3] may be appropriate to answer this question. In their analysis, each patient's ambulatory blood pressure was measured with four different treatment modalities. For each individual separately, the effects of time of day, activity (sleeping, resting, standing) and treatment were estimated while simultaneously controlling for the other effects. These effects were then combined across individuals to arrive at summary estimates for the sample. This method of first estimating the treatment effects for each individual and then combining the results may be preferable to the alternative method of comparing the aggregate pre- and post-treatment values.

Summary and conclusions

The methods by which ambulatory recordings of blood pressure should be analysed largely depend on the purpose for which the readings were made. For the clinician interested primarily in the patient's true blood pressure, the average day, night and 24-hour levels may be all that are required. For the researcher interested in factors influencing blood pressure variability, much more detailed and sophisticated procedures are needed.

For any analysis, the first question to be addressed is the extent to which suspected artefacts in the data should be eliminated. Most ambulatory blood pressure software packages incorporate some editing of physiologically improbable readings, which we believe to be appropriate. Beyond this, however, we recommend that data editing should be kept to a minimum. Eliminating outliers is likely to have a much greater effect on the estimate of the variability of blood pressure than the mean level.

It is appropriate to consider ambulatory blood pressure data as a combination of the mean or steady-state level and the phasic variations about the mean. Both can be estimated statistically. Several measures of centrality have been proposed for estimating the mean level. Since the distribution of blood pressure data is approximately normal, use of the median has no clear advantage over the arithmetical mean. However, the intervals between consecutive readings are likely to vary, so that the estimate can be improved by time weighting. Other measures which have been advocated include the AUC and blood pressure load. Both these methods suffer conceptually from being influenced by variability as well as the mean level, and blood pressure load makes the unwarranted assumption that there is a threshold level for the harmful effects of blood pressure.

Because any measure of blood pressure is profoundly influenced by the circumstances in which the readings are taken, and ambulatory monitoring is normally carried out in relatively uncontrolled conditions, any estimate of the mean level of pressure should ideally be related to factors such as location, posture, physical activity and mood. Many of these factors are correlated with each other (for example, lying while sleeping), so that care must be taken in the analysis to control for potential confounders. Furthermore, the circumstances of recording and the number of readings are unlikely to be the same for all individuals; this should be considered when different individuals' data are combined or compared.

Blood pressure variability can be expressed either in absolute or in relative terms. Because variability is not independent of the mean level (i.e. it is heteroscedastic), we recommend using absolute measures. For most purposes, the standard deviation is adequate. As with the mean level, comparison of the variability of different individuals is best done by controlling for differences in activity.

A special case of blood pressure variability is the diurnal rhythm of blood pressure. Two approaches have been used to analyse this: one based on time and the other on activity. The most widely used time-based measure is the cosinor method, which assumes that blood pressure varies in a sinusoidal fashion over 24 h. We believe that this is an oversimplification of the changes, and do not recommend it. Variants on this theme are Fourier analysis and spline models, which may be statistically more correct but are of limited physiological relevance. Activity-based analysis rests on the assumption that the primary determinant of the diurnal rhythm of blood pressure is the level of physical activity and arousal. The simplest method is the comparison of sleeping and waking values.

References

1. PICKERING TG, HARSHFIELD GA, KLEINERT HD, ET AL.: Blood pressure during normal daily activities, sleep, and exercise. Comparison of values in normal and hypertensive subjects. *JAMA* 1982, 247:992–996.

2. CLARK L, DENBY L, PREGIBON D, ET AL.: A data-based method for bivariate outlier detection: application to automatic blood pressure recording devices. *Psychophysiology* 1987, 24:199–225.

3. MARLER M, JACOB R, LEHOCZKY J, SHAPIRO A: The statistical analysis of treatment effects in 24-hour ambulatory blood pressure recordings. *Stat Med* 1988, 76:697–716.

4. COOK R, WEISBERG S: *Residuals and Influence in Regression.* New York: Chapman & Hall, 1982.

5. STAESSEN J, FAGARD R, LIJNEN P, ET AL.: The use of ambulatory blood pressure monitoring in clinical trials. *J Hypertens* 1991, 9 (suppl 1):S13–S19.

6. LORD F, NOVICK M: *Statistical Theories of Mental Test Scores.* Reading, MA: Addison-Wesley, 1968.

7. CRONBACH L, GLESER C, NANDA L, RAJARATNAM N: *The Dependability of Measures.* New York: Academic Press, 1982.

8. GERIN W, PIEPER C, MARCHESE L, PICKERING T: Measurement reliability of cardiovascular reactivity change scores: a comparison of intermittent and continuous methods of assessment. *Psychophysiology* (in press).

9. LLABRE M, IRONSON GH, SPITZER SB, GELLMAN MD, WEIDLER DJ, SCHNEIDERMAN N: How many blood pressure measurements are enough? An application of generalizability theory to the study of blood pressure reliability. *Psychophysiology* 1988, 25:97–106.

10. CATES EM, SCHLUSSEL YR, JAMES GD, PICKERING TG: A validation study of the Spacelabs 90207 ambulatory blood pressure monitor. *J Amb Mon* 1990, 3:149–154.

11. RADAELLI A, COATES AJS, CLARK SJ, BIRD R, SLEIGHT P: The effects of posture and activity in the accuracy of ambulatory blood pressure recording: a validation of the Oxford Medilog system. *J Amb Mon* 1990, 3:155–161.

12. SWALES JD: *Platt versus Pickering.* London: Keynes Press, 1986.

13. ZACHARIAH PK, SHEPS SG, ILSTRUP DM, ET AL.: Blood pressure load — a better determinant of hypertension. *Mayo Clin Proc* 1988, 63:1085–1091.

14. WHITE WB, DEY HM, SCHULMAN P: Assessment of the daily blood pressure load as a determinant of cardiac function in patients with mild-to-moderate hypertension. *Am Heart J* 1989, 188:782–795.

15. DAWBER TR: *The Framingham Study. The Epidemiology of Atherosclerotic Disease.* Cambridge: Harvard University Press, 1980.

16. MCMAHON S, PETO R, CUTLER J, ET AL.: Blood pressure, stroke, and coronary heart disease. Part I. Prolonged differences in blood pressure: prospective observational studies correlated for the regression dilution bias. *Lancet* 1990, 335:765–774.

17. WHITE WB: Analysis of ambulatory blood pressure data in antihypertensive drug trials. *J Hypertens* (in press).

18. CLARK L, DENBY L, PREGIBON D, ET AL.: A quantitative analysis of the effects of activity and time of day on diurnal variations of blood pressure. *J Chron Dis* 1987, 40:671–681.

19. VAN EGEREN L, MADARASMI S: A computer-assisted diary (CAD) for ambulatory blood pressure monitoring. *Am J Hypertens* 1988, 1:179s–185s.

20. GELLMAN M, SPITZER S, IRONSON G, ET AL.: Posture, place and mood effects an ambulatory blood pressure. *Psychophysiology* (in press).

21. PIEPER C: *The Analysis of Data from 24 Hour Ambulatory Blood Pressure Monitoring: An Application of Hierarchal Linear Models.* Doctoral Dissertation, Columbia University School of Public Health, Division of Biostatistics, 1990.

22. JAMES G, YEE L, HARSHFIELD G, BLANK S, PICKERING T: The influence of happiness, anger and anxiety on the blood pressure of borderline hypertensives. *Psychosom Med* 1986, 48:502–508.

23. JAMES GD, PICKERING TG, SCHLUSSEL YR, CLARK LA, DENBY L, PREGIBON D: Measures of reproducibility of blood pressure variability measured by non-invasive ambulatory blood pressure monitors. *J Amb Mon* 1990, 3:139–147.

24. HEDGES L, OLKIN I: *Statistical Methods for Meta-Analysis.* Orlando: Academic Press, 1985.

25. JUDGE G, GRIFFITHS W, HILL R, LURKEPOHL H, LEE T: *The Theory and Practice of Econometrics.* 2nd Edn. New York: Wiley, 1985.

26. STREITBERG B, MEYER-SABELLEK, BAUMGART P: Statistical analysis of circadian blood pressure recordings in controlled clinical trials. *J Hypertens* 1989, 7 (suppl 3):S11–S17.

27. SCHACHINGER H, LANGEWITZ W, SCHMIEDER R, RUDDELL H: Comparison of parameters and heart rate variability from non-invasive twenty-four hour blood pressure monitoring. *J Hypertens* 1989, 7 (suppl 3):S81–S85.

28. FLEISS J: *Statistical Methods for Rates and Proportions.* 2nd Edn. New York: Wiley, 1981.

29. BOCK D: *Multivariate Statistical Methods in Behavioral Research.* New York: McGraw-Hill, 1975.

30. MANCIA G, FERRARI A, GREGORINI L, ET AL.: Blood pressure and heart rate variabilities in normotensive and hypertensive human beings. *Circ Res* 1983, 53:96–104.

31. BOX G, HILL W: Correcting inhomogeneity of variance with power transformation weighting. *Technometrics* 1974, 16:395–389.

32. HARSHFIELD GA, PICKERING TG, BLANK S, LARAGH JH: How well do casual blood pressures reflect ambulatory blood pressures? In *Blood Pressure Recording in the Clinical Management of Hypertension* edited by Germano G. Rome: Edizioni L Pozzi, 1985, pp 50–54.

33. VAN EGEREN LF, SPARROW AW: Ambulatory monitoring to assess real-life cardiovascular reactivity in type A and type B subjects. *Psychosom Med* 1990, 52:297–306.

34. BINGHAM C, ARBIGAST B, CORNELLISSEN G, LEE J, HALBERG F: Inferential statistical methods for estimating and comparing cosinor parameters. *Chronobiologia* 1982, 9:397–439.

35. LIBRETTI A, LATTUADA S, RINDI M, GRILLO A, SALVAGGIO A: Temporal analysis of blood pressure by ambulatory 24 hour blood pressure monitoring. *Clin Exp Hypertens [A]* 1985, 2:463–467.

36. VAN CAUTER E, HUYBERECHTS S: Problems in the statistical analysis of biological time series: the cosinor test and the periodogram. *J Interdisc Cycle Res* 1973, 4:41–57.

37. VAN CAUTER E: Method for characterization of 24-h temporal variation of blood components. *Am J Physiol* 1979, 237:E255–E264.

38. BRYK A, RAUDENBUSH S: Application of hierarchical linear models to assessing change. *Psychol Bull* 1987, 101:147–158.

39. FLORAS JS, JONES JV, HASSAN MO, SLEIGHT P: Ambulatory blood pressure during once-daily randomized double-blind administration of atenolol, metoprolol, pindolol, and slow-release propranolol. *Br Med J* 1982, 285:1387–1392.

40. BALASUBRAMANIAM V, MANN S, RAFTERY EB, *ET AL*: **Effect of labetalol on continuous ambulatory blood pressure.** *Br J Clin Pharmacol* 1979, 8:1195–1235.

41. DRAYER JIM, WEBER MA, DEYOUNG JL, BREWER DD: **Long-term BP monitoring in the evaluation of antihypertensive therapy.** *Arch Intern Med* 1983, 143:898–901.

Index